AF705390

Thieme

Biomechanics of Spine Stabilization

Self-Assessment and Review

Maxwell Boakye, MD, MPH, MBA
Professor, Vice Chair and Chief of Spinal Surgery
Department of Neurological Surgery
University of Louisville
Louisville, Kentucky, USA

Edward Benzel, MD
Emeritus Chair of Neurosurgery
Department of Neurosurgery
Center for Spine Health
Cleveland Clinic
Cleveland, Ohio, USA

Zoher Ghogawala, MD
Professor
Department of Neurosurgery
Tufts University School of Medicine;
Chairman of Neurosurgery
Lahey Hospital and Medical Center
Burlington, Massachusetts, USA

Darrel S. Brodke, MD
Professor and Chair
Department of Orthopaedics
University of Utah
Salt Lake City, Utah, USA

Jens R. Chapman, MD
Complex Spine Surgeon
Director of Research
Swedish Neuroscience Institute
Swedish Medical Center
Seattle, Washington, USA

468 Illustrations

Thieme
New York • Stuttgart • Delhi • Rio de Janeiro

Library of Congress Cataloging-in-Publication Data is available with the publisher.

Important note: Medicine is an ever-changing science undergoing continual development. Research and clinical experience are continually expanding our knowledge, in particular our knowledge of proper treatment and drug therapy. Insofar as this book mentions any dosage or application, readers may rest assured that the authors, editors, and publishers have made every effort to ensure that such references are in accordance with **the state of knowledge at the time of production of the book**.

Nevertheless, this does not involve, imply, or express any guarantee or responsibility on the part of the publishers in respect to any dosage instructions and forms of applications stated in the book. **Every user is requested to examine carefully** the manufacturers' leaflets accompanying each drug and to check, if necessary, in consultation with a physician or specialist, whether the dosage schedules mentioned therein or the contraindications stated by the manufacturers differ from the statements made in the present book. Such examination is particularly important with drugs that are either rarely used or have been newly released on the market. Every dosage schedule or every form of application used is entirely at the user's own risk and responsibility. The authors and publishers request every user to report to the publishers any discrepancies or inaccuracies noticed. If errors in this work are found after publication, errata will be posted at www.thieme.com on the product description page.

Some of the product names, patents, and registered designs referred to in this book are in fact registered trademarks or proprietary names even though specific reference to this fact is not always made in the text. Therefore, the appearance of a name without designation as proprietary is not to be construed as a representation by the publisher that it is in the public domain.

Thieme addresses people of all gender identities equally. We encourage our authors to use gender-neutral or gender-equal expressions wherever the context allows.

© 2025. Thieme. All rights reserved.

Thieme Publishers New York
333 Seventh Avenue, 18th Floor
New York, NY 10001, USA
www.thieme.com
+1 800 782 3488, customerservice@thieme.com

Cover design: © Thieme
Cover image source: Biomechanics of Spine Stabilization: Third Edition, © 2015 Thieme Medical Publishers, Inc.
Typesetting by TNQ Tech Private Limited, India

Printed in India by Replika Press Pvt. Ltd. 5 4 3 2 1

MIX
Paper | Supporting responsible forestry
FSC™ C016779

DOI: 10.1055/b000000887

ISBN: 978-1-68420-579-0

Also available as an e-book:
eISBN (PDF): 978-1-68420-580-6
eISBN (epub): 978-1-68420-582-0

This book, including all parts thereof, is legally protected by copyright. Any use, exploitation, or commercialization outside the narrow limits set by copyright legislation, without the publisher's consent, is illegal and liable to prosecution. This applies in particular to photostat reproduction, copying, mimeographing or preparation of microfilms, and electronic data processing and storage.

I dedicate this book to my wife Pet, for her kindness, patience, love, and support.

Maxwell Boakye

I dedicate this book to my wife, Mary. I cannot accomplish what I do without her perpetual support.

Edward Benzel

I dedicate this book to my wife Tasneem, who represents all that is good in the world.

Zoher Ghogawala

I dedicate this book to my wife, Anne, for her love and support. She is my strength.

Darrel S. Brodke

To Ed for inspiration and guidance and to family and friends for love and support.

Jens R. Chapman

Contents

Part IX: Synthesis: Putting it All Together

Videos

Foreword

French Jesuit philosopher, scientist, and paleontologist, Teilhard de Chardin, has stated that "future generations stand on the shoulders of the previous leaders." That comment has always resonated with me.

I am of the vintage that allows a longitudinal perspective of the history of modern spine surgery. I was fortunate to be at the right place at the right time and be immersed in the growth and development of current techniques and philosophies in the treatment of spinal disorders. Ed Benzel was the spearhead.

Dr. Benzel, with a background in engineering and the experience of studying under Dr. Sanford Larson, led the way in promulgating the importance of biomechanics in the treatment of spinal pathologies.

Ed and I were engaged with our fellow orthopaedists at a time when such interaction was too often frowned upon by the reigning political powers. With a cadre of like-minded spinal neurosurgeons and orthopaedists, the foundation of modern spinal reconstruction was advanced. Dr. Benzel taught biomechanics to all of us—three-point bending, fixed rigid cantilevers, compression, distraction, rotation, etc.

At the time, and prior, I had to refer to numerous orthopaedic texts to learn these terminologies and how to apply these principles to spinal reconstruction. I was exposed to Harrington rods, sublaminar wires, the Luque technique, Edward's sleeves, etc., via my post Neurosurgery Fellowship in Orthopaedic Spine. But it was my exposure to a talk at Harvard about the derotation principles of the Cotrel-Dubousset instrumentation that stimulated my interest in full force. I realized that neurosurgeons at that time were fairly ignorant of these principles, and thus a tremendous opportunity was afforded.

Luckily, I became friends with Ed Benzel, and along with a few other stalwarts (Ron Apfelbaum, Volker Sonntag, Paul Cooper), we taught each other, learned, and partnered with our orthopaedic colleagues.

Ed led the way in biomechanics—every spine course included a lecture on the principles. His textbooks and chapters paved the way for this new edition of *Biomechanics of Spine Stabilization: Self-Assessment and Review* by Drs. Boakye, Benzel, Ghogawala, Brodke, and Chapman. All of these authors are colleagues and well-established experts in this field. They are building upon the broad shoulders of Ed Benzel.

However, this book is more than biomechanics. It encompasses anatomy, pathophysiology, surgical decision-making and technique selection, nonsurgical care, and nonoperative management. It includes the history of stabilization, modes of implant failure, bone healing, bone graft extenders, and biologics.

It is clear, concise, and VERY INSTRUCTIVE.

Each elegant chapter has learning objectives, a question-and-answer format, with fabulous elucidation of the correct answer, key principles to be gleaned, and a list of the most important references.

It was enjoyable to read, re-learn, learn anew, and refresh some long-forgotten principles.

This book is a MUST for every resident in training and fellow in spine surgery. It should be read by every practitioner of the art and science of spinal surgery. It includes case discussions, philosophical approaches to both operative and nonoperative care, with a focus on optimization of treatment. The difference between good and great outcomes is attention to detail. This book will aid every surgeon in becoming a better doctor.

On a personal note, it is meaningful to me to be a colleague of Ed, and to have been taught by him. It is equally important to have my friends, Zo, Darrel, and Jens, contribute to this effort. Lastly, to have a former fellow of mine, Max, also contribute to this provides hope that our educational endeavors will continue to prosper and enhance the care of our patients.

Respectfully submitted,
Regis Haid, MD
Past President
American Association of Neurological Surgeons
Past Chair
AANS/CNS Spine Section
Atlanta, Georgia, USA

Preface

In 1992, Dr. Benzel's first Spine Fellow, Perry Ball, inspired him to write a biomechanics book to simplify the complex existing literature. This led to the first edition of *The Biomechanics of Spine Stabilization* in 1995, followed by two more editions that expanded upon the original. Single-handedly authoring these editions was a monumental task, so after the 2015 third edition, Dr. Benzel chose not to continue. However, a serendipitous conversation with Dr. Max Boakye sparked a new project. Dr. Boakye suggested a question-and-answer format for the book, which the team found to be ideal. Dr. Boakye along with his co-editors, Drs. Ed Benzel, Darrel Brodke, Jans Chapman, and Zoher Ghogawala, and the chapter authors, worked diligently to bring this book to life—the one you're now holding.

This book reflects an important realization: while the fundamental principles of mathematics and physics are constant, their application in spinal biomechanics has evolved, especially with new surgical technologies altering the landscape. As you delve into this book, consider the principles as they stood in the mid-2010s, juxtaposed with the advancements in technology that have since improved surgical outcomes. It is essential to understand both the old and new techniques to fully appreciate the biomechanical foundations of spine surgery.

As spine surgery continues to advance, this book may not cover every aspect of this dynamic field. However, it is our hope that it will lay a lasting foundation and provide an enjoyable learning experience for all. This book is designed not just to inform, but also to make biomechanics accessible and routinely and practically applicable in clinical practice, thereby enhancing the proficiency and confidence of spine surgeons in their craft. We hope that you will find the book to be a valuable resource.

The Editors

Acknowledgments

I extend my deepest gratitude to all the authors and my co-editors, whose tireless efforts have made this book a reality. Special thanks are due to Dr. Benzel for his enthusiasm, unwavering support, and responsiveness. His profound knowledge and inspirational teaching, combined with his approachability and meticulous attention to detail, have been invaluable in emphasizing the key principles of spinal biomechanics.

Additionally, I would like to express my sincere appreciation to Karen Edmonson (Thieme) for her steadfast belief, dedication, and vision, which were instrumental in bringing this book to life. My gratitude also extends to Judith Tomat (Thieme) for her exceptional organization skills and commitment to working with the authors, managing every aspect from the inception to the completion of this product.

Maxwell Boakye, MD

I extend my deepest gratitude to Max, Darrel, Jens, Zo, and all the authors for revitalizing my original work and for their invaluable contributions. Their dedication has breathed new life into my initial concepts, and for this, I am profoundly thankful.

Edward Benzel, MD

Contributors

Muhammad Abd-El-Barr, MD
Associate Professor of Neurosurgery
Department of Orthopaedics
Duke University School of Medicine
Duke Health Center
Morrisville, North Carolina, USA

Shawn W. Adams, MD
Neurosurgeon
Norton Neuroscience Institute
Leatherman Spine
Louisville, Kentucky, USA

Owoicho Adogwa, MD, MPH
Assistant Professor
Department of Neurological Surgery
University of Cincinnati College of Medicine
Cincinnati, Ohio, USA

Nitin Agarwal, MD
Associate Professor of Neurological Surgery and Director
Minimally Invasive Spine and Robotics Surgery;
Associate Program Director
Neurological Surgery Residency
Co-Director
Complex and Minimally Invasive Spine Deformity Fellowship
Department of Neurological Surgery
University of Pittsburgh School of Medicine
Pittsburgh, Pennsylvania, USA

Paul M. Arnold, MD, FACS
Professor of Neurosurgery
Carle Illinois College of Medicine
Chairman
Department of Neurosurgery
Associate Medical Director
Director of Research
Carle Neuroscience Institute
Adjunct Research Professor of Electrical and Computer Engineering
Grainger Illinois College of Engineering
Urbana, Illinois, USA

Stephen M. Bergin, MD
Neurosurgery Resident
Department of Neurosurgery
Duke University
Durham, North Carolina, USA

Mark Bilsky, MD
Neurosurgeon and Director
Multidisciplinary Spine Tumor Service
Memorial Sloan Kettering Cancer Center
New York, New York, USA

Maxwell Boakye, MD, MPH, MBA
Professor, Vice Chair and Chief of Spinal Surgery
Department of Neurological Surgery
University of Louisville
Louisville, Kentucky, USA

Thomas J. Buell, MD
Assistant Professor of Neurological Surgery
Department of Neurological Surgery
University of Pittsburgh School of Medicine
Pittsburgh, Pennsylvania, USA

Mohamad Bydon, MD
Professor of Neurosurgery
Department of Neurologic Surgery
Mayo Clinic
Rochester, Minnesota, USA

Fabian Carballo Madrigal, MD
Neurosurgeon
University of Louisville Health
Louisville, Kentucky, USA

Joseph A. Carnevale, MD
Chief Resident
Department of Neurosurgery
NewYork-Presbyterian/Weill Cornell Medical Brain and Spine Center
New York, New York, USA

Vikram B. Chakravarthy, MD
Assistant Professor
Department of Neurological Surgery
Wexner Medical Center
Ohio State University
Columbus, Ohio, USA

Joseph Cheng, MD, MS
Frank H. Mayfield Professor and Chair
Department of Neurosurgery
University of Cincinnati College of Medicine
Cincinnati, Ohio, USA

Theodore J. Choma, MD, FAAOS
J. Vernon Luck, Sr Distinguished Professor and Vice Chairman;
Director
Spine Division
Department of Orthopaedic Surgery;
Chairman
University Physicians
University of Missouri
Columbia, Missouri, USA

Ian Connolly, MD
Neurosurgery Resident
Department of Neurosurgery
Massachusetts General hospital
Harvard Medical School
Boston, Massachusetts, USA

Andrew T. Dailey, MD
Professor
Department of Neurosurgery
Clinical Neurosciences Center
University of Utah
Salt Lake City, Utah, USA

Sarah Danehower, MD
Resident
Department of Neurological Surgery
University of Louisville
Louisville, Kentucky, USA

Harel Deutsch, MD
Associate Professor
Department of Neurosurgery
Rush University Medical Center
Chicago, Illinois, USA

Joravar Dhaliwal, MD
Resident
Department of Neurosurgery
The Ohio State University Wexner School of Medicine
Columbus, Ohio, USA

Sanjay Dhawan, MD
Neurosurgery Resident
Department of Neurosurgery
University of Minnesota
Minneapolis, Minnesota, USA

Doniel Drazin, MD, MA
Neurosurgeon
Department of Neurosurgery
Providence Regional Medical Center
Everett, Washington, USA

Daniel Farivar, MD
Research Fellow
Department of Orthopedics, Spine Center
Cedars-Sinai Medical Center
Los Angeles, California, USA

Megan Finneran, DO
Neurosurgical Resident
Carle Neuroscience Institute
Carle BroMenn Medical Center
Normal, Illinois, USA

Patrick M. Flanigan, MD
Spine Fellow
Department of Neurosurgery
Mayo Clinic
Rochester, Minnesota, USA

David Freeman, MD
Assistant Professor
Department of Neurological Surgery
University of Miami Miller School of Medicine
Miami, Florida, USA

Jacob L. Goldberg, MD
Chief Resident
Department of Neurosurgery
Weill Cornell Medicine Brain & Spine Center
NewYork-Presbyterian/Weill Cornell Medical Center
New York, New York, USA

Glenn A. Gonzalez, MD
Post-Doctoral Research Fellow
Department of Neurosurgery
Thomas Jefferson University
Philadelphia, Pennsylvania, USA

Garret Greeneway, MD
Resident
Department of Neurosurgery
University of Wisconsin-Madison School of Medicine
Madison, Wisconsin, USA

Muhamed Hadzipasic, MD, PhD
Clinical Fellow in Neurosurgery
Department of Neurosurgery
Massachusetts General Hospital
Boston, Massachusetts, USA

Ghani Haider, MD
Post Doctoral Scholar in Neurosurgery
Department of Neurosurgery
Stanford University
Palo Alto, California, USA

D. Kojo Hamilton, MD
Professor of Neurological Surgery
Director
UPMC Neurosurgical Spine Services
Director
Residency Training Program
Co-Director
Spine Fellowship Program
Department of Neurological Surgery
University of Pittsburgh School of Medicine
Pittsburgh, Pennsylvania, USA

James S. Harrop, MD
Professor
Neurological Surgery and Orthopedic Surgery
Thomas Jefferson University
Philadelphia, Pennsylvania, USA

Roger Härtl, MD
Hansen-MacDonald Professor of Neurological Surgery
Director of Neurosurgery Spine
Weill Cornell Medicine
Director
Weill Cornell Medicine Center for Comprehensive Spine Care;
Co-director
New York Presbyterian OCH SPINE
Weill Cornell Medicine Center for Comprehensive Spine Care
New York, New York, USA

Andrew M. Hersh, MD
Resident
Department of Neurosurgery
Johns Hopkins University School of Medicine
Baltimore, Maryland, USA

Kevin Hines, MD
Assistant Professor
Department of Neurosurgery
Thomas Jefferson University
Philadelphia, Pennsylvania, USA

Joseph S. Hudson, MD
Chief Resident
Department of Neurological Surgery
University of Pittsburg School of Medicine
Pittsburg, Pennsylvania, USA

Ibrahim Hussain, MD
Assistant Professor
Department of Neurosurgery
Weill Cornell Medicine Brain & Spine Center
New York, New York, USA

Nikhil Jain, MD
Assistant Professor of Orthopaedics
Missouri Orthopaedic Institute
University of Missouri
Columbia, Missouri, USA

Karl Janich, MD
Neurosurgeon
Indiana University Health
Lafayette, Indiana, USA

J. Patrick Johnson, MD
Professor
Cedars Sinai Spine Center
Director
Neurosurgery Spine Fellowship
President and CEO
Spine Institute Foundation
Los Angeles, California, USA

Sarah E. Johnson, MBBS
Postdoctoral Research Fellow
Neuro-Informatics Laboratory
Department of Neurological Surgery
Mayo Clinic
Rochester, Minnesota, USA

Rafid Kasir, MD
Spine Surgeon
San Diego, California, USA

Ryan Khanna, MD
Fellow
Department of Neurosurgery
Memorial Sloan Kettering Cancer Center
New York, New York, USA

Leo J.Y. Kim, MD, PhD
Resident
Department of Neurosurgery
Clinical Neurosciences Center
University of Utah
Salt Lake City, Utah, USA

Terrence T. Kim, MD
Associate Professor
Cedars-Sinai Medical Center
Director of Education
Cedars-Sinai Spine Center
Los Angeles, California, USA

Rakesh Kumar, MD
Complex Spine Fellow
Virginia Mason Hospital & Medical Center
Seattle, Washington, USA

Raj Swaroop Lavadi, MBBS
Postdoctoral Research Fellow
Department of Neurological Surgery
University of Pittsburgh School of Medicine
Pittsburgh, Pennsylvania, USA

Brandon D. Lawrence, MD
Professor;
Chief of Spine Surgery
Department of Orthopaedics
University of Utah
Salt Lake City, Utah, USA

Jean-Christophe Leveque, MD
Head of Neurosurgery
Virginia Mason Medical Center
Seattle, Washington, USA

Mohamed Macki, MD, MPH
Spine Surgeon
Cleveland Clinic Foundation
Mayfield Heights, Ohio, USA

Neelan Joseph Marianayagam, MD
Neurosurgeon
Stanford Hospital
Palo Alto, California, USA

Rohit Mauria, MD
Complex Spine Fellow
Case Western/University Hospitals Cleveland Medical Center
Cleveland, Ohio, USA

Juan C. Mejia, MD
Complex Spinal Surgery fellow
Department of Neurosurgery
University of Cincinnati College of Medicine
Cincinnati, Ohio, USA

Eric Mong, MD
Neurosurgery Resident
Oakland University William Beaumont
Royal Oak, Michigan, USA

Benjamin Motley, MD
Assistant Professor
Department of Neurosurgery
University of Cincinnati Medical Center
Cincinnati, Ohio, USA

Praveen V. Mummaneni, MD, MBA
Professor and Vice Chair
Department of Neurosurgery
University of California San Francisco
San Francisco, California, USA

Venu Nemani, MD
Staff Spinal Neurosurgeon
Virginia Mason Hospital & Seattle Medical Center
Seattle, Washington, USA

David O. Okonkwo, MD, PhD
Professor
Department of Neurological Surgery
University of Pittsburgh
Pittsburgh, Pennsylvania, USA

Thomas A. Pieters, MD
Assistant Professor
Department of Neurosurgery
University of Massachusetts Memorial Health,
Worcester, Massachusetts, USA

Guilherme Bastos Ferreira Porto, MD
Fellow
Department of Neurosurgery
Thomas Jefferson University
Philadelphia, Pennsylvania, USA

Daniel Resnick, MD
Professor
Department of Neurosurgery
University of Wisconsin-Madison
Madison, Wisconsin, USA

James Rizkalla, MD
Spine Fellow
Department of Orthopaedic Surgery
Spine Surgery Division
University of Utah
Salt Lake City, Utah, USA

Brett Rocos, MD, FRCS
Assistant Professor
Duke Orthopaedic Surgery
Division of Spine Surgery;
Assistant Professor of Neurosurgery
Duke University
Durham, North Carolina, USA

Clayton L. Rosinski, MD
Neurosurgery Resident
Department of Neurosurgery
University of Iowa Hospitals and Clinics
Iowa City, Iowa, USA

Timothy C. Ryken, MD
Adjunct Professor
Department of Neurosurgery
University of Iowa Hospitals and Clinics
Iowa City, Iowa, USA

Rajiv Saigal, MD
Associate Professor
Neurological Surgery
University of California
San Francisco, California, USA

Gabrielle Santangelo, MD
Assistant Professor
Department of Neurosurgery
University of Rochester
Rochester, New York, USA

Bradley Schmidt, MD
Assistant Professor
Department of Neurosurgery
University of Wisconsin-Madison
Madison, Wisconsin, USA

Daniel M. Sciubba, MD, MBA
Chair
Department of Neurosurgery
Northwell Health
Great Neck, New York, USA

Rajiv Sethi, MD
Executive Medical Director
Center of Neuroscience and Spine
Virginia Mason Hospital & Seattle Medical Center
Seattle, Washington, USA

Mayur Sharma, MD
Assistant Professor
Department of Neurosurgery
University of Minnesota
Minneapolis, Minnesota, USA

India Shelley
BA Medical Student
Medical Student
Sidney Kimmel Medical College
Thomas Jefferson University
Philadelphia, Pennsylvania, USA

Kylee Shivok, BS
Medical Student
Sidney Kimmel Medical College | *Class of 2026*
Thomas Jefferson University
Philadelphia, Pennsylvania, USA

Emily Payne Sieg, MD, MS, FAANS
Director of Neurotrauma
Department of Neurological Surgery
University of Louisville Health;
Chief of Neurosurgery
University Hospital
Louisville, Kentucky, USA

Christopher A. Sy, MD
Spine Surgery Fellow
Department of Neurosurgery
Cedars-Sinai Medical Center
West Hollywood, California, USA

Bobby Tay, MD
Professor
Department of Orthopaedic Surgery
University of California
San Francisco, California, USA

Khoi D. Than, MD
Professor of Neurosurgery
Department of Neurosurgery
Duke University
Durham, North Carolina, USA

Nicholas Theodore, MD
Professor of Neurosurgery
Department of Neurosurgery;
Orthopaedics and Biomedical Engineering Director
Neurosurgical Spine Program
Johns Hopkins University School of Medicine
Baltimore, Maryland, USA

Luis M. Tumialán, MD
Professor of Neurosurgery
Department of Neurosurgery
Barrow Neurological Institute
Phoenix, Arizona, USA

Anand Veeravagu, MD
Associate Professor
Department of Neurosurgery
Stanford Medicine
Palo Alto, California, USA

John V. Wainwright, MD
Neurosurgeon
Westchester Medical Center
Valhalla, New York, USA

Marjorie C. Wang, MD
Professor of Neurological Surgery
Department of Neurosurgery
Medical College of Wisconsin
Milwaukee, Wisconsin, USA

Michael Wang, MD
Neurosurgeon
University of Miami Health System
Miami, Florida, USA

Joseph Weiner, MD
Assistant Professor
Department of Orthopaedic Surgery
University of Kansas Health Systems
Kansas City, Kansas, USA

Brian J. Williams, MD
Neurosurgeon
University of Louisville Health
Louisville, Kentucky, USA

John Williams, MD
Assistant Professor of Neurosurgery
Department of Neurosurgery
The University of Texas Health Science Center
Houston, Texas, USA

Theresa Williamson, MD, MPH
Assistant Professor of Neurosurgery
Harvard Medical School;
Mass General Neurosurgery
Boston, Massachusetts, USA

Kelly H. Yoo, MD, PhD
Postdoctoral Scholar
Department of Neurosurgery
Stanford University School of Medicine
Stanford, California, USA

Introduction

Several years ago, I embarked on a journey to deepen my understanding of how adults learn through courses in health professions education, a pursuit that began nearly two decades after my initial appointment as an attending physician. My medical career had been significantly shaped during my residency in the 1990s, a crucial period when I chose to specialize in neurosurgery and later complex spine surgery. It was around this time that the authoritative textbook by Dr. Benzel on biomechanics was published, marking a new era in the field.

For over two decades, I committed myself to mastering the content of this text, yet found its complexities challenging to grasp fully. Despite my growing conviction of its vital importance to my practice in spine surgery, the concepts often felt elusive. My efforts to understand this material were steadfast, but I consistently felt a deeper connection was missing.

All this changed when I completed some pivotal courses in health professions education that shed light on the art of learning. The course revealed the importance of retrieval practice and demonstrated how repeated testing and review could transform a passive recipient of information into an active, engaged learner. This epiphany in learning principles finally enabled me to comprehend the nuances of biomechanics in a way I had previously been unable to achieve.

This personal journey and breakthrough inspired me to create the idea of a companion question and answer book to Dr. Benzel's original textbook on the biomechanics of spinal stabilization, for which I sought and received his permission.

Maxwell Boakye, MD

Part I

Overview of Fundamental Concepts

I

1 Biomechanically Relevant Anatomy and Material Properties of the Spine and Associated Elements

Ghani Haider, Kelly H. Yoo, Neelan Joseph Marianayagam, Anand Veeravagu

Learning Objectives

- Understand the distinctive anatomical features present in the cervical, thoracic, and lumbar regions of spine.
- Understand the intricate functional interplay and structural aspects of the spine including the craniocervical junction.
- Analyze the clinical significance of divergent vertebral anatomies and their associated joints and ligaments, discerning their implications in the onset, progression, and management of spinal pathologies, thereby informing tailored treatment approaches.

Questions

▸▸ Question 1

From which part of the cervical vertebra do foraminal osteophytes most commonly emerge?

- A. Lamina
- B. Facet joints
- C. Uncinate process
- D. Vertebral body
- E. Pedicle

▸▸ Question 2

In which region of the spine does the spinal canal have the minimum cross-sectional area, providing minimal room for neural element protection?

- A. Cervical
- B. Upper thoracic
- C. Lower thoracic
- D. Lumbar
- E. Sacral

▸▸ Question 3

With regard to the size of pedicles, where is pedicle screw instrumentation safest?

- A. Cervical
- B. Upper thoracic
- C. Lower thoracic
- D. Lumbar
- E. Sacral

▸▸ Question 4

In cervical and thoracic spine pedicle screw instrumentation, a small breach is most likely to involve which spinal tract?

- A. Spinothalamic tract
- B. Corticospinal tract
- C. Dorsal columns
- D. Rubrospinal tract
- E. Spino-cerebellar tract

▸▸ Question 5

From which junction do the transverse processes of the vertebrae emerge?

- A. Pedicle and vertebral body
- B. Pedicle and lamina
- C. Lamina and facet joint
- D. Two lamina
- E. Spinous process and lamina

▸▸ Question 6

Which structure primarily bears the axial load of the spine?

- A. Vertebral body
- B. Facet joints
- C. Lamina
- D. Spinous process
- E. Transverse process

▸▸ Question 7

Which spinal ligament, due to its relatively long moment arm, provides significant resistance to forward flexion of the spine?

- A. Anterior longitudinal ligament
- B. Posterior longitudinal ligament
- C. Ligamentum flavum
- D. Capsular ligament
- E. Interspinous ligament

▸▸ Question 8

Of all the ligaments in the spine, which one has the highest proportion of elastic fibers, surpassing any other human tissue?
- A. Anterior longitudinal ligament
- B. Posterior longitudinal ligament
- C. Ligamentum flavum
- D. Capsular ligament
- E. Interspinous ligament

▸▸ Question 9

Among the following regions of the spine, where is resistance to pedicle screw pullout the least?
- A. Cervical spine
- B. Sacrum
- C. Upper thoracic spine
- D. Lumbar spine
- E. Lower thoracic spine

▸▸ Question 10

At which level does the vertebral artery typically enter the transverse foramen?
- A. C5
- B. C6
- C. C7
- D. C1
- E. C2

▸▸ Question 11

The relatively steep orientation of lumbosacral junction predisposes the lumbosacral region to what kind of injury?
- A. Translational
- B. Rotational
- C. Compression
- D. Distraction
- E. Flexion-extension

▸▸ Question 12

Which form of sacro-iliac fixation provides the most robust construct when fixing the lumbar spine to the pelvis?
- A. S-rods
- B. Sacro-iliac screws
- C. Sacral screws
- D. Anterior plating
- E. Posterior trans-iliac plating

▸▸ Question 13

Weakness of cortical bone at the vertebral end plate can lead to the formation of which of the following?
- A. Schmorl's node
- B. Schuerman's kyphosis
- C. Klippel Feil anomaly
- D. Hemi-vertebrae
- E. Vertebral fusion

▸▸ Question 14

Compared to the coronal orientation of facet joints in the cervical spine, the sagittal orientation of facet joints in the lumbar spine limits what kind of motion?
- A. Flexion
- B. Extension
- C. Rotation
- D. Lateral bending
- E. Translation

▸▸ Question 15

In the cervical spine, which joint allows for maximum rotation?
- A. Occiput–C1 joint
- B. C1–C2 joint at odontoid process
- C. Combined rotation of C3–C6 joint
- D. C2–C3 facet joint
- E. Lateral atlanto-axial joint

▸▸ Question 16

During placement of trans-facet screws at C1–C2, which nerve should be kept in mind and protected?
- A. Occipital nerve
- B. Accessory nerve
- C. Hypoglossal nerve
- D. C2 nerve root
- E. C3 nerve root

▸▸ **Question 17**

Which of the following structures have the highest strength to resist failure in the cervical spine?
- A. Alar and transverse ligaments
- B. Posterior longitudinal ligament
- C. Anterior longitudinal ligaments
- D. Tectorial membrane
- E. Interspinous ligaments

▸▸ **Question 18**

In which region are herniated disks most common due to deficiency of ligaments?
- A. Ventral
- B. Dorsal
- C. Lateral
- D. Dorsolateral
- E. Anterolateral

▸▸ **Question 19**

On eccentric axial loading of the spine, the annulus fibrosus on the convex side is under tension while the nucleus pulposus tends to migrate in which direction?
- A. Convex side
- B. Concave side
- C. Cranially
- D. Caudally
- E. Does not move

▸▸ **Question 20**

In the lumbar spine, which ligament has the highest strength to resist failure?
- A. Anterior longitudinal ligament
- B. Posterior longitudinal ligament
- C. Ligamentum flavum
- D. Capsular ligament
- E. Interspinous ligament

Answers

▸▸ **Answer 1**

Correct answer is C

The uncinate process forms the walls of the neural foramen in the cervical spine. Consequently, osteophytes arising from the uncinate process have a propensity to grow into the foramen and impinge on the exiting nerve root.[1] Osteophytes emerging from other anatomical structures listed would not project into the neuro-foramina.

▸▸ **Answer 2**

Correct answer is B

The upper thoracic spine exhibits the smallest cross-sectional area within the spinal canal, primarily occupied by the spinal cord. This configuration predisposes the spinal cord to a higher risk of injury compared to other spinal regions, as there is relatively less epidural space and cerebrospinal fluid providing cushioning (see ▸ Fig. 1.1).[1,2,3,4]

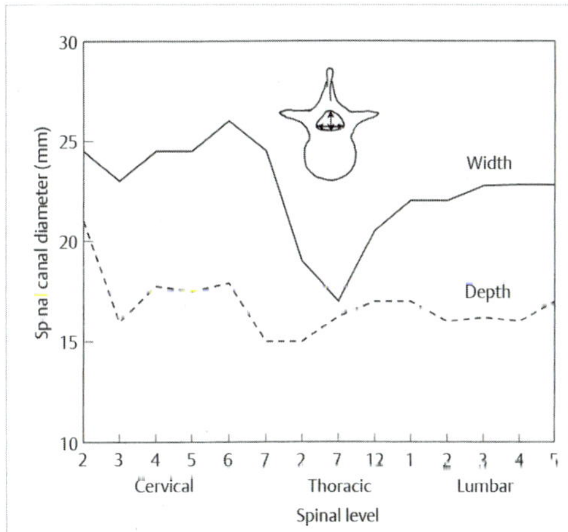

Fig. 1.1 Spinal canal diameter versus spinal level. Source: Data obtained from Berry et al,[1] Panjabi et al,[2] Reynolds et al,[3] McCormack et al.[4]

▸▸ **Answer 3**

Correct answer is D

The lumbar spine features the largest pedicle diameters, making it the safest region for pedicle screw instrumentation placement. (see ▸ Fig. 1.2).[6,7,8,9] In contrast, the upper thoracic and upper cervical spine have smaller pedicle diameters, leaving little margin for error. Any medial or inferior breach in these regions poses a significant risk of damaging neurological structures. The angle of the pedicles varies along the spine, necessitating careful consideration during instrumentation placement.

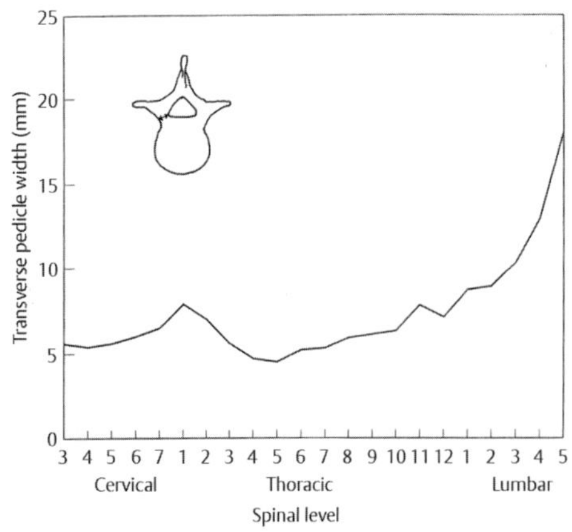

Fig. 1.2 Transverse pedicle width versus spinal level. Source: Data obtained from Panjabi et al,[1] Krag et al,[2] Zindrick et al,[3] Bernard and Seibert.[4]

▸▸ Answer 4

Correct answer is A

During pedicle screw instrumentation, patients are typically positioned prone, with the spinal cord resting on the dorsal aspect of the vertebral body. In the event of a small medial breach, the anterolateral region of the spinal cord, where the spinothalamic tracts are located, is most susceptible.[10] The spinal long tracts and the nerves of the cauda equina are somatotropically arranged so that specific parts of the body are arranged in particular areas in both sensory and motor tracts. The lower elements are situated most medially and those preparing to exit the spinal canal are more lateral. Awareness of these arrangements is crucial for neurosurgeons to minimize the risk of damage.

▸▸ Answer 5

Correct answer is B

Anatomically, the transverse processes of the vertebrae emerge from the junction of the pedicle and lamina. The spinous process arises from the point where the two lamina meet.

▸▸ Answer 6

Correct answer is A

The vertebral bodies, comprised of cortical and cancellous bones, constitute the main bulk of the vertebrae and bear the majority of applied loads. While the posterior elements, such as the spinous process, transverse process, lamina, and facet joints, also participate in load-bearing their smaller size relative to the vertebral body limits their contribution to weight-bearing significantly.

▸▸ Answer 7

Correct answer is E

The interspinous ligaments are present between the spinous processes and have the longest moment arm during forward flexion of the spine. This configuration allows them to exert significant resistance against forward bending. While the posterior longitudinal ligament, ligamentum flavum, and capsular ligaments also contribute to the stability, their moment arms are comparatively shorter. The anterior longitudinal ligament primarily resists extension of the spine.

▸▸ Answer 8

Correct answer is C

The ligamentum flavum possesses the highest proportion of elastic fibers among spinal ligaments. This unique composition enables the ligamentum flavum to accommodate maximum flexion of the spine. During spinal flexion, the ligamentum flavum expands, contributing to the spinal flexibility. In contrast, the anterior and posterior longitudinal ligaments, as well as the capsular and interspinous ligaments, exhibit lesser elasticity compared to the ligamentum flavum.

▸▸ Answer 9

Correct answer is B

The ratio of cancellous to cortical bone affects the resistance to pedicle screw pullout. There is a higher ratio of cortical bone in the pedicles of the cervical, thoracic, and lumbar spine compared to the sacrum. Hence, the lower bone density correlates with increased susceptibility to problems with pedicle screw pullout in the sacral region.

▸▸ Answer 10

Correct answer is B

The vertebral arteries typically enter the transverse foramina of the C6 vertebra. Although the C7 vertebral body possesses a transverse foramen, it usually does not accommodate arterial vessels.[11,12,13] The vertebral artery passes through the foramina of all other cervical vertebrae.

▸▸ **Answer 11**

Correct answer is A

The steep orientation of the lumbosacral junction results in the pelvis sitting at an angle to the lumbar spine. This configuration makes the lumbosacral region most susceptible to translational injuries, often leading to anterior listhesis of L5 over S1. Such injuries involve a forward displacement of the vertebra relative to the one below it, as depicted in ▸ Fig. 1.3.

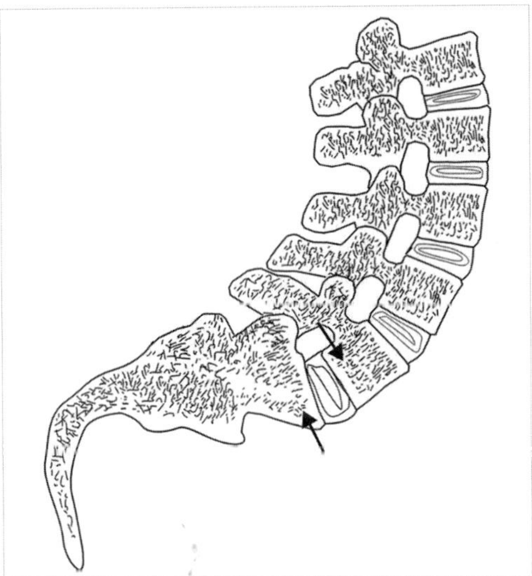

Fig. 1.3 Orientation of the lumbar and the lumbosacral joints. Arrows depict the translational forces resulting from the assumption of upright posture. (Source: Biomechanics of Spine Stabilization: Third Edition, © 2015 Thieme Medical Publishers, Inc.)

▸▸ **Answer 12**

Correct answer is B

The sacro-iliac screws provide the most robust construct for fixing the lumbar spine to the pelvis, offering secure fixation least likely to fail under stress, such as weight-bearing.[14] The other forms of fixation listed are comparatively less robust and therefore more prone to failure.

▸▸ **Answer 13**

Correct answer is A

Weakness of cortical bone at vertebral end plates most commonly leads to the formation of Schmorl's nodes. These are herniations of the nucleus pulposus through the vertebral end plate into the adjacent vertebral body. Vertebral fusion, hemi-vertebrae, and Klippel Feil anomaly are typically congenital anomalies of bone formation. Scheuermann's kyphosis primarily involves anterior wedging of multiple thoracic vertebrae with normal vertebral end plates.

▸▸ **Answer 14**

Correct answer is C

The sagittal orientation of facet joints in the lumbar spine restricts rotational motion in this region, as the joint surfaces are aligned in the sagittal plane. Conversely, the coronal orientation of facet joints in the cervical spine permits rotational movements but limits flexion and extension motions due to their alignment.[15,16,17]

▸▸ **Answer 15**

Correct answer is B

The C1–C2 joint at the odontoid process allows for maximum rotation of the head from side to side (see ▸ Table 1.1).[18,19] This joint is pivotal in enabling rotational movements of the head, such as head nodding and shaking. While the occiput–C1 joint contributes to head nodding motion, and combined rotation of C3–C6 joints facilitates general cervical spine rotation, the C1–C2 joint is specifically responsible for maximal rotation.

Table 1.1 Joint Mobility in the Cervical Spine

Joint	Motion	Range of motion (degrees)
Occiput–C1	Combined flexion-extension	25
	Lateral bending (unilateral)	5
	Axial rotation (unilateral)	5
C1–C2	Combined flexion-extension	20
	Lateral bending (unilateral)	5
	Axial rotation (unilateral)	40

(Source: Biomechanics of Spine Stabilization: Third Edition, © 2015 Thieme Medical Publishers, Inc.)

▸▸ Answer 16

Correct answer is A

The occipital nerve courses dorsal to the atlanto-axial joint and must protected to avoid injury while placing C1–C2 trans-facet screws. This nerve is in close proximity to the surgical site and therefore at risk of injury during the procedure. Other nerves mentioned are further away from the C1–C2 joint and thus less prone to injury.

▸▸ Answer 17

Correct answer is A

The alar and transverse ligaments, two among the strongest ligaments in the body, are responsible for holding the C1 vertebral body close to the odontoid process. Failure of these ligaments can result in significant spinal cord injury. Other ligaments mentioned are relatively less strong and may not provide the same level of stability.

▸▸ Answer 18

Correct answer is D

Herniated disks are most common in the dorsolateral region due to deficiencies in spinal ligaments in this area. Under axial load and flexion, the nucleus pulposus is more likely to migrate posteriorly and herniate through the relatively narrow and weak posterior longitudinal ligament. This predisposes the dorsolateral region to herniated disks, especially under conditions of excessive loading.

▸▸ Answer 19

Correct answer is A

During eccentric loading, the nucleus pulposus shifts to the area of least stress, which is typically on the convex side.[20] This movement allows the annulus fibrosus on the convex side to be under tension, while the nucleus pulposus acts as a shock absorber by migrating away from the area of increased stress.

▸▸ Answer 20

Correct answer is A

The anterior longitudinal ligament is highly developed in the lumbar spine and has the highest strength to resist failure. It plays a crucial role in preventing translational injury to the spine by providing stability and limiting excessive movement. While the anterior longitudinal ligament has a greater capacity to withstand forces, it is less elastic compared to other ligaments such as the ligamentum flavum.

Key Principles

- The spine exhibits a distinctive design, providing both rigidity for tasks like maintaining an erect posture and protecting neural elements, and flexibility for motor tasks such as movement.
- The spine segmented into various regions, each sharing general structural and functional similarities.
- Constructs used in spinal procedures should align with the natural requirements of the spine. Additionally, spinal procedures and instrumentation should prioritize avoiding damage to neurovascular structures to optimize patient outcomes and minimize complications.

References

[1] Tubbs RS, Rompala OJ, Verma K, et al. Analysis of the uncinate processes of the cervical spine: an anatomical study. J Neurosurg Spine 2012;16:402–407

[2] Berry JL, Moran JM, Berg WS, Steffee AD. A morphometric study of human lumbar and selected thoracic vertebrae. Spine 1987;12:362–367

[3] Panjabi MM, Duranceau J, Goel V, Oxland T, Takata K. Cervical human vertebrae. Quantitative three-dimensional anatomy of the middle and lower regions. Spine 1991;16:861–869

[4] Reynolds AF Jr, Roberts PA, Pollay M, Stratemeier PH. Quantitative anatomy of the thoracolumbar epidural space. Neurosurgery 1985;17:905–907

[5] McCormack BM, Benzel EC, Adams MS, Baldwin NG, Rupp FW, Maher DJ. Anatomy of the thoracic pedicle. Neurosurgery 1995;37:303–308

[6] Panjabi MM, Duranceau J, Goel V, Oxland T, Takata K. Cervical human vertebrae. Quantitative three-dimensional anatomy of the middle and lower regions. Spine 1991;16:861–869

[7] Krag MH, Weaver DL, Beynnon BD, Haugh LD. Morphometry of the thoracic and lumbar spine related to transpedicular screw placement for surgical spinal fixation. Spine 1988;13:27–32

[8] Bernard TN, Seibert CE. Pedicle diameter determined by computed tomography. Its relevance to pedicle screw fixation in the lumbar spine. Spine 1992;17 Suppl:S160–S163

[9] Zindrick MR, Wiltse LL, Doornik A, et al. Analysis of the morphometric characteristics of the thoracic and lumbar pedicles. Spine 1987;12:160–166

[10] Wall EJ, Cohen MS, Massie JB, Rydevik B, Garfin SR. Cauda equina anatomy. I: Intrathecal nerve root organization. Spine 1990;15:1244–1247

[11] Johnson H, Rauschning WP. Surgical anatomy of the cervical spine. Tech Orthop 1994;9:18–29

[12] Tubbs RS, Rompala OJ, Verma K, et al. Analysis of the uncinate processes of the cervical spine: an anatomical study. J Neurosurg Spine 2012;16:402–407

[13] Ebraheim NA, Reader D, Xu R, Yeasting RA. Location of the vertebral artery foramen on the anterior aspect of the lower cervical spine by computed tomography. J Spinal Disord 1997;10:304–307

[14] Vaccaro AR, Ring D, Scuderi G, Garfin SR. Vertebral artery location in relation to the vertebral body as determined by two-dimensional computed tomography evaluation. Spine 1994;19:2637–2641

[15] Van Schaik JPJ, Verbiest H, Van Schaik FDJ. The orientation of laminae and facet joints in the lower lumbar spine. Spine 1985;10:59–63

[16] White AA, Panjabi MM. Clinical Biomechanics of the Spine. 2nd ed. Philadelphia, PA: J. B. Lippincott; 1990:1–125

[17] Van Schaik JPJ, Verbiest H, Van Schaik FDJ. The orientation of laminae and facet joints in the lower lumbar spine. Spine 1985;10:59–63

[18] White AA III, Panjabi MM. The basic kinematics of the human spine. A review of past and current knowledge. Spine 1978;3:12–20

[19] White AA, Panjabi MM. Clinical Biomechanics of the Spine. 2nd ed. Philadelphia, PA: J. B. Lippincott; 1990:1–125

[20] Panjabi M, Dvorak J, Duranceau J, et al. Three-dimensional movements of the upper cervical spine. Spine 1988;13:726–730

[21] Krag MH, Seroussi REW, Wilder DG, Pope MH. Internal displacement distribution from in vitro loading of human thoracic and lumbar spinal motion segments: experimental results and theoretical predictions. Spine 1987;12:1001–1007

2 Physical Principles and Kinematics

Mohamad Bydon, Sarah E. Johnson, Patrick M. Flanigan

An understanding of the physical principles and kinematics involved in the discipline of spine surgery allows the surgeon to appreciate actions and reactions, force vectors, related component vectors, and the movements and/or deformations that they cause, enabling them to apply these concepts to clinical practice.

Learning Objectives

- Understand the importance of the instantaneous axis of rotation (IAR) and the effect of different loads on the IAR.
- Understand Newton's laws of motion and Hooke's law.
- Understand the relationship between stress, bending moment, and section modulus.
- Understand the stress–strain curve, the modulus of elasticity, the moment of inertia, and the coupling effect.

Questions

▸▸ Question 1

Where is the IAR located?

- A. Vertebral body
- B. The location is variable
- C. Facet joint
- D. Pedicle
- E. Neural foramen

▸▸ Question 2

How many degrees of freedom exist around each axis of rotation?

- A. 6
- B. 8
- C. 10
- D. 12
- E. 14

▸▸ Question 3

In the equation $M = F \times D$, what does M represent?

- A. Section modulus
- B. Loading force
- C. Bending moment
- D. Torque
- E. Momentum

▸▸ Question 4

The time rate of momentum of a body is equal in magnitude and direction to the vector sum of the forces acting upon it. Which of the following does this statement best describe?

- A. The law of inertia
- B. Newton's first law of motion
- C. Hooke's law
- D. Newton's second law of motion
- E. Newton's third law of motion

▸▸ Question 5

When rotation is superimposed on translation, what is the resultant component of movement called?

- A. Torque
- B. Bending moment
- C. Helical axis of motion
- D. Momentum
- E. Coupling

▸▸ Question 6

Which of the following statements regarding paradoxical spinal motion is correct?

- A. It is the movement that occurs during the application of flexion only
- B. It is the movement that occurs during the application of extension only
- C. It is the movement that occurs during the application of flexion and extension
- D. It is the movement that occurs during the application of rotation stress only
- E. It is the movement that occurs during the application of flexion, extension, and rotation stress

▸▸ Question 7

Which of the following statements best describes Newton's third law of motion?

- A. If a body is subjected to no net external influence, it has a constant velocity, either zero or nonzero
- B. Interactions between objects result in no net change in momentum
- C. The time rate of momentum of a body is equal in magnitude and direction to the vector sum of the forces acting upon it
- D. Momentum is the product of mass and velocity
- E. An object responds to the summation of the forces applied to it

▸▸ Question 8

Which of the following statements best defines the physical principle of a couple?

- A. The phenomenon by which a movement of the spine along or about an axis obligates another movement along or about another axis (of the Cartesian coordinate system)
- B. A structure acted on by a couple can be kept in equilibrium only by another couple of the same moment and the opposite direction
- C. A couple is a pair of forces applied to a structure that are of equal magnitude and opposite direction, having two lines of action that ultimately coincide
- D. A couple is a pair of forces applied to a structure that are of equal magnitude and opposite direction, having lines of action that are parallel but do not coincide
- E. A couple is a pair of forces applied to a structure that are of unequal magnitude but in the same direction, having lines of action that are parallel but do not coincide

▸▸ Question 9

An axial load applied to a vertebral body at the point of the IAR results, by definition, in an equal (in magnitude) but opposite (in direction) reaction force. This pair of forces may result in deformation or failure of the vertebral body, resulting in which of the following?

- A. Fracture-dislocation
- B. Wedge fracture
- C. Burst fracture
- D. Chance fracture or flexion-distraction fracture
- E. No change in the vertebral body

▸▸ Question 10

For small displacements, the size of the deformation is proportional to the deforming force. Which law does this statement describe?

- A. Hooke's law
- B. Newton's first law of motion
- C. Newton's second law of motion
- D. Newton's third law of motion
- E. The law of superimposition of forces

▸▸ Question 11

A couple is a pair of forces applied to a structure that are of equal magnitude and opposite direction, having lines of action that are parallel but do not coincide. ▸ Fig. 2.1 illustrates a couple consisting of two forces, each of magnitude F, acting upon a structure and separated by a perpendicular distance D. What does the following equation represent?

$$x_1F - x_2F = x_1F - (x_1 + D)F = -DF$$

- A. Bending moment
- B. Section modulus
- C. Momentum
- D. Loading force
- E. Torque

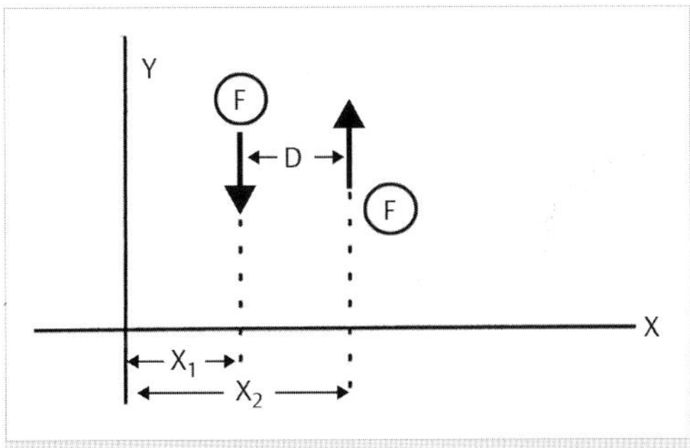

Fig. 2.1 A couple acting on a structure of width D. In this case, translation will not occur, but rotation will occur if the couple is unopposed. (Source: Biomechanics of Spine Stabilization: Third Edition, © 2015 Thieme Medical Publishers, Inc.)

▸▸ Question 12

In this typical stress–strain curve for a biological tissue, such as a ligament, what does CD represent (see ▸ Fig. 2.2)?

- A. Elastic limit
- B. Elastic zone
- C. Neutral zone
- D. Point of failure
- E. Plastic zone

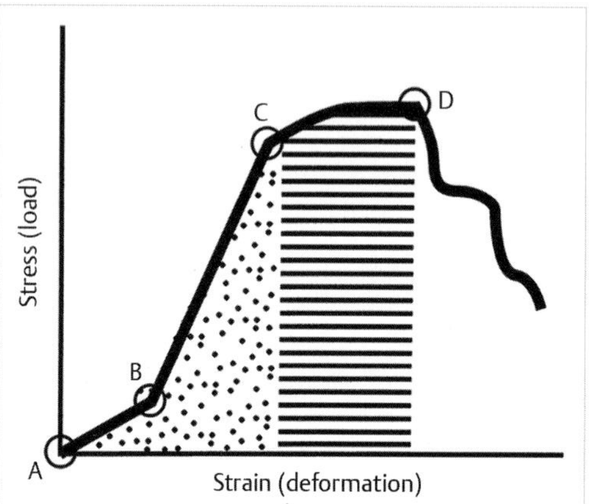

Fig. 2.2 (Source: Biomechanics of Spine Stabilization: Third Edition, © 2015 Thieme Medical Publishers, Inc.)

▸▸ Question 13

Elastic modulus or the modulus of elasticity, which is a constant that is characteristic of a given material, is defined by which of the following equations?

- A. Elastic modulus = stress × strain
- B. Elastic modulus = stress/strain
- C. Elastic modulus = strain/stress
- D. Elastic modulus = stress − strain
- E. Elastic modulus = stress + strain

▸▸ Question 14

In the equation $\theta = M/Z$, what does Z represent?

- A. Loading force
- B. Section modulus
- C. Momentum
- D. Bending moment
- E. Torque

▸▸ Question 15

Which of the following is the section modulus proportional to?

- A. Third power of the outer diameter of a screw
- B. Second power of the outer diameter of a screw
- C. Third power of the inner diameter of a screw
- D. Second power of the diameter of the rod
- E. Fifth power of inner diameter of a screw

▸▸ Question 16

Which of the following is stiffness or the moment of inertia (*I*) proportional to?

- A. Second power of the outer diameter of a screw
- B. Third power of the outer diameter of a screw
- C. Fourth power of the diameter of the rod
- D. Fifth power of the diameter of the rod
- E. Fifth power of inner diameter of a screw

▸▸ Question 17

Which of the following statements best describes Newton's first law of motion?

- A. For small displacements, the size of the deformation is proportional to the deforming force
- B. The time rate of momentum of a body is equal in magnitude and direction to the vector sum of the forces acting upon it
- C. For every action, there is an equal but opposite reaction
- D. If a body is subjected to no net external influence, it has a constant velocity, either zero or nonzero
- E. Interactions between objects result in no net change in momentum

▸▸ Question 18

Which of the following phenomena demonstrate the "coupling" effect? Select the best answer.

- A. A pair of forces applied to a structure that are of equal magnitude and opposite direction, having lines of action that are parallel but do not coincide
- B. Spinal rotation
- C. Screw motion when a screw is placed through the bone graft
- D. Spinal burst fracture
- E. Failure of constructs due to use of variable screws in traumatic spine fracture

▸▸ Question 19

How can momentum be best defined? Select the best answer.

- A. Stress/strain
- B. For small displacements, the size of the deformation is proportional to the deforming force
- C. Bending moment/section modulus
- D. Mass × velocity
- E. The ability of an object to resist bending

▸▸ Question 20

The area under the stress–strain curve is proportional to the energy absorbed before failure (point of failure). What is this a measure of?

- A. Resilience
- B. Strength
- C. Stress
- D. Strain
- E. Momentum

Answers

▸▸ Answer 1

Correct answer is B

Forces applied to the spine can be broken down into component vectors. A vector is defined here as a force oriented in a fixed and well-defined direction in three-dimensional space. A force vector may act on a lever (moment arm), causing a bending moment. The bending moment applied to a point in space causes rotation, or a tendency to rotate, about an axis. This axis, regarding the spine, is termed the instantaneous axis of rotation (IAR). The IAR is the axis about which each vertebral segment rotates at any given instant. The word instantaneous is included to emphasize that the axis of rotation varies depending on the loads and forces applied. Multiple factors, such as degenerative disease, fractures, ligamentous injuries, instrumentation and/or fusion placement, and segmental motion, can affect its position (see ▸ Fig. 2.3). The IAR should be considered dynamic. As spinal movement occurs, the IAR of each involved spinal segment moves. The IAR is clinically derived from dynamic radiographs (i.e., flexion and extension radiographs). For example, the IAR is affected by the extent of degeneration and deformation in the spondylotic spine with a lysis of the pedicle (spondylolysis). The IAR migrates rostrally as the extent of the pars defect advances and the wedge deformity progresses.[1] In a sense, the IAR is a fulcrum. For example, if the spine is flexed, all points ventral to the IAR come closer together and all points dorsal to the IAR move farther apart (see ▸ Fig. 2.4). It is important to note that these considerations are clinically important. For example, both cervical spine flexion and extension can decompress the neuroforamina, depending on the location of the IAR. In the case in which the IAR is located in the region of the facet joint, flexion causes neuroforaminal compression and extension causes neuroforaminal decompression. Its location

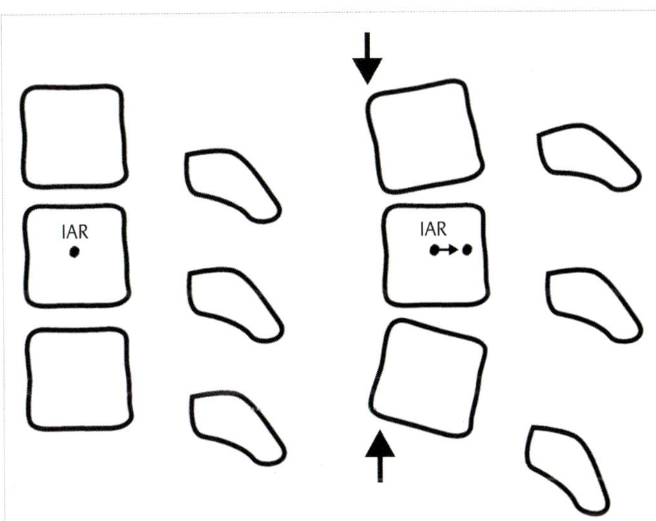

Fig. 2.3 A depiction of an applied bending moment altering the location of the IAR (*dot*) from the (A) preload situation to the (B) postload situation. Because a ventral bending moment was applied, the IAR, as is often the case, moved dorsally. *IAR*, instantaneous axis of rotation. (Source: Biomechanics of Spine Stabilization: Third Edition, © 2015 Thieme Medical Publishers, Inc.)

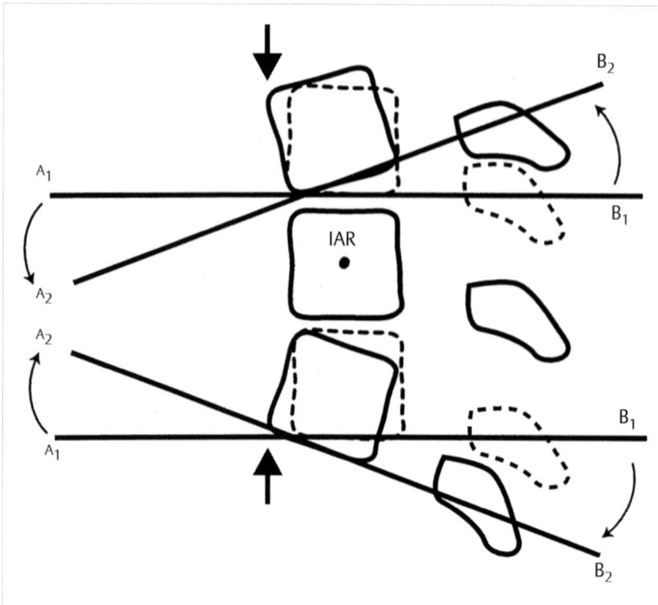

Fig. 2.4 A depiction of the fulcrum-like nature of the IAR (*dot*). If spinal flexion occurs, as depicted, all points ventral to the IAR come closer to one another and all points dorsal to the IAR spread farther apart, as depicted by the curved arrows. A_1 and B_1 designate ventral and dorsal points aligned with the vertebral end plates in the neutral position. A_2 and B_2 represent ventral and dorsal points aligned with the vertebral end plates following flexion. *IAR*, instantaneous axis of rotation. (Source: Biomechanics of Spine Stabilization: Third Edition, © 2015 Thieme Medical Publishers, Inc.)

is variable, depending on the intrinsic curvature of the spine, as well as other factors,[2,3] which is why option B is correct and options A, C, D, and E are incorrect.

▸▸ Answer 2

Correct answer is A

To make things easier, the standard Cartesian coordinate system has been applied to the spine. In this system, there are three axes: the x-, y-, and z-axes. For simplicity, the terms rostral, caudal, ventral, dorsal, right, and left are used. Rotational and translational movements can occur about these axes, resulting in 12 potential movements about the IAR: 2 translational movements along each of the 3 axes (1 in each direction) and 2 rotational movements around each of the axes (1 in each direction). These potential movements may also be considered in terms of degrees of freedom; thus, six degrees of freedom exist about each IAR (see ▸ Fig. 2.5); hence, option A is the correct answer and options B, C, D, and E are incorrect.

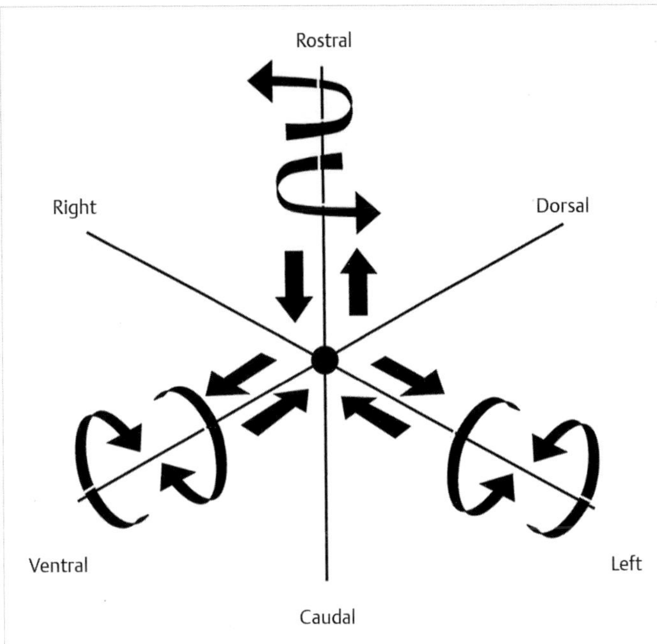

Fig. 2.5 The Cartesian coordinate system with the instantaneous axis of rotation as the center. Translation and rotation can occur in both of their respective directions about each axis. (Source: Biomechanics of Spine Stabilization: Third Edition, © 2015 Thieme Medical Publishers, Inc.)

▸▸ Answer 3

Correct answer is C

The bending moment (M) is defined as the product of the force (F) applied to the lever arm and the length of the lever arm (D), where D is equal to the perpendicular distance from the force vector to the IAR (see ▸ Fig. 2.1). Therefore, option C is correct, and options A, B, D, and E are incorrect.

▸▸ Answer 4

Correct answer is D

Newton's second law of motion, the law of superimposition of forces, can be stated as: the time rate of momentum of a body is equal in magnitude and direction to the vector sum of the forces acting upon it. In other words, an object responds to the summation of the forces applied to it. Therefore, option D is the correct answer, and options A, B, C, and E are incorrect.

▸▸ Answer 5

Correct answer is C

When rotation is superimposed on translation, the resultant component of movement described by the translational movement vector is called the helical axis of motion. Thus, option C is the correct answer. It is oriented in the direction of the translational movement. A screw motion can be defined, in part, by this parameter. It must be emphasized that the determination of these axes is subject to error. Torque is a measure of the force that can cause an object to rotate about an axis; thus, option A is incorrect. The bending moment (M) is defined as the product of the force (F) applied to the lever arm and the length of the lever arm (D), where D is equal to the perpendicular distance from the force vector to the IAR. The bending moment is effectively the torque applied by the force (circular force). More correctly, torque is a moment with magnitude; thus, option B is incorrect. Momentum is defined as the product of mass and velocity of an object, which is why option D is incorrect. Coupling is defined as the phenomenon by which a movement of the spine along or about an axis obligates another movement along or about another axis; hence, option E is incorrect.

▸▸ Answer 6

Correct answer is E

Paradoxical spinal motion is the unexpected and potentially untoward segmental spinal movement

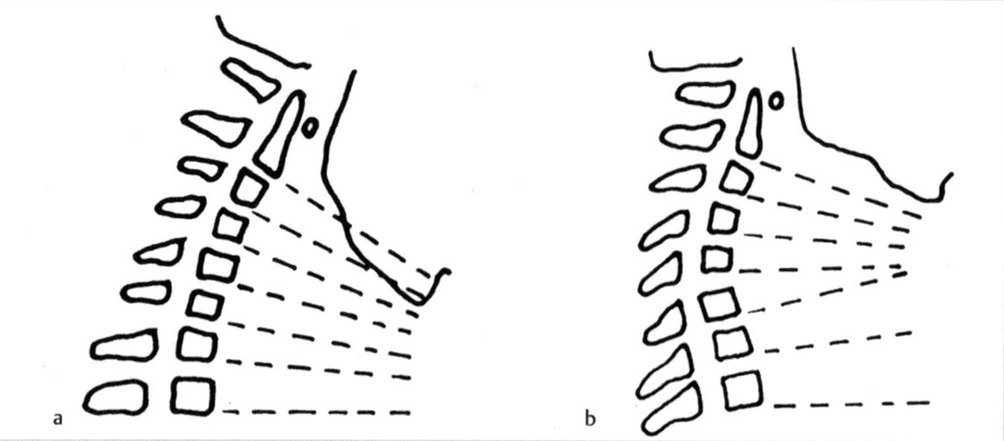

Fig. 2.6 Paradoxical spinal motion is the phenomenon whereby an intended motion, such as flexion, is accompanied by an unintended motion, such as extension, at one or more motion segments. Paradoxical motion can occur when at least two intervertebral discs are suspended between fixation points (either via external splinting or via spinal instrumentation). **(a)** Unobstructed cervical flexion results in uniform segmental flexion in the nonpathologic situation. If restriction of movement at the termini of a brace (e.g., halo) is significant, paradoxical spinal motion may occur. **(b)** Spinal snaking is a manifestation of the paradoxical spinal motion phenomenon. It is depicted here in the case of a rigid external spinal splint. (Source: Biomechanics of Spine Stabilization: Third Edition, © 2015 Thieme Medical Publishers, Inc.)

that occurs during the application of flexion, extension, or rotation stresses to the involved spinal segment and adjacent segments. Thus, option E is correct and option A, B, C, and D are incorrect statements. This motion occurs in two circumstances: (1) in cases of segmental spine instability and (2) in cases in which stabilization techniques (spinal implants or external splints) are used that limit motion between two nonadjacent vertebrae with at least two intervertebral discs located between the termini of the implant or splint (see ▶ Fig. 2.6). In segmental spine instability, paradoxical movement can occur at the index and adjacent levels. In the case of stabilization techniques, the suspension of vertebral body segments between rigidly immobilized segments allows segmental muscular attachments to cause segmental movement in a paradoxical manner (snaking). Snaking is a characteristic type of movement of spinal segments in response to external force applications. With such movement, the sum of the movements of individual spinal motion segments is greater than the overall spinal movement observed.[4] In some clinical circumstances, it can be objectively assessed.[5] In these cases, it can be quantified by measuring the overall movement between the rigidly immobilized rostral and caudal components. This is subtracted from the sum of the absolute values of each of the individual intervening segmental movements.[1] The paradoxical motion phenomenon may become significant with external spinal splinting or in cases in which an instrumented spine is not instrumented at every segmental level (e.g., only at the termini of the construct). In either case, movement of the suspended spinal segments can occur (between the extremes of the fixation).

▸▸ Answer 7

Correct answer is B

The law of conservation of momentum, or Newton's third law of motion, can be stated thus: interactions between objects result in no net change in momentum. When two objects interact via a collision, the first body exerts a force on the second. The overall momentum of the two bodies remains constant—i.e., any momentum lost by one body is gained by the other. In other words, for every action there is an equal (in magnitude) but opposite (in direction) reaction. Option B best describes Newton's third law of motion; thus, it is the correct answer. For example, when a force is applied to a vertebral body by the application of an axial load, the force applied by the vertebral body on its neighboring vertebral bodies is equal in magnitude

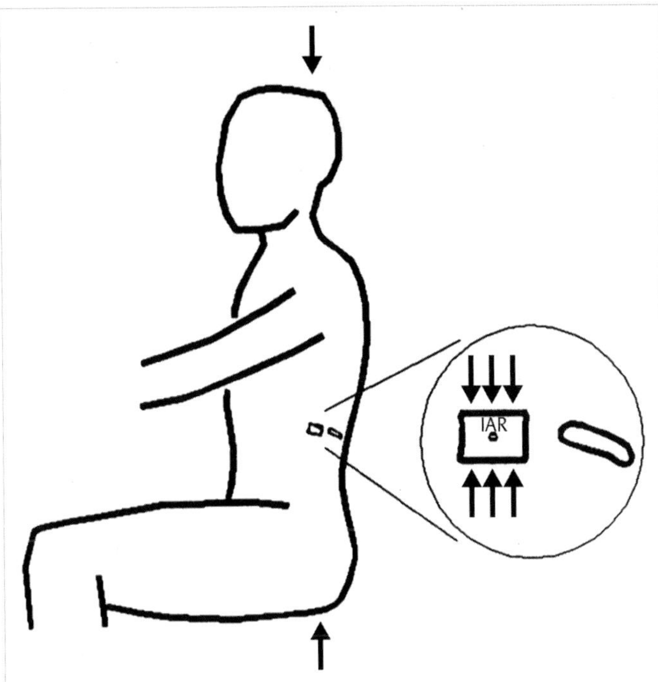

Fig. 2.7 Forces always occur in pairs. For every action, there is an equal but opposite reaction (Newton's third law). If an axial load is applied to a vertebral body, the forces impinging on the rostral and caudal portions of the vertebral body are equal. (Source: Biomechanics of Spine Stabilization: Third Edition, © 2015 Thieme Medical Publishers, Inc.)

but opposite in direction to the applied force (see ▶ Fig. 2.7). This is a manifestation of Newton's third law of motion. This may subsequently result in deformation, or failure of integrity, of the vertebral body. Option A is incorrect as it represents Newton's first law of motion, the law of inertia, which may be stated as: if a body is subjected to no net external influence, it has a constant velocity, either zero or nonzero. As long as there is no force acting on an object, its speed and direction of motion do not change. Newton's second law of motion, the law of superimposition of forces, can be stated thus: the time rate of momentum of a body is equal in magnitude and direction to the vector sum of the forces acting upon it. In other words, an object responds to the summation of the forces applied to it. Therefore, options C and E are both incorrect. Option D describes momentum, which is the product of mass and velocity.

▸▸ Answer 8

Correct answer is D

A couple is a pair of forces applied to a structure that are of equal magnitude and opposite direction, having lines of action that are parallel but do not coincide. Thus, option D is the correct answer, and options C and E are incorrect. ▶ Fig. 2.1 illustrates a couple consisting of two forces, each of magnitude F, acting upon a structure and separated by a perpendicular distance D. The resultant force is zero ($F - F = 0$). Option B describes the effect of a couple on a structure; however, it is not the correct definition of this phenomenon. Option A describes coupling, which is the phenomenon by which a movement of the spine along or about an axis obligates another movement along or about another axis (of the Cartesian coordinate system), which is not to be confused with the physical principle of a couple.

▸▸ Answer 9

Correct answer is C

This pair of forces may result in deformation or failure of the vertebral body, resulting in a burst fracture; hence, option C is the correct answer and options A, B, D, and E are incorrect (see ▶ Fig. 2.8a). If the load is applied in a plane at some distance from the IAR, a bending moment is created (see ▶ Fig. 2.9). If this bending moment is matched with an equal (in magnitude) but opposite (in direction) reaction bending moment, this pair of forces may similarly result in deformation or failure of the vertebral body, resulting in a wedge compression fracture (see ▶ Fig. 2.8b). In this case, the ventral concentration of stress "facilitated" the ventral vertebral body failure. This type of deformation or failure may occur in any plane, depending on the point of application of the force vector (load). This is illustrated for a lateral bending component (see ▶ Fig. 2.10a) and for a combination ventral and lateral bending component (see ▶ Fig. 2.10b).

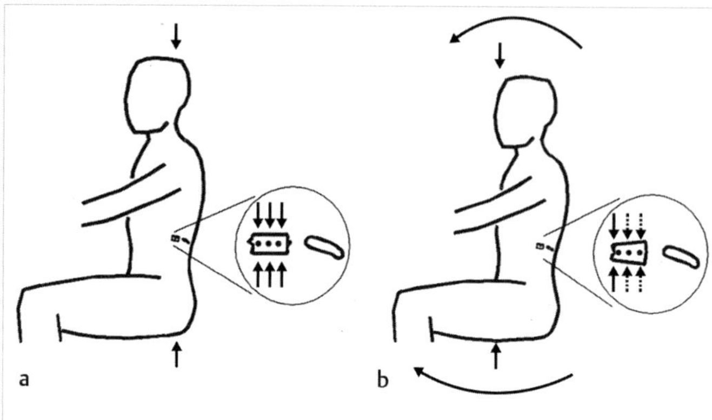

Fig. 2.8 **(a)** If a load is sufficient to result in vertebral body failure, the failure is of a burst fracture nature. **(b)** If, however, a load is applied in a plane ventral to the instantaneous axis of rotation (IAR), an asymmetric force pair and bending moment (*curved arrows*) will be applied to the IAR, resulting in a wedge compression fracture. Dots, IAR; *straight arrows*, loads; *curved arrows*, bending moments. (Source: Biomechanics of Spine Stabilization: Third Edition, © 2015 Thieme Medical Publishers, Inc.)

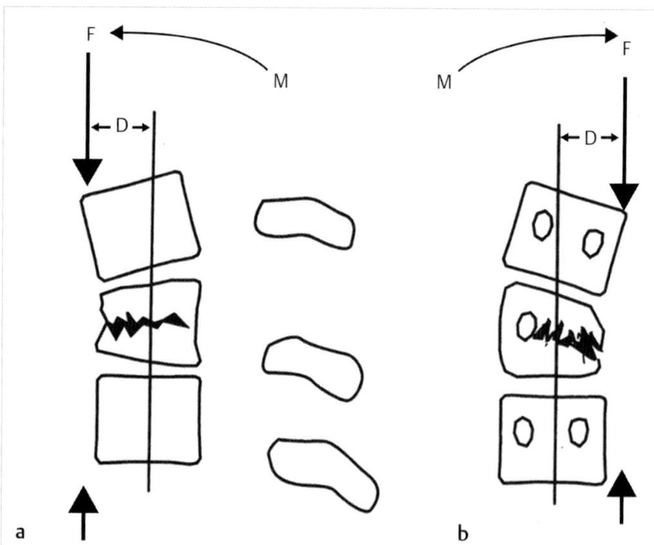

Fig. 2.9 The bending moment (*M*, depicted by a *curved arrow*) is the product of the force (*F*) and the length of the moment arm (*D*). The maximum bending moment is located at the center of the circle defined by the radius of the bending moment's arc (i.e., the instantaneous axis of rotation). **(a)** Lateral view. **(b)** Anteroposterior view. (Source: Biomechanics of Spine Stabilization: Third Edition, © 2015 Thieme Medical Publishers, Inc.)

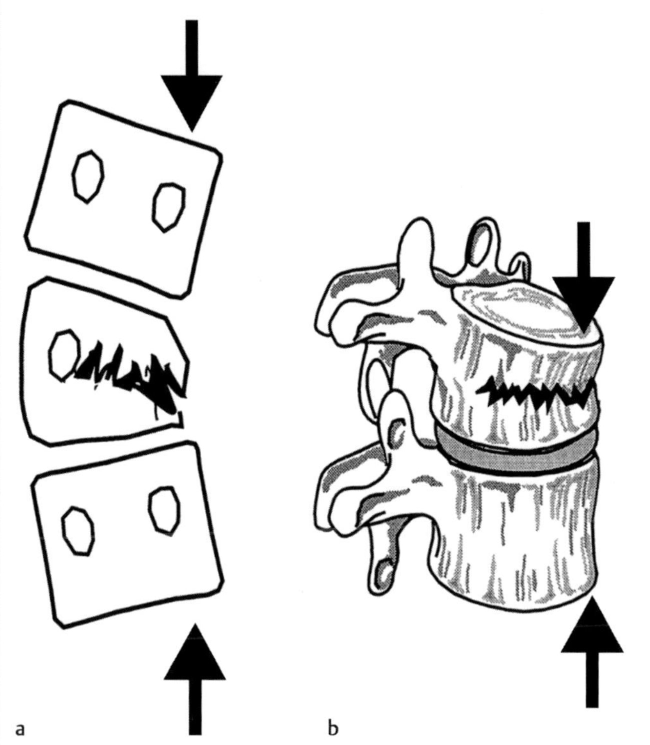

Fig. 2.10 The bending moment generated by the force pair may occur in any plane. **(a)** Lateral bending. **(b)** A combination of flexion and lateral bending. (Source: Biomechanics of Spine Stabilization: Third Edition, © 2015 Thieme Medical Publishers, Inc.)

▸▸ Answer 10

Correct answer is A

Hooke's law states that for small displacements, the size of the deformation is proportional to the deforming force; hence, A is the correct answer, and options B, C, D, and E are incorrect. No solid is perfectly rigid. When several external forces act on a solid at rest and the resultant net force is zero, the solid will be deformed. This linear relationship pertains only to solids that are deformed within their elastic zone (see ▸ Fig. 2.11). Elastic deformation (in the elastic zone) occurs whenever a strain totally recovers following the removal of a stress. This law is important when one considers the forces applied to the spine by a spinal instrumentation construct, as well as the response of the construct to these forces. For larger displacements, however, the elastic zone is exceeded, and the elastic limit (or yield point) is reached. This is the point at which the force departs from the linear relationship between the extent of deformation and the deforming force (i.e., Hooke's law no longer applies).

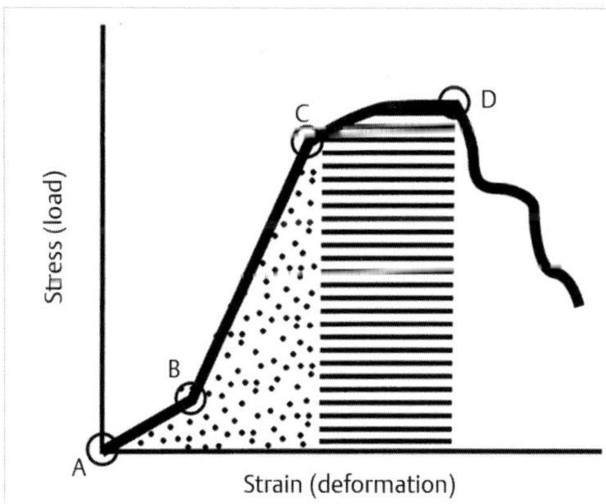

Fig. 2.11 A typical stress–strain curve for a biological tissue, such as a ligament. AB represents the neutral zone. BC represents the elastic zone. When the elastic limit (yield point (C) is reached, permanent deformation can occur (permanent set). CD represents the plastic zone where a permanent set occurs. Past D, failure occurs and the load diminishes. Striped area plus dotted area represent strength, whereas the dotted area represents resilience. (Source: Biomechanics of Spine Stabilization: Third Edition, © 2015 Thieme Medical Publishers, Inc.)

▸▸ Answer 11

Correct answer is E

This equation defines the resultant torque (bending moment) about any arbitrary point. In this case as illustrated in ▸ Fig. 2.1, translation will not occur, but rotation will occur if the couple is unopposed. Because x_1 and x_2 do not appear in the result, the torque of the couple is the same about all points in the plane of the forces forming the couple and is equal to the product of the magnitude of either force and the perpendicular distance between their lines of action. The concept of the couple is important, particularly regarding the complex forces applied by instrumentation constructs. Thus, option E is correct, and options A, B, C, and D are incorrect.

▸▸ Answer 12

Correct answer is E

When the elastic limit (yield point [C]) is reached, permanent deformation can occur (permanent set). CD represents the plastic zone where a permanent set occurs, so option E is correct and options A, B, C, and D are incorrect. Past point D, failure occurs, and the load diminishes. The striped area plus dotted area represent strength, whereas the dotted area represents resilience. AB represents the neutral zone. BC represents the elastic zone. For most materials, the elastic limit occurs close to the point where a permanent set is reached. The area under the stress–strain curve is proportional to the energy absorbed before failure (point of failure). This is a measure of strength. The removal of a stress recovers energy. The energy expended (area under the stress–strain curve up the yield point C) is a measure of an object's resilience. In vivo, most solids (e.g., bones) subjected to external forces are buffered from these forces by ligaments, tendons, and other soft tissues. Therefore, before the elastic zone is "reached," a zone of nonengagement (neutral zone) is passed. Within the neutral zone (AB in ▸ Fig. 2.2), the application of a small force results in relatively large displacement.

▸▸ Answer 13

Correct answer is B

The elastic modulus is defined by stress/strain, where the elastic modulus (modulus of elasticity) is a constant that is characteristic of a given material. The modulus of elasticity essentially should be thought of as a measure of the deformability of an object (i.e., stiffness). Stress is defined as the force applied to an object (load), whereas strain is defined as the response of the object to the force (deformation). Strain is the change in length or angle of a material subjected to a load. Strain may be either normal (linear) or shear (angular) in nature. Normal strain reflects tensile or compressive force–resisting abilities of a material; shear strain reflects angular deformation–resisting abilities of a material. Three types of elastic moduli exist: Young's modulus, a measure of the elastic properties of a body that is stretched or compressed; shear modulus, a measure of the shear deformation experienced by a body that is subjected to transverse forces of equal and opposite direction, applied at opposite faces of the body; and bulk modulus, the elastic deformation of a solid when it is squeezed.

▸▸ Answer 14

Correct answer is B

Stress (θ) applied to an implant is a function of two factors: bending moment (M) and section modulus (Z). The relationship is described by the equation $\theta = M / Z$. Therefore, option B is correct, and options B, C, D, and E are incorrect.

▸▸ Answer 15

Correct answer is C

Section modulus (Z) defines the ability of an object, such as a screw or rod, to resist bending.

$Z \propto \pi \times D^3/32$

It is proportional to the third power of the diameter of a rod or the third power of the inner diameter of a screw. Option C is correct, and options A, B, D, and E are incorrect.

▸▸ Answer 16

Correct answer is C

The moment of inertia essentially defines stiffness. Stiffness is proportional to the fourth power of the diameter of a rod or the fourth power of the inner diameter of a screw.

Stiffness $\propto \pi \times D^4/32$

Therefore, as the diameter of a rod is increased, the stiffness increases more rapidly than the strength, as strength is proportional to the diameter cubed, while stiffness is proportional to the diameter to the fourth power. Hence, larger diameter rods are more stiff than they are strong, when compared with smaller diameter rods.

▸▸ Answer 17

Correct answer is D

Newton's first law of motion, the law of inertia, can be stated as: if a body is subjected to no net external influence, it has a constant velocity, either zero or nonzero. As long as there is no force acting on an object, its speed and direction of motion do not change. Option A describes Hooke's law, option B describes Newton's second law of motion, and options C and E describe Newton's third law of motion and are therefore all incorrect answers.

▸▸ Answer 18

Correct answer is B

Coupling is defined as the phenomenon by which a movement of the spine along or about an axis obligates another movement along or about another axis (of the Cartesian coordinate system); thus, option B is the correct answer. In the cervical region, for example, lateral bending results in rotation of the spinous processes away from the concave side of the curvature (the direction of the bend). This is due, in part, to the orientation of the facet joints as well as to the presence of the uncovertebral joints. In the lumbar region, however, the coupling movements associated with the lateral bending are in the opposite direction, with the spinous processes rotating in the same direction as the concave side of the direction of the bend. The phenomenon of coupling also explains the association of the obligatory rotatory component associated with degenerative scoliosis of the lumbar spine. A describes the physical principle of a couple, which is different from the coupling effect; therefore, A is wrong. Placing a screw through a bone graft weakens the construct but is not associated with rotation or the coupling effect; option C is incorrect. A burst fracture may result when an axial load is applied to a vertebral body at the point of the IAR resulting in an equal (in magnitude) but opposite (in direction) reaction force; thus, option D is wrong. Using variable angle (nonfixed moment arm) screws in traumatic spine fractures may lead to construct failure, but this does not demonstrate the coupling effect. Therefore, E is incorrect.

▸▸ Answer 19

Correct answer is D

Momentum is the product of the mass and velocity of an object. Thus, option D is correct. Momentum, therefore, is defined in part by direction; it demonstrates its vector component in this manner. To appropriately appreciate the stresses withstood by the spine, the surgeon must understand the fundamental action–reaction phenomenon, and an appreciation of the concept of momentum is integral to this process. Option A describes the elastic modulus, option B is the definition of Hooke's law, option C defines stress, and option E describes section modulus; hence, options A, B, C, and E are incorrect.

▸▸ Answer 20

Correct answer is B

The area under the stress–strain curve is proportional to the energy absorbed before failure (point of failure) and this is a measure of strength; hence, option B is correct. The removal of a stress recovers energy. The energy expended (area under the stress–strain curve up the yield point) is a measure of an object's resilience; thus, option A is incorrect. Stress is defined as the force applied to an object (load), whereas strain is defined as the response of the object to the force (deformation); therefore, options C and D are incorrect. Option E is incorrect, as momentum is the product of the mass and velocity of an object.

Key Principles

- IAR is dynamic and depends on the different loads and forces applied.
- Hooke's law states that for small displacements, the size of the deformation is proportional to the deforming force.
- Stress = bending moment/section modulus.
- Elastic modulus = stress/strain.

References

[1] Sakamaki T, Katoh S, Sairyo K. Normal and spondylolytic pediatric spine movements with reference to instantaneous axis of rotation. Spine (Phila Pa 1976) 2002;27:141–145

[2] Brod JJ. The concepts and terms of mechanics. Clin Orthop Relat Res 1980;146:9–17

[3] Caruso SA, Marguilies JY, Gorup J, et al. Instrumented fusions of the lumbosacral spine: a technical overview. In: Margulies JY, ed. Lumbosacral and Spinopelvic Fixation. Philadelphia, PA: Lippincott-Raven Publishers; 1996:199–211

[4] Benzel EC, Hadden TA, Saulsbery CM. A comparison of the Minerva and halo jackets for stabilization of the cervical spine. J Neurosurg 1989;70:411–414

[5] Caruso SA, Marguilies JY, Gorup J, et al. Instrumented fusions of the lumbosacral spine: a technical overview. In: Margulies JY, ed. Lumbosacral and Spinopelvic Fixation. Philadelphia, PA: Lippincott-Raven Publishers; 1996:199–211

3 Stability and Instability of the Spine

James Rizkalla, Joseph Weiner, Brandon D. Lawrence

Learning Objectives

- Understand the definitions of spinal stability and instability.
- Understand the various scoring systems available for defining acute spinal instability.
- Describe the types of chronic instability including glacial and dysfunctional segmental motion.
- Describe the role of the rib cage and core musculature in spinal stability.
- Understand how deformity impacts spinal stability.

Questions

▸▸ Question 1

How is spinal instability generally defined?

- A. The association of pain with movement of the spine
- B. Balance and gait dysfunction
- C. Weakness of muscle function within a specified nerve distribution
- D. Neural element injury
- E. The inability to limit excessive or abnormal spinal displacement

▸▸ Question 2

What is the White and Panjabi "stretch" test?

- A. A test used to assess range of motion in the axial plane
- B. A method of assessing acute cervical spine stability
- C. The association of lumbar radicular pain with extension of the lower extremity
- D. The contact forces identified in the facet joints with extension of a spinal segment
- E. Transient sensation of an electric shock radiating into the extremities with flexion of the cervical spine

▸▸ Question 3

Which of the following is NOT a component of the posterior column of the spine?

- A. Pedicles
- B. Spinous process
- C. Posterior longitudinal ligament
- D. Posterior ligament complex
- E. Facets

▸▸ Question 4

What is the definition of the "neutral axis" of the spine?

- A. The longitudinal region of the spine that bears a significant portion of the axial load
- B. The area of the spine that protects the spinal elements
- C. The region of the spine synonymous with the posterior ligamentous complex
- D. The area of the spine that carries minimal axial load
- E. The region of the spine determined by the apex of sagittal curvature

▸▸ Question 5

What is the definition of glacial instability and what is its importance to spinal stability?

- A. The inability of the spine to support the torso during normal activity
- B. Instability that involves neither the overt disruption of spinal integrity nor deformity progression
- C. The loss of either ventral or dorsal spinal integrity with preservation of the other, which is sufficient to support some normal activities
- D. Spinal instability that is not overt and that does not pose a significant risk for the rapid development or progression of kyphotic, scoliotic, or translational deformity
- E. Instability that involves all three columns of the spine and results in high risk of deformity progression

▸▸ Question 6

What types of injuries are associated with "limited instability"?
- A. Obvious overtly unstable injuries
- B. Injuries that result in loss of integrity of the ventral and dorsal columns
- C. Injuries that result in loss of integrity of either the ventral or dorsal column
- D. Injuries that frequently require surgical intervention
- E. Injuries that are not commonly mistaken for overt instability

▸▸ Question 7

Is it always necessary to "see" movement on dynamic radiographs (flexion–extension X-rays) to establish the presence of dysfunctional segmental motion?
- A. Yes, movement of dynamic radiography is essential to defining instability
- B. Yes, as all instability can be exposed by weight-bearing radiographs
- C. No, flexion–extension radiographs are not useful in the setting of instability
- D. No, the patient may be guarding due to pain, limiting the motion seen on radiographs
- E. No, but if movement is not seen on dynamic films, it will be evident in advanced radiographic imaging

▸▸ Question 8

Which of the following is true regarding muscular contribution to spine stability?
- A. Muscles provide stability by virtue of the orientation of their attachments to the spine
- B. Imbalance of muscle forces improves functional stability of the spine
- C. Muscles work individually, with no other anatomical counterbalance
- D. Muscles are a negligible contribution to the overall stability of the spine
- E. Muscles play a minimal role in affecting overall spinal movement

▸▸ Question 9

How are Cobb angles of the spine related to structural deformity and deformity progression of the spine?
- A. The Cobb angle describes the overall stability of the spine
- B. The Cobb angle is unrelated to curve progression
- C. The Cobb angle affects only the coronal deformity of the spine
- D. All patients with the same Cobb angle have the same risk of deformity progression
- E. As the Cobb angle increases, an increased moment arm length is applied to the spine, often resulting in deformity progression

▸▸ Question 10

Why is a different scheme for quantitating upper cervical instability (as contrasted with subaxial instability) necessary?
- A. Assessment of the stability of the upper cervical spine is complicated by the complex anatomy of this region and by the relative success of the nonsurgical management of injuries in this region
- B. In contrast to the subaxial cervical spine, the definition of upper cervical instability tends to be more clear cut
- C. Because of the frequency of injury, upper cervical spine instability warrants a separate evaluating schema
- D. Due to the more complex anatomy of the subaxial cervical spine, the definition of an unstable spine is more uncertain than in the upper cervical trauma patient
- E. Historically, different schemes were used to evaluate subaxial and upper cervical trauma patients; however, with advanced imaging, a single scheme for quantitating instability is sufficient for all cervical trauma

▸▸ Question 11

How does the instantaneous axis of rotation (IAR) change following the loss of ventral axial load-bearing ability?

- A. Shifts the IAR in a ventral direction
- B. Shifts the IAR in a proximal direction
- C. Shifts the IAR in a lateral direction
- D. Shifts the IAR in a dorsal direction
- E. Shifts the IAR in a distal direction

▸▸ Question 12

In what region of the spine is the IAR routinely found?

- A. In the anterior column
- B. In the posterior column
- C. Within the neutral axis
- D. Lateral to the spinal canal
- E. At the anterior longitudinal ligament

▸▸ Question 13

What anatomical features uniquely contribute to the stability of the thoracic spine?

- A. Erector spinae and rectus abdominus muscles
- B. Nuchal ligament
- C. Iliopsoas
- D. Ribs and sternum
- E. Sagittally oriented facet joints

▸▸ Question 14

Which of the following is not indicative of C0–C1–C2 instability?

- A. > 1 mm of C0–C1 translation in the sagittal plane
- B. < 4 mm of C1–C2 translation in the sagittal plane
- C. > 7 mm of overhang C1–C2 (total right and left)
- D. > 8 degrees of axial rotation C0–C1 to one side
- E. Avulsed transverse ligament of the atlas

▸▸ Question 15

Which of the following is necessary for overt instability to exist?

- A. > 40% height loss of vertebral body
- B. Disruption of the posterior ligamentous complex
- C. > 1.5 cm of anterolisthesis on flexion–extension radiographs
- D. Acute fracture involving two columns of the spine
- E. Loss of integrity of the vertebral body and/or disc with associated loss of integrity of the dorsal elements

▸▸ Question 16

Which of the following deformity scenarios is at highest risk for progressive instability?

- A. 15-degree Cobb with large radius of curvature
- B. 15-degree Cobb with small radius of curvature
- C. 50-degree Cobb with large radius of curvature
- D. 30-degree Cobb with small radius of curvature
- E. 50-degree Cobb with small radius of curvature

▸▸ Question 17

Which of the following describes the risk for spinal deformity in a patient with a neuromuscular disorder, such as Duchenne's muscle dystrophy?

- A. Decreased risk due to genetic mutation leading to improved bone quality
- B. Increased risk due to aberrations in truncal muscle control leading to decreased secondary spinal stability
- C. Decreased risk due to reduced ambulation
- D. Increased risk due to intrinsic segmental motion defects
- E. Increased risk due to ligamentous laxity

▸▸ Question 18

A 69-year-old woman has a mobile degenerative L4–L5 spondylolisthesis and stenosis that requires fusion. There is 6 mm of dynamic anterolisthesis from extension to flexion. What type of instability is this pathologic motion an example of?

- A. Overt instability
- B. Acute limited instability
- C. Glacial instability
- D. Dysfunctional segmental motion
- E. Fixed instability

▸▸ Question 19

Which of the following is not a characteristic of mechanical back pain?

- A. Deep and agonizing in nature
- B. Worse with spinal loading
- C. Relieved with unloading
- D. Leads to radicular pain
- E. Associated with mechanical instability

▸▸ Question 20

Why has discography fallen out of favor?

- A. Decreased iatrogenic disc degeneration
- B. High specificity
- C. High false-positive rates
- D. More helpful than less invasive imaging techniques
- E. Decreases surgical rates

Answers

▸▸ Answer 1

Correct answer is E

The definition of instability, generally speaking, is the inability to limit excessive or abnormal spinal displacement. The use of the word excessive reflects the difficulty of clinical quantitation as various anatomic locations are associated with varying anatomic stability.

▸▸ Answer 2

Correct answer is B

The stretch test, as described by White and Panjabi, involves the progressive addition of cervical traction weight (to 33% of the patient's weight) with serial radiographic and clinical assessments. A positive test (indicating the presence of instability) shows a disc interspace separation of more than 1.7 mm or a change in angle between vertebrae of more than 7.5 degrees between the prestretch and poststretch conditions. It should be noted that the merits of this test are uncertain. In addition, this test poses potential risks to the patient.

▸▸ Answer 3

Correct answer is C

The posterior column of the spine, as described by Denis, is comprised of the pedicles, facets, ligamentum flavum, spinous process, and posterior ligament complex. The posterior longitudinal ligament is a component of the middle column of the spine.

▸▸ Answer 4

Correct answer is A

The neutral axis is that longitudinal region of the spinal column that frequently bears a significant portion of the axial load and about which spinal element distraction or compression does not excessively occur with flexion or extension. Usually, the neutral axis is located in the region of the middorsal aspect of the vertebral body—that is, the middle column of Denis (see ▸ Fig. 3.1).

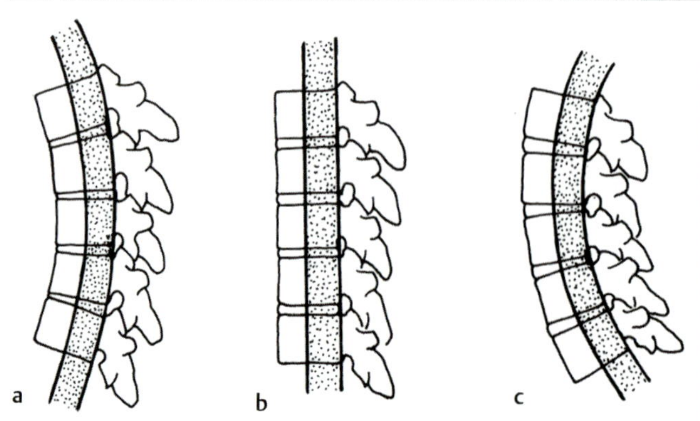

Fig. 3.1 Depiction of the neutral axis (*shaded areas*). The neutral axis is the longitudinal region of the spinal column that bears much of the axial load and about which spinal element distraction or compression does not significantly occur with the assumption of **(a)** flexed, **(b)** neutral, or **(c)** extension postures. This is a dynamic and theoretical concept. (Source: Biomechanics of Spine Stabilization: Third Edition, © 2015 Thieme Medical Publishers, Inc.)

▸▸ **Answer 5**

Correct answer is D

Glacial instability is defined as spinal instability that is not overt and that does not pose significant risk for the rapid development or progression of kyphotic, scoliotic, or translational deformities; however, like the motion of a glacier, the deformity progresses gradually, although substantial external forces do not cause immediate movement or progression of deformity.[1]

▸▸ **Answer 6**

Correct answer is C

Limited instability is defined as the loss of either ventral or dorsal spinal integrity with preservation of the other, which is sufficient to support some normal activities. If both ventral loss and dorsal loss of integrity are present, overt instability usually exists. The ventral type is often associated with an isolated end plate or vertebral body fracture. A true burst fracture resulting in collapse of the vertebra should be considered to be such an injury. The dorsal type is either ligamentous (a spinal strain of sorts) and/or bony (the result of laminar or facet fracture) in nature.

▸▸ **Answer 7**

Correct answer is D

Dynamic radiographs (flexion and extension radiographs) may be useful to establish the diagnosis of an associated dysfunctional motion segment (see the following). For example, they may demonstrate excessive or atypical movement. As previously emphasized, if excessive movement is not present on dynamic imaging, the absence of instability cannot be assumed. Pain and guarding may result in a protection from movement that might have been demonstrated if the pain and guarding were not present. This is true for all subcategories of instability.

▸▸ **Answer 8**

Correct answer is A

Muscles provide stability to the spine due to their direct attachment and play a critical role in spinal movement and stability. In general, any imbalance of muscular forces causes movement about a motion segment. Conversely, a balancing of muscle and other intrinsic forces about a motion segment results in no net movement (Newton's second law) and a stable spinal segment.

▸▸ **Answer 9**

Correct answer is E

As the Cobb angle increases, an increased moment arm length is applied to the spine. In the case of a kyphotic deformation, the dorsal ligamentous structures are stressed excessively because their main function is to resist tensile loads. Simultaneously, the ventral structures (vertebral body, etc.) are also stressed, but in compression (axial loading). These concepts apply to angular deformations in any plane.

▸▸ **Answer 10**

Correct answer is A

Ligamentous or bony disruption, with a resultant loss of translation-resisting integrity, constitutes an overtly unstable spine. Ligamentous or bony disruption that does not result in overt loss of translation-resisting integrity constitutes limited instability. This interpretation of the unstable upper cervical spine, although vague, should suffice if the clinician uses the principles presented earlier as well as common sense.

▸▸ **Answer 11**

Correct answer is D

The loss of ventral axial load-bearing ability generally shifts the IAR in a dorsal direction. Conversely, the loss of dorsal axial load-bearing ability generally shifts the IAR in a ventral direction. The IAR is shifted in a predictable manner, usually toward the region of the nonpathologic neutral axis.

▸▸ **Answer 12**

Correct answer is C

Denis' three column theory, which adds the concept of a middle column to the two-column theories, allows specific assessment of that component of the spinal column in the region of the neutral axis. The neutral axis is that longitudinal region of the spinal column that bears a significant portion of the axial load and about which spinal element distraction or compression does not excessively occur with flexion or extension. Usually, the neutral axis is located in the region of the middorsal aspect of the vertebral body—that is, the middle column of Denis. Usually, the IARs in the sagittal plane are located close to or within the neutral axis.[2,3]

▸▸ Answer 13

Correct answer is D

The ribs and sternum make an important contribution to the stability of the middle and upper thoracic spine. They function together to enhance stability. The costovertebral and costosternal joints play a pivotal role in this stabilization process. The stiffness of the spine is greatly increased if all components of the rib cage–spine unit are intact. An intact rib cage augments the axial load-resisting ability fourfold.

▸▸ Answer 14

Correct answer is B

Of the answers listed, < 4 mm of C1–C2 translation in the sagittal plane would be indicative of stability at the C1–C2 junction. > 4 mm of translation, however, would be indicative of C1–C2 stability of this spinal segment.

▸▸ Answer 15

Correct answer is E

Overt instability is defined as the inability of the spine to support the torso during normal activity. This leads to the sudden development of spinal deformity, which can impinge on the spinal cord or nerve roots. For overt instability to exist, there must be circumferential loss of spinal integrity, typically resulting from injury to all three columns of the spinal column.[4]

▸▸ Answer 16

Correct answer is E

"Deformity begets deformity." The greater the deformity, the greater the moment arm length. This results in axial loads causing the application of a progressively larger bending moment. However, the Cobb angle alone can be deceptive as the radius of curvature plays a major role in determining the amount of force applied to a particular level. More acute curves with shorter radii of curvature exert increased segmental force and are more likely to lead to progressive instability (see ▸ Fig. 3.2).

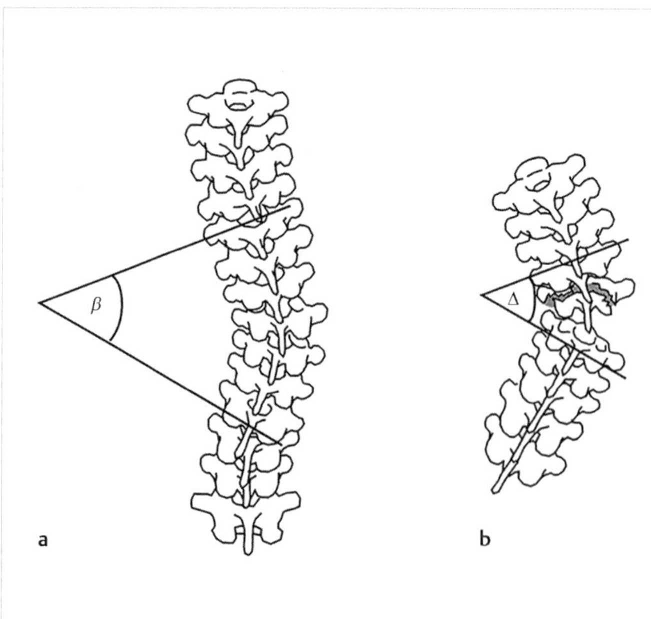

Fig. 3.2 (a) The determination of the Cobb angle (β) in a spine with a moderate scoliotic deformity is depicted. This illustrates the importance of spinal deformity in the determination of acute spinal instability. The Cobb angle is measured from neutral vertebra to neutral vertebra. The neutral vertebra is located between curves that are concave toward opposite directions, as depicted. The radii of the curvatures of two spinal deformities may be widely disparate despite their having the same Cobb angle. **(b)** A lesser radius of curvature is observed at the injured segment in a situation in which an acute segmental angulation occurs, **(c)** compared with less acute, multisegmental angulations. Note that each has the same Cobb angle. (Source: Biomechanics of Spine Stabilization: Third Edition, © 2015 Thieme Medical Publishers, Inc.)

▸▸ Answer 17

Correct answer is B

Muscles provide stability to the spine due to their direct attachment and play a critical role in spinal movement and stability. Patients with neuromuscular disorders often have dysfunctional truncal muscles, leading to loss of the muscular stabilizing effects (see ▸ Fig. 3.3).

▸▸ Answer 18

Correct answer is D

Dysfunctional segmental motion is defined as a type of instability related to segmental degenerative changes that result in pathologic motion. In degenerative spondylolisthesis, degenerative changes to the intervertebral disc and facet joints lead to pathologic motion and subsequent neurologic compression. Despite knowing that degenerative spondylolisthesis results from dysfunctional segmental motion, the definition of what represents pathologic motion remains controversial.[5]

▸▸ Answer 19

Correct answer is D

Mechanical back pain is the pain that is associated with mechanical instability. Mechanical pain is pain that is deep and agonizing in nature, worsened by spinal loading, and relieved by spinal unloading. Mechanical back pain is not generally characterized by radicular pain; rather, radicular pain is secondary to neurologic compression.

▸▸ Answer 20

Correct answer is C

The specificity of discography is dramatically affected by the characteristics of the patient examined.

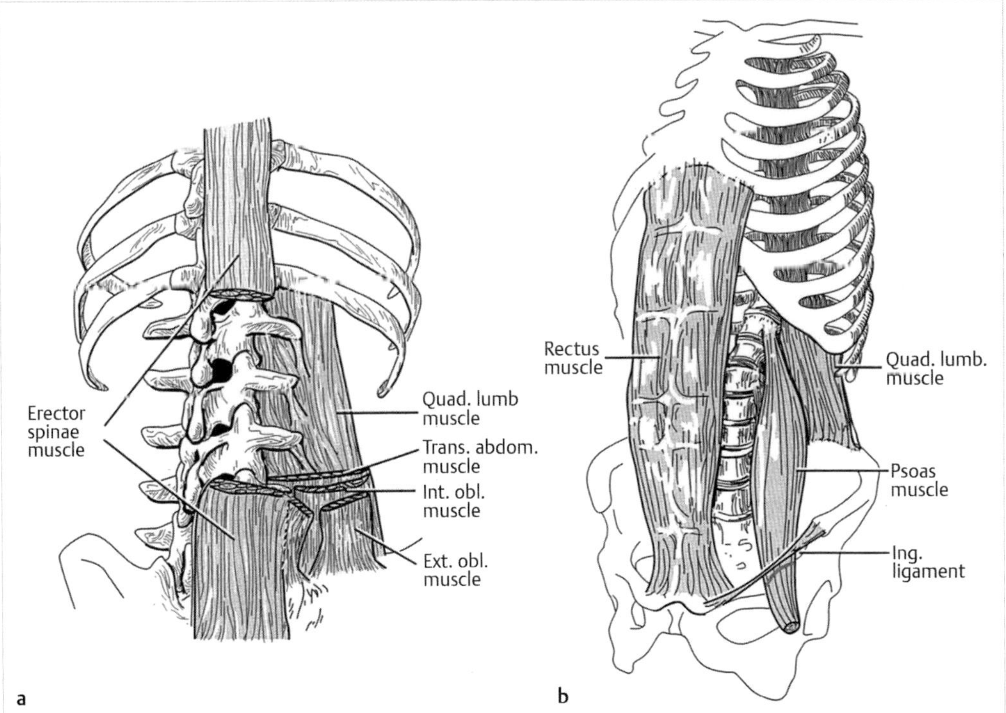

Fig. 3.3 The effects of muscles on stability. **(a)** Muscles provide stability by virtue of the orientation of their attachments to the spine. **(b)** In some situations, as with the rectus abdominis muscle, the muscle may influence spinal movement indirectly (i.e., without direct attachment to the spine). Similarly, this muscle may stabilize the spine by balancing opposing muscle function, resulting in no movement. Stability is thus provided. Lateral bending is achieved via the contraction of muscles attached to the lateral aspect of the spine—for example, the quadratus lumborum muscle. (Source: Biomechanics of Spine Stabilization: Third Edition, © 2015 Thieme Medical Publishers, Inc.)

In a patient with chronic pain states and psychiatric risk factors, the specificity was determined to be low, at most 20%. The ability of a patient to determine reliably the concordance of pain provoked during discography is poor and therefore has high false-positive rates.[6,7]

Key Principles

- Instability is the inability to limit excessive or abnormal spinal displacement.
- For overt instability to exist, a loss of integrity of the vertebral body and/or disc must be associated with a loss of integrity of the dorsal elements.
- Glacial instability progresses gradually, but external forces do not cause immediate movement or progression of deformity.
- "Deformity begets deformity." The larger the deformity, the large the moment arm of the force applied to the spine and the greater the likelihood for progression and glacial instability.

References

[1] Benzel EC. Biomechanics of lumbar and lumbosacral spine fracture. In: Rea GL, Miller CA, eds. Spinal Trauma: Current Evaluation and Management. Park Ridge, IL: American Association of Neurological Surgeons; 1993:165–195

[2] Gertzbein SD, Holtby R, Tile M, Kapasouri A, Chan KW, Cruickshank B. Determination of a locus of instantaneous centers of rotation of the lumbar disc by moiré fringes. A new technique. Spine 1984;9:409–413

[3] Haher TR, Bergman M, O'Brien M, et al. The effect of the three columns of the spine on the instantaneous axis of rotation in flexion and extension. Spine 1991;16(Suppl):S312–S318

[4] Rea GL, Miller CA, eds. Spinal Trauma: Current Evaluation and Management. Park Ridge, IL: American Association of Neurological Surgeons; 1993:165–195

[5] Spina N, Schoutens C, Martin BI, Brodke DS, Lawrence B, Spiker WR. Defining instability in degenerative spondylolisthesis: surgeon views. Clin Spine Surg 2019;32(10):E434–E439

[6] Carragee EJ, Alamin TF. Discography. A review. Spine J 2001;1(5):364–372

[7] Harada GK, Siyaji ZK, Younis S, Louie PK, Samartzis D, An HS. Imaging in spine surgery: current concepts and future directions. Spine Surg Relat Res 2019;4(2):99–110

Part II

Spine and Neural Element Pathology

II

▸▸ Question 6

Which of the following is true regarding osteoporosis?

- A. Osteoporosis is a fixed process that cannot be altered
- B. Low bone mineral density is associated with a lower risk of fractures
- C. Exercise, vitamin D and K supplements, and antiresorptive agents are viable strategies for preventing or managing osteoporosis
- D. Due to low side effect profile, bisphosphonates are appropriate for all patients with osteoporosis
- E. There are currently no Food and Drug Administration (FDA)-approved medications to stimulate bone formation

▸▸ Question 7

Which of the following correctly lists important factors that affect fixation of a spinal implant in bone?

- A. Number of bone–implant interfaces, anchor choice, anchor design, and screw geometry
- B. Anchor design, muscle strength, facet fluid, and slip angle
- C. Screw geometry, pelvic incidence–lumbar lordosis (PI-LL) mismatch, and pelvic tilt (PT)
- D. Anchor choice, anchor design, disc desiccation, and vacuum phenomenon
- E. Number of implants, paraspinal muscle geometry, and disc height

▸▸ Question 8

Which of the following is correct regarding anchor choice?

- A. The most popular anchor choices currently in practice are cables, nails, clamps, and pins
- B. Screws have better pullout resistance than hooks
- C. Screws best resist loads parallel to their long axis
- D. Hooks and screws fail with the same applied force in normal bone
- E. Compared with screws, hooks have better pullout resistance and resist loads in line with the spine's long axis

▸▸ Question 9

Which of the following statements is correct regarding factors that affect screw pullout resistance?

- A. Tapping before screw placement increases likelihood of screw pullout
- B. Larger screw major diameter decreases pullout resistance
- C. Screw material has no impact on pullout resistance
- D. Screw pullout resistance is improved by increased thread depth and decreased pitch
- E. Screw pullout resistance is improved by increased thread pitch and decreased thread depth

▸▸ Question 10

Which of the following is the correct relationship that governs screw pullout resistance?

- A. $F = mA$
- B. $PI = PT + SS$
- C. F_s is directly proportional to $S \times L \times D_{major}$
- D. $F_s = SVA - PI - LL$
- E. $PI = PT/SS$

▸▸ Question 11

Which of the following is screw pullout resistance mainly a function of?

- A. The Cobb angle between the upper instrumented vertebra and the lower instrumented vertebra
- B. Speed of screw placement
- C. Screw hydrophobicity
- D. Size of vertebral body
- E. Volume of bone between screw threads

▸▸ Question 12

Placement of a pilot hole prior to screw placement _____

- A. Increases pullout resistance
- B. Decreases insertional torque
- C. Should be long to create the screw trajectory
- D. Should be wide to allow sufficient space for the screw
- E. Has no effect on pullout resistance

▸▸ Question 13

Tapered inner diameter screws _____

- A. Decrease pullout resistance.
- B. Do not affect insertional torque
- C. Increase insertional torque
- D. Decrease insertional torque
- E. Have no effect on pullout resistance

▸▸ Question 14

What is the effect of removing and replacing screws?

- A. Increases fixation integrity
- B. Replacing with the same diameter screw increases fixation integrity
- C. Length of rescue screw, compared with the initial screw, has the biggest impact on fixation
- D. Rescue screws with larger diameter than original screw increase fixation
- E. Shims augment fixation

▸▸ Question 15

What is the impact of increasing thread depth?

- A. Increased thread depth with decreased inner screw diameter leads to decreased fixation
- B. Increased thread depth with decreased inner screw diameter increases the risk of screw fracture
- C. Decreased thread depth improves bony fixation
- D. Changes in thread depth offset any changes in inner screw diameter
- E. Increased thread depth increases pullout resistance even if bone volume between screw threads decreases

▸▸ Question 16

Which of the following is correct regarding screw triangulation?

- A. Screw triangulation improves pullout resistance
- B. Cross fixation is unrelated to the triangulation effect
- C. The triangulation effect can be achieved by a medial trajectory (i.e., toeing in) but not by a lateral trajectory (i.e., toeing out)
- D. A fixation plate has no impact on the triangulation effect
- E. Fixation plates decrease pullout resistance from triangulation

▸▸ Question 17

Prior to screw placement, tapping has important effects on bone that must be considered. Which of the following is correct?

- A. Tapping increases the bone compression effect in cancellous bone
- B. Tapping decreases the bone compression effect in cortical bone
- C. Tapping creates threads in bone that the screw can follow
- D. Tapping and drilling are equally effective in cortical and cancellous bone
- E. Bone fracture is more likely in cancellous bone if there is no tapping prior to screw placement

▸▸ Question 18

Which of the following is correct regarding the surface area of interbody implants?

- A. The surface areas of the vertebral body and interbody implant do not matter as long as the interbody implant is large
- B. Small surface areas of contact can be adequately compensated by increasing morselized bone graft placement in the disc space
- C. Smaller struts better support axial loads
- D. The corpectomy wall does not influence the biomechanical advantage of the strut
- E. Surface area mismatch leads to subsidence or a gap

▸▸ Question 19

Which of the following is correct regarding the boundary effect?

- A. A hollow implant can resist force equally anywhere along its upper and lower boundaries
- B. There is most resistance to distortion along the perimeter of a hollow cylindrical implant
- C. Bone morphogenetic proteins are most effective at the boundary of the fusion surface
- D. An interbody cage placed centrally has the best load bearing
- E. Overlap with the perimeter of an end plate increases the likelihood of subsidence

▸▸ **Question 20**

Which of the following is correct regarding the impact of interbody implant shape on subsidence?

- A. Femoral ring allografts are likely to subside due to peripheral end plate contact
- B. Round-faced implants best match the curved end plate
- C. Round implants are best for dynamic loading during motion
- D. Flat surfaces are best for resisting subsidence and bearing axial loads
- E. Round and flat interbody implants have equivalent risk of pseudarthrosis and subsidence

Answers

▸▸ **Answer 1**

Correct answer is B

The general population of the United States is aging, with approximately 55 million Americans over 65 years in 2020. This number is expected to grow to 72 million by 2030. Therefore, B is correct. The population of older Americans has not yet peaked and is expected to continue to grow.

▸▸ **Answer 2**

Correct answer is D

It is important to understand how implant fixation strength relates to bone quality. With an aging population, many elderly patients are osteopenic or osteoporotic. In the osteopenic spine, fixation strength is one-fourth that of normal bone. Therefore, D is correct. Fixation strength is even worse in osteoporotic bone.

▸▸ **Answer 3**

Correct answer is C

As shown in ▸ Fig. 4.1, intradiscal pressure goes from being uniform in youth (**part a**) to asymmetrical, with most pressure located on the lateral edges. This is due to desiccation of the nucleus pulposus and its resulting inability to withstand pressure. C is correct.

▸▸ **Answer 4**

Correct answer is E

Wolff's law relates to bone remodeling, not muscle or supportive soft tissues. It states that bone remodels in response to stress. E is correct. Osteoporosis leads to bone loss, effectively competing against bone formation in response to Wolff's law.

▸▸ **Answer 5**

Correct answer is D

Height loss occurs during aging starting in midlife, with changes in the axial spine being the primary cause. Vertebral collapse and spinal deformity can both contribute to height loss. Therefore, D is correct.

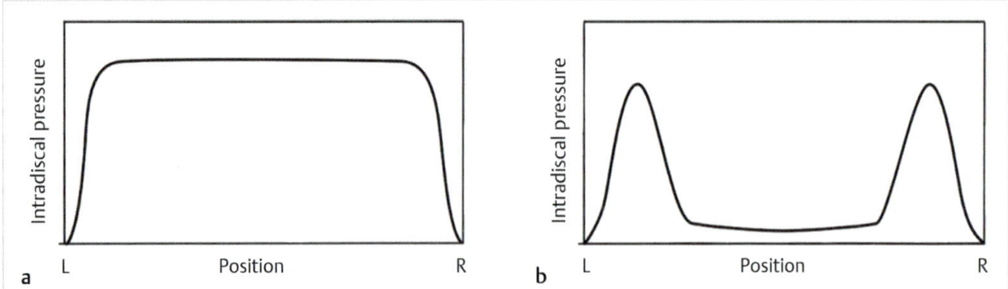

Fig. 4.1 The degenerative process in the intervertebral disc is associated with pressure changes within the disc interspace. **(a)** In youth, the pressures within the central portion of the intervertebral disc are relatively high and uniform across the diameter of the disc space during axial loading. As aging and degeneration continue, **(b)** the pressure in the nucleus region falls even farther and can fall below zero in some conditions. (Source: Biomechanics of Spine Stabilization: Third Edition, © 2015 Thieme Medical Publishers, Inc.)

▸▸ Answer 6

Correct answer is C

Osteoporosis can be altered by both pharmaceutical and nonpharmaceutical means. Regarding the former, a number of medications are approved for preventing bone resorption, such as bisphosphonates, and promoting bone formation, such as parathyroid hormone analogs. Weight-bearing exercise and vitamin D and K supplements can also help prevent bone loss. Therefore, C is correct.

▸▸ Answer 7

Correct answer is A

The critical factors affecting spine fixation include number of bone–implant interfaces, anchor choice, anchor design, and screw geometry. A is correct. Nonbony elements do not affect implant fixation in bone. Spinopelvic parameters are important in planning fixation, but any effect on fixation is secondary.

▸▸ Answer 8

Correct answer is E

Hooks have better pullout resistance than screws but fail at lower applied force in normal bone. E is correct. Since axial loads are common when humans are upright, pedicle screws frequently resist loads perpendicular to their long axis. In comparison, hooks resist loads in the spine's long axis. Fixation failure in osteopenic bone is more related to bone mineral density than anchor choice.

▸▸ Answer 9

Correct answer is D

Multiple factors affect screw pullout resistance. Decreased screw pitch (distance between threads), increased thread depth, and larger diameter screws all have stronger pullout resistance. The mechanism by which pitch, depth, and screw outer diameter improve pullout resistance is by increasing thread surface area. Thus, D is correct.

▸▸ Answer 10

Correct answer is C

The predicted shear failure force, F_S, is directly proportional to the material ultimate shear stress (S) times the length of thread engagement (L) times the screw major diameter (D_{major}). Therefore, C is correct. PI, PT, sacral slope (SS), and sagittal vertical axis (SVA) are not directly related to screw pullout; therefore, B and D are incorrect. While force (F) is equal to mass (m) times acceleration (A), this equation does not describe the important factors in screw failure; thus, A is incorrect. Shear failure force is directly proportional to length and screw major diameter, not inversely proportional; thus, D is incorrect.

▸▸ Answer 11

Correct answer is E

The volume of bone between screw threads is the primary driver of screw pullout resistance; thus, E is correct. A smaller pitch increases contact area with bone, with more threads per unit length of the screw. This results in a greater surface area of the screw being in contact with the bone. More threads in contact with the bone lead to increased friction between the screw and the bone. With a decreased pitch, the threads can engage more effectively with the trabecular structure of the bone. A screw with a smaller pitch can distribute the stress applied to it over a larger area of bone. As shown in ▸ Fig. 4.2, volume of bone can be influence by thread pitch (**a, b**). Volume between threads is improved by increasing thread length (**c**) and screw triangulation (**e**). The Cobb angle does not affect screw pullout resistance; thus, A is incorrect. The speed of screw placement does not affect pullout resistance; thus, B is incorrect. Screw material properties related to shear stress do affect pullout, but hydrophobicity is not a significant driver of failure; thus, C is incorrect. Placing screws in smaller vertebrae may be more challenging, but the size of the vertebral body itself is not the main factor for screw pullout; thus, D is incorrect.

▸▸ Answer 12

Correct answer is B

Pilot holes decrease insertional torque; thus, B is correct. The pilot hole should be of smaller diameter than the screw and should be short; thus, C and D are incorrect. Pilot holes do decrease pullout resistance; thus, A and E are incorrect.

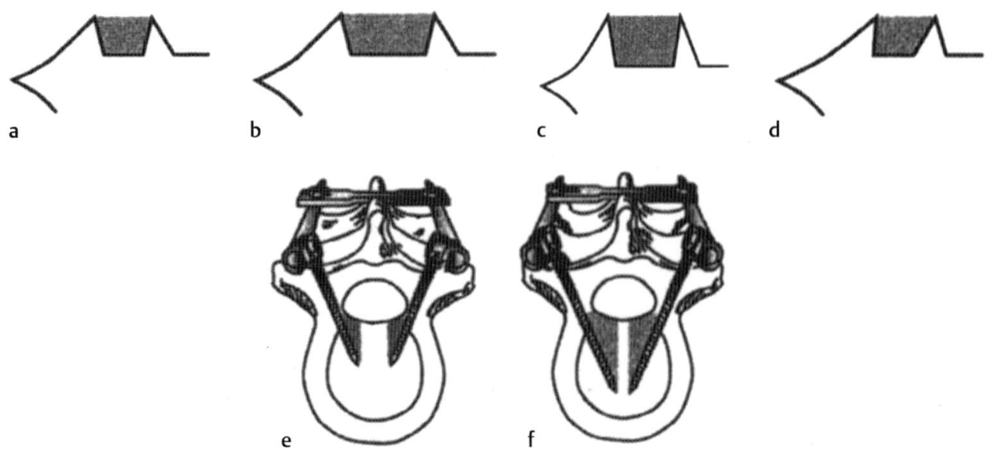

Fig. 4.2 Methods of minimizing screw pullout. **(a)** Screw pullout resistance is mainly a function of the volume of bone (*shaded area*) between screw threads. **(b)** Thread pitch affects this by altering interthread distance. **(c)** Thread depth affects this by altering thread penetration into bone. Thread shape affects this by altering the amount of bone volume directly. If the pitch and depth are unchanged, the only factor that can affect bone volume is screw thread volume (metal volume). **(d)** Decreasing screw thread volume (metal volume) increases bone volume. The triangulation of pedicle screws provides additional resistance to pullout (*shaded area*). **(e)** Pullout resistance is proportional not only to the volume of bone between screw threads but also to the triangular area defined by the screw, the perpendicular, and the dorsal vertebral body surface. **(f)** Although screw length does not routinely contribute significantly to pullout resistance, it contributes significantly when screws are rigidly triangulated. Note the increase in the shaded area. Increasing the screw angle (e.g., toe-in) also increases the size of the shaded area and thus pullout resistance. (Source: Biomechanics of Spine Stabilization: Third Edition, © 2015 Thieme Medical Publishers, Inc.)

▸▸ Answer 13

Correct answer is C

Compared with constant inner diameter screws, tapered inner diameter screws may increase pullout resistance and do increase insertional torque. Therefore, C is correct. This is particularly true if the outer diameter tapers with the inner diameter. A, B, D, and E are incorrect. Tapered inner diameter screws increase insertional torque. Therefore, C is correct and B and D are incorrect.

▸▸ Answer 14

Correct answer is D

If a screw is removed, replacing it with a larger diameter rescue screw increases fixation, but increased length does not necessarily. Increased length technically increases thread surface area and increases strength slightly, albeit less than increasing diameter. Shims also do not augment fixation. D is correct, and B, C, and E are incorrect. Removing and replacing screws decrease fixation integrity unless a larger diameter screw is used; therefore, A is incorrect.

▸▸ Answer 15

Correct answer is B

Increasing thread depth on its own does increase fixation and pullout resistance. However, smaller inner diameter leads to risk of screw fracture and susceptibility to axial loads. Therefore, B is correct, and A, C, and D are incorrect. Larger bone volume between threads is a major factor in pullout resistance; therefore E is incorrect.

▸▸ Answer 16

Correct answer is A

Screw triangulation increases pullout resistance, as shown in ▸ Fig. 4.3. Therefore, A is correct. The shaded area is defined by the screw, horizontal and vertical line. When triangulating, longer screws do add to pullout resistance. A fixation plate or cross connector is needed for rigid fixation in order to achieve the benefit of triangulation; therefore, B, D, and E are incorrect. The effect of triangulation can be achieved by toeing in or out; thus, C is incorrect.

▸▸ Answer 17

Correct answer is C

Tapping and drilling have different effects on cortical and cancellous bone; therefore, D is incorrect. For cancellous bone, compression of the medullary bone is important for good bone purchase and increasing pullout resistance. Therefore, A, B, and E are incorrect. In cortical bone, tapping creates threads that the screw can follow, decreasing the likelihood of fracture. C is correct.

▸▸ Answer 18

Correct answer is E

It is important that the surface area of the interbody implant (strut) match the vertebral body interface (mortise) as well as possible. Surface area mismatch leads to a piston effect that can cause subsidence or a gap; therefore, E is correct. The effect of different size struts is shown in ▶ Fig. 4.4 (**a, b**). By matching the implant to the corpectomy wall, biomechanical advantage is increased (**c, d**); therefore, D is incorrect. Morselized bone lacks mechanical strength; therefore, B is incorrect. Larger interbody implants can support larger axial loads, but surface area match still plays an important role in biomechanics; therefore, A is incorrect.

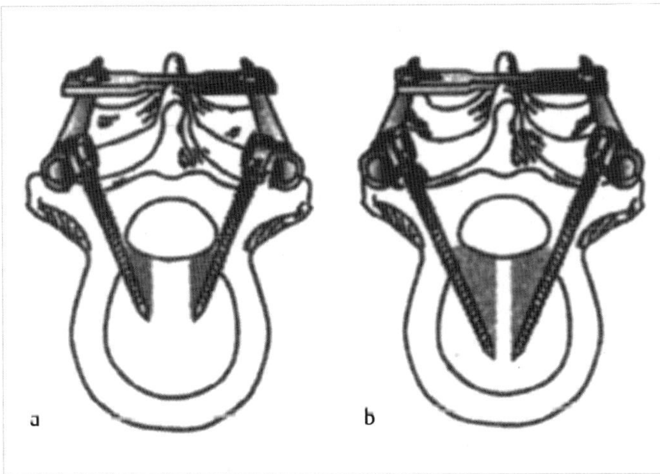

Fig. 4.3 (a) Pullout resistance is proportional not only to the volume of bone between screw threads but also to the triangular area defined by the screw, the perpendicular, and the dorsal vertebral body surface. **(b)** Although screw length does not routinely contribute significantly to pullout resistance, it contributes significantly when screws are rigidly triangulated. Note the increase in the shaded area. Increasing the screw angle (e.g., toe-in) also increases the size of the shaded area and thus pullout resistance. (Source: Biomechanics of Spine Stabilization: Third Edition, © 2015 Thieme Medical Publishers, Inc.)

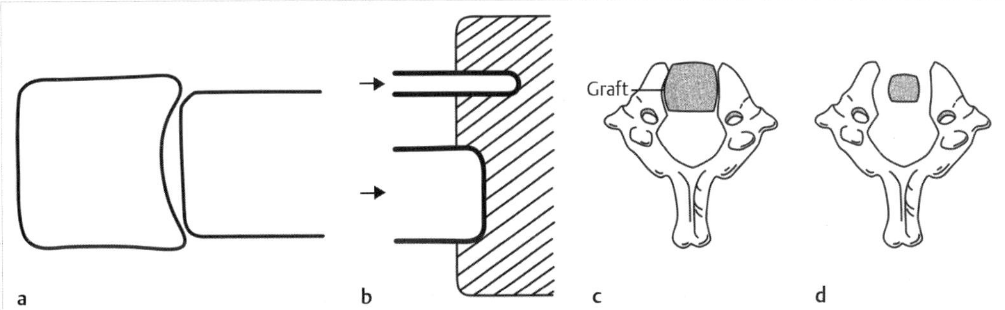

Fig. 4.4 (a) A mismatch between the strut and mortise geometry obligates subsidence or the persistence of a gap. **(b)** A strut with a large surface area of contact will support axial loads more effectively than a strut with small surface area of contact. **(c)** A large strut can also be "bolstered" by the corpectomy wall, thus providing increased biomechanical advantage. **(d)** A lesser-diameter strut can provide neither of these advantages. (Source: Biomechanics of Spine Stabilization: Third Edition, © 2015 Thieme Medical Publishers, Inc.)

▸▸ **Answer 19**

Correct answer is B

Hollow cylindrical structures best resist forces at their periphery, as shown in the model of a tin can in ▸ Fig. 4.5. B is correct, and A, D, and E are incorrect. This phenomenon is termed the boundary effect. Bone morphogenetic protein is not related to this phenomenon; therefore, C is incorrect.

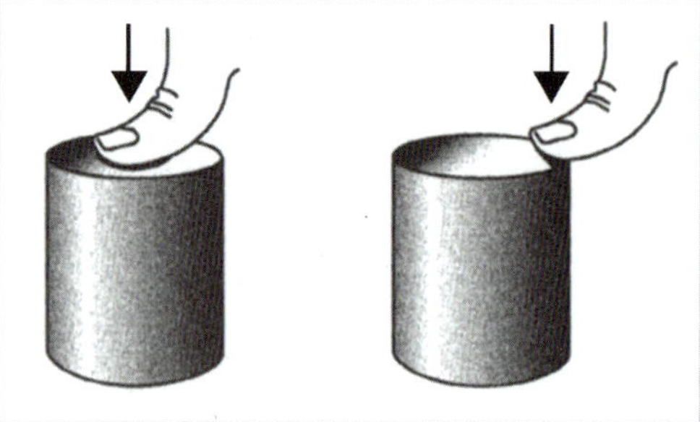

Fig. 4.5 (A) If one pushes on the center of the end of an empty tin can, the surface is easily distorted, whereas such does not occur when the same force is applied to the perimeter of the can. This phenomenon is termed the *boundary effect*. (B) Hence, interbody cages that are placed near the center of the endplate have a suboptimal mechanical effect. If placed near the perimeter, their axial load-bearing ability is much greater. (Source: Biomechanics of Spine Stabilization: Third Edition, © 2015 Thieme Medical Publishers, Inc.)

▸▸ **Answer 20**

Correct answer is D

As shown in ▸ Fig. 4.6 (**a**), numerous choices exist for interbody implant shape. The shape of the interbody implant is important for maximizing load bearing and minimizing risk of subsidence. As shown in (**b**), a flat-faced implant best matches the end plate and can resist subsidence, especially when overlapping the strong cortical bone at the periphery. Thus, D is correct, and A is incorrect. A round-faced implant is likely to make contact at the weaker central part of the end plate (**c**) and is at high risk of subsidence. B, C, and E are incorrect.

Key Principles

- Consideration of bone quality is key to successful arthrodesis.
- The aging process changes load bearing of the disc and vertebral body.
- Multiple aspects of screw geometry affect pullout resistance.
- Interbody shape and surface area have significant effects on axial load bearing and risk of subsidence.

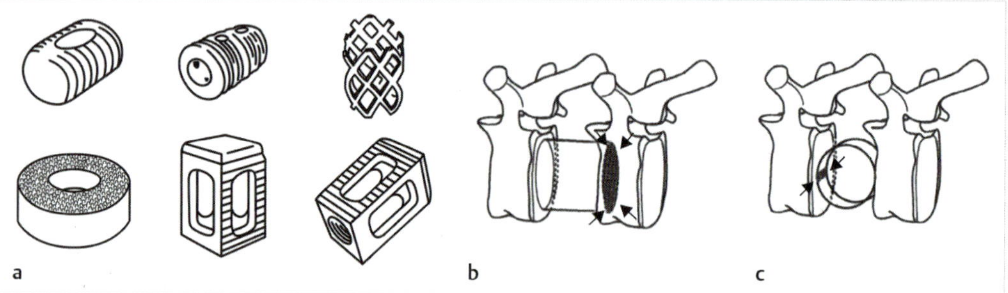

Fig. 4.6 **(a)** Interbody cages are available in a variety of shapes and sizes. **(b)** If they present a flat surface to the endplate, they are able to bear and resist axial loads and subsidence much more effectively than **(c)** if they present a round surface to the endplate. (Source: Biomechanics of Spine Stabilization: Third Edition, © 2015 Thieme Medical Publishers, Inc.)

5 Degenerative and Inflammatory Diseases of the Spine

Eric Mong, Glenn A. Gonzalez, James S. Harrop

Patients with degenerative and inflammatory diseases of the spine make up a large majority of the treatment population for spine surgeons. A foundational and thorough understanding of the pathophysiology of these disease processes is essential to creating effective conservative and surgical treatment plans in this vast patient population.

Learning Objectives

- To understand the pathogenesis of inflammatory and degenerative diseases of the spine and its implications in surgical and conservative management.
- To properly assess and differentiate the different etiologies of axial spine pain.
- To understand the factors that contribute to both preoperative and postoperative spinal stability in degenerative and inflammatory spine pathologies.

Questions

▸▸ Question 1

Which of the following is the impetus for lumbar spondylosis?
- A. Facet hypertrophy
- B. Disc degeneration
- C. Hypertrophy of the ligamentum flavum
- D. Osteophyte formation
- E. End plate sclerosis

▸▸ Question 2

Which of the following movements of the disc interspace is most effectively prevented by the 30-degree orientation of the annular fibers relative to the end plates?
- A. Subluxation
- B. Distraction
- C. Torsion
- D. Compression
- E. Lateral flexion

▸▸ Question 3

The vertebral bodies must be able to continuously adapt to the stress of repetitive axial loading. Which of the following best describes the structural integrity of the vertebral body that is formed by the continuous bony remodeling process?
- A. Trabecular bone oriented in a vertical fashion
- B. Trabecular bone oriented in a horizontal fashion
- C. Cortical bone oriented in a vertical fashion
- D. Cortical bone oriented in a horizontal fashion
- E. Trabecular bone oriented in both horizontal and vertical fashion

▸▸ Question 4

The coupling phenomenon discussed in the chapter regarding the structural physiology of the lumbar spine and progression of deformity can be attributed to which of the following?
- A. Coronal orientation of the lumbar facet joints and asymmetric disc degeneration progressing to a coronal deformity with a rotary component
- B. Sagittal orientation of the lumbar facet joints and symmetrical disc degeneration progressing to coronal and kyphotic deformity with a rotary component
- C. Sagittal orientation of the lumbar facet joints and asymmetric disc degeneration progressing to a coronal and kyphotic deformity with a rotary component
- D. Coronal orientation of the facet joints with symmetrical disc degeneration leading to kyphotic deformity
- E. Sagittal orientation of the lumbar facet joints and asymmetrical disc degeneration progressing to kyphotic deformity

▸▸ Question 5

The chapter discusses the biomechanics of disc herniation and how certain laboratory studies have attempted to elucidate the exact mechanism. Based on the discussion in the chapter, a high percentage of posterolateral disc herniations are thought to arise from which of the following mechanisms?

- A. Flexion followed by extension of the disc space
- B. Lateral bending, rotation, and axial loading of the disc space
- C. Extension and axial loading of the disc space
- D. Flexion, lateral bending, and axial loading of the disc space
- E. Axial loading with rotation of the disc space

▸▸ Question 6

Scheuermann's disease is a complex clinical condition affecting many patients of adolescent age. The physiologic process from which the disease develops is thought to arise from which of the following?

- A. Asymmetrically high dorsal intradiscal pressures
- B. Asymmetrically high ventral intradiscal pressures
- C. Congenital malformation of the anterior and middle columns of the thoracic vertebral bodies
- D. Ligamentous laxity
- E. Insufficiency of the posterior column

▸▸ Question 7

Basilar impression, also known as basilar invagination or cranial settling, is a common pathology seen at the craniocervical junction that may lead to myelopathy and lower cranial nerve deficits if not treated appropriately. In rheumatoid arthritis, the most common cause of this process originates from which of the following?

- A. Insufficiency of the atlantal condyles with microfractures at the C0–C1 joints
- B. Atlantoaxial instability
- C. Repetitive microtrauma to the dens
- D. Insufficiency of the alar ligaments
- E. Insufficiency of the tectorial membrane and clivus

▸▸ Question 8

Distinguishing different etiologies of axial spine pain is critical in deciding the best treatment for patients. A patient with a history of L4–L5 open laminectomy and posterolateral fusion 1 year ago presents with persistent aching and burning pain in his back as well as burning pain down his legs bilaterally, which has been present since the surgery. He states he is severely debilitated and has depression and low energy levels. He has taken high doses of gabapentin with no success. Dynamic X-rays of the lumbar spine show fusion across the disc space and facet complex with no dynamic subluxation. Magnetic resonance imaging (MRI) of the lumbar spine shows peridural scarring around the L4 and L5 nerve roots with no foraminal, lateral recess or central canal stenosis. MRI shows no fluid collection or findings consistent with infection. The disc and end plates appear normal above and below the previous fusion, with minimal degenerative changes. What is the most appropriate treatment option?

- A. Surgical exploration of the previous surgery with revision decompression
- B. Referral to pain management specialist for consideration of spinal cord stimulator trial
- C. Extension of fusion to the lumbosacral junction
- D. Increase gabapentin dosage
- E. Lumbosacral orthosis brace with physical therapy

▸▸ Question 9

Ankylosing hyperostosis, also known Forestier disease or diffuse idiopathic skeletal hyperostosis (DISH), is a distinct axial spondyloarthropathy variant of ankylosing spondylitis. Which of the following is a radiographic feature of ankylosing hyperostosis that is not seen in ankylosing spondylitis?

- A. Loss of intervertebral disc height
- B. Circumferentially bridging syndesmophytes
- C. Fusion across the facet joints
- D. Preservation of the vertebral end plates
- E. Involvement of the sacroiliac joints

▸▸ Question 10

A 78-year-old patient with a history of rheumatoid arthritis and severe mechanical neck pain presents with a 3-month history of worsening difficulty with ambulation, including equilibrium and balance. Additionally, the patient has had significant difficulty using her hands, causing her to drop objects on several occasions. On physical exam, she is very weak in both the upper and lower extremities and is diffusely hyperreflexic in her upper and lower extremities. MRI of the cervical spine shows a large pannus at the tip of the odontoid with severe ventral compression of the cervical spinal cord with associated cord signal change. Computed tomography (CT) of the cervical spine does not reveal any calcification in the pannus. What are the viable treatment options?

- A. C1–C2 posterior fusion or occipital cervical fusion
- B. Ventral approach for odontoidectomy alone
- C. Either C1–C2 posterior fusion or combination of ventral odontoidectomy and posterior fusion
- D. Ventral odontoidectomy with posterior cervical laminectomy
- E. Posterior cervical laminectomy

▸▸ Question 11

Enthesitis, a key process involved in the pathogenesis of ankylosing spondylitis, is defined by which of the following?

- A. Inflammation and ossification of the anterior and posterior vertebral end plates
- B. Circumferential inflammation and ossification of the vertebral bodies and facet joints
- C. Inflammation and ossification of the posterior tension band
- D. Inflammation and ossification of the ligamentous insertion sites on bone
- E. Inflammation and ossification of the sacroiliac joints

▸▸ Question 12

A 72-year-old man with a 50-year smoking history and hypertension presents with 1 year of difficulty ambulating and using his hands. He has chronic neck pain that has significantly worsened during this time and is often worse with turning the head to either side. MRI of the cervical spine shows subtle cord signal change at the level of C1–C2 but no significant central canal stenosis at this level. There is mild ligament flavum hypertrophy with no significant central canal or lateral recess stenosis in the subaxial cervical spine. CT of the cervical spine shows mild posterior osteophytes at several levels. What additional test could be ordered to delineate the cause of the patient's symptoms?

- A. CT myelogram
- B. Electromyogram (EMG) and nerve conduction studies
- C. Flexion and extension X-rays of the cervical spine
- D. MRI of the brain with and without contrast
- E. Lumbar puncture with work-up for autoimmunity

▸▸ Question 13

Compared with a normal lordotic posture in the cervical spine, the cervical kyphosis secondary to degenerative cervical spondylosis involves what biomechanical processes?

- A. A decrease in moment arm ventral to the IAR causing an increased bending moment with axial forces perpendicular to the moment arm
- B. An increase in moment arm dorsal to the IAR causing an increased bending moment with axial forces parallel to the moment arm
- C. A decreased moment arm dorsal to the IAR causing an increased bending moment with axial loads parallel to the moment arm
- D. An increased moment arm ventral to the IAR causing an increased bending moment with axial forces perpendicular to the moment arm
- E. An increased moment arm ventral to the IAR causing an increased bending moment with axial forces parallel to the moment arm

▸▸ Question 14

Pelvic parameters effect mechanical stresses at the lumbosacral junction. Which of the following set of pelvic parameters are most likely to lead to an isthmic pars defect and increased shear stress leading to spondylolisthesis at the lumbosacral junction?

- A. Pelvic incidence of 34 degrees; sacral slope of 20 degrees; lumbar lordosis of 29 degrees
- B. Pelvic incidence of 40 degrees; sacral slope of 31 degrees; lumbar lordosis of 35 degrees
- C. Pelvic incidence of 60 degrees; lumbar lordosis of 49 degrees; sacral slope of 40 degrees
- D. Pelvic incidence of 48 degrees; lumbar lordosis of 43 degrees; sacral slope of 45 degrees
- E. Pelvic incidence of 65 degrees; lumbar lordosis of 55 degrees; sacral slope of 43 degrees

▸▸ Answer 3

Correct answer is A

In response to axial loading, the vertebral bodies respond by reinforcing itself along the lines of stress by developing columnar-like trabeculation aligned in a vertical direction (see ▶ Fig. 5.2). This columnar orientation allows support of the spine analogous to pillars of a building and allows maximum strength with minimal mass. Trabecular bone oriented in a horizontal fashion would not be biomechanically advantageous, as the trabecular bone would be oriented perpendicular to the force vector and predispose to compression fractures. The interior of the vertebral body is composed of trabecular bone, whereas the outer rim of the vertebral body is composed of cortical bone, which makes up a minority of the total mass of the entire vertebral body and therefore does not provide the majority of stress resistance to axial loads (answers C and D are incorrect).

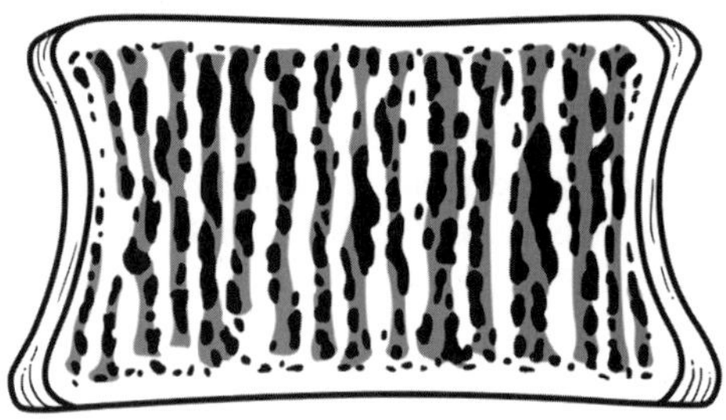

Fig. 5.2 Bone structure forms and matures in response to loading to provide maximum strength with minimum mass. For example, trabecular bone in the vertebral body is aligned in a vertical direction, as depicted. Such trabeculation supports the spine as pillars may support a building. (Source: Biomechanics of Spine Stabilization: Third Edition, © 2015 Thieme Medical Publishers, Inc.)

▸▸ Answer 4

Correct answer is C

The lumbar spine is subject to coronal deformity due to increased flexibility compared with the thoracic spine combined with sagittally oriented facet joints that allow for the progression of coronal deformities, especially in the setting of asymmetric disc degeneration. There is a rotatory component of lumbar degenerative scoliosis that often stabilizes when the osteophyte forms at the concave side of the coronal imbalance (see ▶ Fig. 5.3); therefore, C is the correct answer.

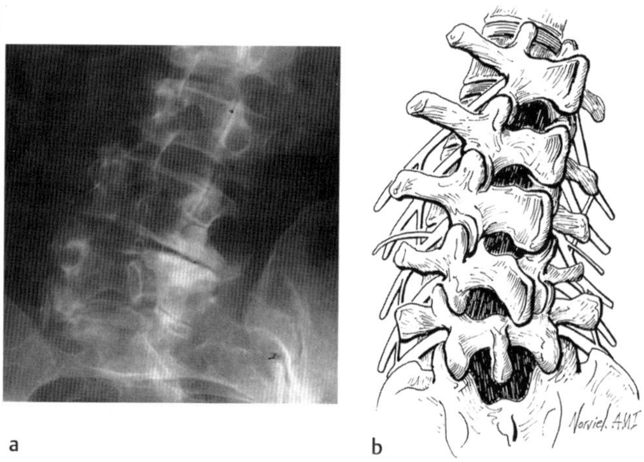

a b

Fig. 5.3 **(a)** The obligatory rotation of the spine (rotatory component of scoliosis resulting from the coupling phenomenon), as illustrated on an anteroposterior radiograph. Note that the low lumbar spinous processes are rotated to the right, toward the concave side of this scoliotic curve. This is associated with a propensity for nerve root injury during dissection along the transverse process on the concave side of the curvature. **(b)** This is because of the juxtaposition of the exiting nerve root to the overlying transverse process created by spinal rotation. The nerve roots exiting on the concave side of the curve can be injured by stretching associated with surgical deformity correction. The proximal (intradural) nerve roots are much less tolerant of stretching than their more distal peripheral nerve counterparts because of their deficient perineurium. (Source: Biomechanics of Spine Stabilization: Third Edition, © 2015 Thieme Medical Publishers, Inc.)

▸▸ Answer 5

Correct answer is D

The force pattern of disc herniation has been postulated to come from a combination of flexion, lateral bending, and axial loading of the disc space in the setting of a degenerated disc and weakened annulus fibrosis. First, when the spine flexes, the nucleus pulposus migrates posteriorly. The posterior longitudinal ligament is stronger relative to the annulus, making purely posterior disc herniations difficult to occur. When combined with lateral bending, the asymmetric increase in intradiscal pressure causes the nucleus pulposus to migrate to the posterolateral annulus, which is under tension and weakened during lateral bending. When axial loading is high enough to increase the intradiscal pressure eccentrically, a posterolateral disc herniation is most likely to occur; therefore, D is the correct answer. Mechanisms involving extension increase stress on the posterior elements, leading to pars defects and facet hypertrophy, rather than disc herniation (A and C are incorrect) (see ▸ Fig. 5.4).

▸▸ Answer 6

Correct answer is B

In a normal developing spine, intradiscal pressure is relatively uniform throughout the intervertebral disc space, allowing normal curvatures of the spine to develop in a balanced fashion. In Scheuermann's kyphosis, the preexisting thoracic kyphosis may cause asymmetrically elevated ventral intradiscal pressures, which may lead to ventrally oriented end plate penetration, resulting in destruction of the growth plate and disproportionate loss of ventral portion of the vertebral body height. Scheuermann's disease is therefore associated with the shortening of the anterior column of the spine, making B the correct answer. It is not caused by insufficiency of the posterior column or ligamentous laxity (D and E are incorrect). Asymmetrically high dorsal intradiscal pressure would affect the middle column of the spine and would not be expected to lead to progressive kyphosis (A is incorrect).

▸▸ Answer 7

Correct answer is B

Basilar impression is thought to be secondary to atlantoaxial facet joint instability, with the migration of the tip of the odontoid through the foramen magnum due to listhesis of the C1–C2 facets.[1] As the dens penetrates through the foramen magnum, it may cause compression of the cervicomedullary junction. Atlantoaxial instability is thought to be a more common etiology of basilar impression than insufficiency of the occipital condyle and atlantal condyle at C0–C1, given that many cases of basilar impression have significantly improved with C1–C2 facet distraction and posterior fixation.[2] The dens itself does not undergo microtrauma during the process of basilar impression; however, atlantoaxial instability may lead to formation of a pannus, causing compression of the upper cervical spinal cord (C is incorrect). The alar ligaments, tectorial membrane, and lower clivus make up key anatomy of the

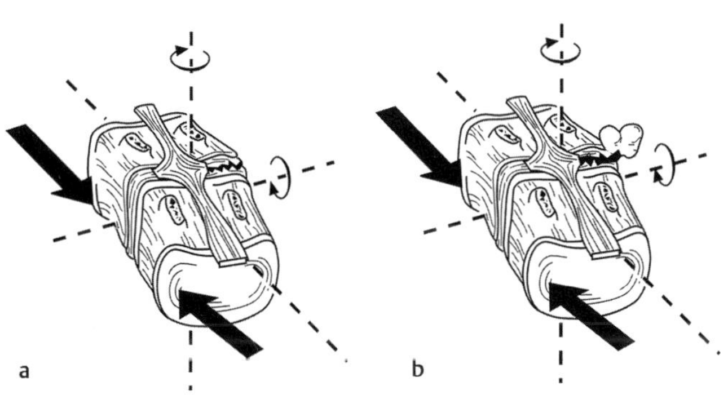

Fig. 5.4 (a) The application of an axial load, lateral bending, and flexion causes the nucleus pulposus to migrate in the direction of the region of the annulus fibrosus that is under tension and prone to tearing. **(b)** This may result in disc herniation in the dorsal paramedian location if the disc is degenerated (and thus predisposed to pathological migration). (Source: Data obtained White AA, Panjabi MM, Eds. Clinical Biomechanics of the Spine. 2d ed. Philadelphia: Lippincott 1990:1–125; Adams MA, Hutton WC. Prolapsed intervertebral disc. A hyperflexion injury 1981 Volvo Award in Basic Science. Spine 1982; 7: 184–191)

craniocervical junction but are not implicated in the process of basilar impression (E is incorrect).

▸▸ Answer 8

Correct answer is B

The patient's axial spine pain with associated radiculopathy in the absence of significant radiographic abnormalities is likely chronic pain with a component of neuropathic pain. The patient is experiencing failed back syndrome and has had persistent axial back pain and radicular pain since the surgery. Radiographic imaging does not suggest pseudoarthrosis or adjacent segment disease, making a mechanical etiology of pain less likely (answer A and C are incorrect). Bracing would not be expected to help due to the lack of evidence to suggest a mechanical instability (E is incorrect). MRI imaging only reveals peridural scarring without nerve root compression. Scarring along the nerve roots in the absence of compression should not be surgically explored (A is incorrect). In the setting of chronic pain from failed back syndrome with no obvious surgical pathology on imaging, evaluation by a pain specialist for treatment options of chronic pain, including consideration of a spinal cord stimulator, would be the most viable option; therefore, B is the correct answer. Chronic pain can be significantly difficult to treat and should not just be treated by increasing gabapentin doses (D is incorrect).

▸▸ Answer 9

Correct answer is D

There are many radiographic similarities and differences between ankylosing spondylitis and DISH. Early and bilateral sacroiliitis and fusion of the sacroiliac joint is a hallmark radiographic finding of ankylosing spondylitis that distinguishes it from DISH (E is incorrect). Ankylosing spondylitis forms broad syndesmophytes that bridge circumferentially around the vertebral body. As these fusions across the disc space occur, they create the "bamboo" appearance of the vertebral body. In DISH, there are anterior bridging osteophytes; however, the vertebral bodies and end plates are largely preserved compared with ankylosing spondylitis, making D the correct answer. The process of spondylodiscitis that occurs in ankylosing spondylitis causes loss of disc space height, compared with DISH where the disc height is preserved (A is incorrect). The facets in ankylosing spondylitis will also fuse and are spared in DISH (C is incorrect).

▸▸ Answer 10

Correct answer is C

The patient has severe cervical myelopathy from pannus formation secondary to C1–C2 instability from rheumatoid arthritis. Resolution of the pannus following posterior C1–C2 fusion alone or occipital cervical fusion supports the theory that a pannus is formed secondary to mechanical instability rather than an acute inflammatory process.[3] In some cases, surgeons may choose to start with a ventral decompression, by means of a transoral or endonasal odontoidectomy due to the severity of ventral compression. This inherently destabilizes the C1–C2 joint and always requires posterior cervical fusion (making B incorrect). Due to the ventral vector of compression, a cervical laminectomy at the C1 and C2 levels is rarely an effective option (making E incorrect). In cases where the pannus is calcified, there is more of a need for ventral decompression followed by posterior stabilization, given that the chance of spontaneous regression of the calcified pannus is much lower with posterior stabilization of the C1–C2 joint alone.

▸▸ Answer 11

Correct answer is D

Enthesitis, or inflammation of the ligamentous and tendinous insertion sites of the vertebral bodies, is a key process in the pathogenesis of ankylosing spondylitis. Early in the disease course, proinflammatory mediators cause inflammation at the entheses, the attachment points of the ligaments to the cartilage in the vertebral bodies, and lead to the formation of syndesmophytes across a disc space. This new bone formation, which begins in the sacroiliac joints, leads to the appearance of the bamboo spine as the disease progress rostrally and is therefore not unique to the sacroiliac joint (E is incorrect).

▸▸ Answer 12

Correct answer is C

The patient has myelopathy in the setting of C1–C2 instability. Patients with instability at this level may have myelopathy from dynamic translation of C1 on C2 due to insufficiency of the transverse ligament. The spinal canal diameter at the C1–C2 level is often large and is not expected to be stenotic in the setting of myelopathy at this level. Dynamic flexion/extension radiographs of the cervical spine should reveal dynamic translation at this level, making C the correct answer. An enlarged predental interval is often seen. Cervical myelopathy in the setting of C1–C2 instability is best treated with a C1–C2 posterior cervical fusion and stabilization. Patients with dynamic instability may appear to have no central canal stenosis on static imaging, even in the setting of myelopathy, making CT myelogram (A) incorrect. The patient is significantly myelopathic, leading to a lower suspicion of peripheral neuropathy or peripheral nerve entrapment unlikely, making EMG (B) incorrect. The patient's symmetric symptoms with both weakness and numbness are more consistent with myelopathy rather than intracranial pathology, which would likely cause more unilateral symptoms, making MRI of the brain (D) incorrect. Lumbar puncture would be considered if other radiographic imaging was inconclusive (E is incorrect).

▸▸ Answer 13

Correct answer is D

The normal configuration of cervical lordosis is in part due to increased disc height in the ventral portion of the disc space. As the cervical discs degenerate with time and become flatter, the cervical spine will develop a straight configuration and eventually a kyphotic posture. As a loss of cervical lordosis occurs, the moment arm is offset ventrally from the IAR of the cervical vertebral body leading to an increased bending moment when gravitational forces perpendicular to the moment arm are applied, which perpetuates cervical kyphosis, making D the correct answer (see ▸ Fig. 5.5).

▸▸ Answer 14

Correct answer is E

The stresses at the lumbosacral junction are highly dependent on pelvic parameters, including sacral slope, lumbar lordosis, and pelvic incidence. Lumbar lordosis is highly influenced by pelvic incidence and sacral slope. A high pelvic incidence correlates with a high sacral slope, which influences a larger lumbar lordosis. This in turn puts higher amounts of stress on the posterior elements at the lumbosacral junction, which may lead to an isthmic pars defect. The larger lumbar lordosis combined with a steep sacral slope and high pelvic incidence will subject the lumbosacral junction to the high sheer stresses, which may lead to translation of L5 on S1 secondary to isthmic pars defect (see ▸ Fig. 5.6). The largest values of pelvic incidence, lumbar lordosis, and sacral slope are seen in Roussouly grade 4 spines; out of the answer choices, E has the largest values, making it the correct answer.[4]

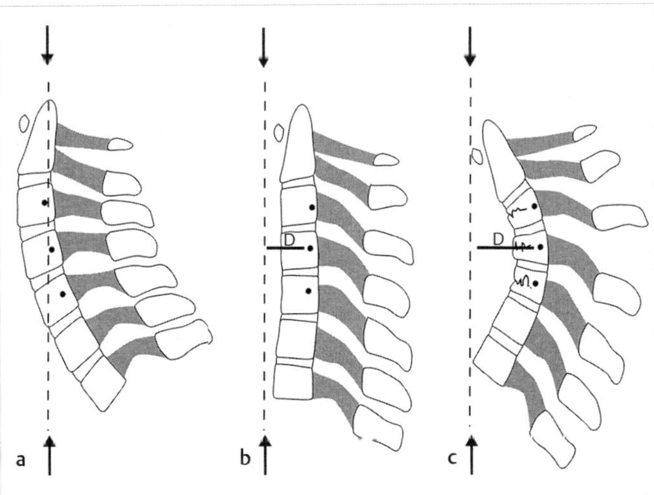

Fig. 5.5 The non-pathological situation in which the dorsal vertebral body height is less than the ventral height. **(a)** This results in the normal lordotic curvature in the cervical spine. **(b)** Ventral disc interspace height loss (via the typical degeneration process) results in the loss of the non-pathological lordotic posture. This causes the creation and elongation of the moment arm applied to the spine, D, leading to ventral vertebral body compression. **(c)** A further exaggeration of a pathological kyphotic posture may then ensue. (Source: Biomechanics of Spine Stabilization: Third Edition, © 2015 Thieme Medical Publishers, Inc.)

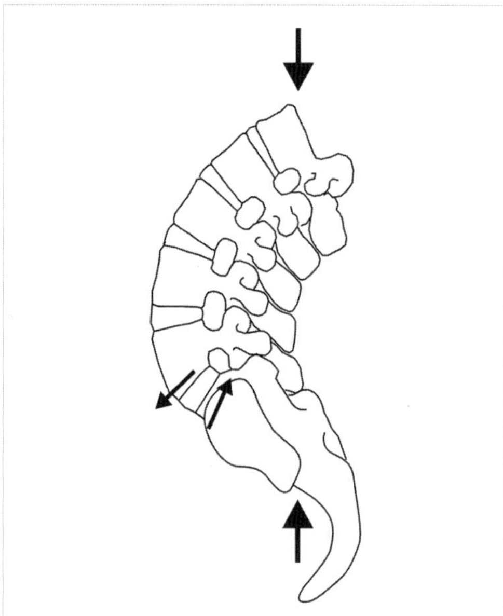

Fig. 5.6 An exaggeration of the normal lumbar lordosis places excessive translational stresses on the lumbosacral junction when the patient is exposed to axial loads (vertical arrows). This may result in a parallelogram-like translational deformation at the lumbosacral junction (diagonal arrows). (Source: Biomechanics of Spine Stabilization: Third Edition, © 2015 Thieme Medical Publishers, Inc.)

▸▸ Answer 15

Correct answer is A

Changes in pressure dynamics with the disc space are essential in understanding the process of degenerative disc disease. The dynamics of intradiscal pressure are described in terms of hydrostatic intradiscal pressure and osmotic intradiscal pressure. The change in water content of the nucleus pulposus with weight bearing contributes to the hydrostatic intradiscal pressure. As a person bears weight, the intradiscal hydrostatic pressure increases, causing water content to exit the disc through a semipermeable membrane. This migration of water out of the disc space results in a net increase in micromolecules within the disc space, thus increasing the intradiscal oncotic pressure. This facilitates the re-entry of water content into the disc space following the cessation of weight bearing. Therefore, both the intradiscal hydrostatic pressure and oncotic pressure within the disc space are increased during normal weight bearing, making A the correct answer (see ▸ Fig. 5.7).

▸▸ Answer 16

Correct answer is E

The majority of elderly patients will have radiographic signs of cervical spondylosis, even in the

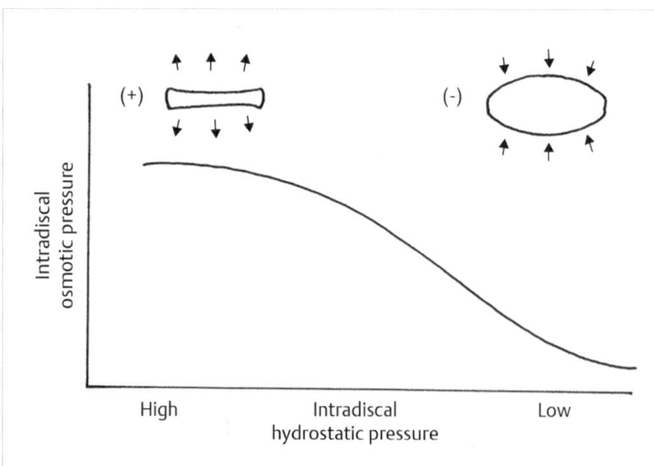

Fig. 5.7 Osmotic and hydrostatic factors affecting the disc interspace. Note that an increased intradiscal pressure, resulting from an increase in weight bearing, causes fluid to migrate out of the intradiscal space (*arrows*). This, in turn, increases the concentration of micromolecules and the oncotic pressure within the disc space (+). Hence, the absorption capacity of the disc is increased. Decreasing intradiscal pressure has the opposite effect. (Source: Data obtained from Kramer J. Intervertebral Disc Disease: Causes, Diagnosis, Treatment, and Prophylaxis, 2d ed: Stuttgart and New York: George Thieme Verlag. 1990:14–47)

absence of clinically symptomatic cervical stenosis or myelopathy. Radiographic findings include degenerative changes in the disc with end plate sclerosis, facet hypertrophy, and hypertrophy of the ligamentum flavum. Facet hypertrophy and ligamentum flavum hypertrophy effectively lower the diameter of the cervical spinal canal and play a key part in cervical stenosis. With extension injuries, buckling of the ligamentum flavum is the most common cause of SCI, making E the correct answer. Spondylolisthesis due to ligamentous laxity contributes to cervical stenosis but is not as common a mechanism with cervical SCI (A is incorrect). Fractures through autofused motion segments are a common cause of neurological injury and mechanical instability in patients with DISH and ankylosing spondylitis and may have concomitant epidural hematoma; however, this is not the most common overall mechanism of SCI in the elderly (D is incorrect). Disc herniation and facet fractures are associated with flexion injury (B and C are incorrect).

▸▸ Answer 17

Correct answer is D

The patient has an acute three-column injury in the setting of ankylosing spondylitis, warranting surgical stabilization via a posterior thoracic fusion. The long lever arm created by autofusion at multiple levels in the spine creates a highly unstable motion segment in the setting of a three-column injury, making patients susceptible to worsening deformity and eventual spinal cord compromise and paralysis. These fractures are best treated with posterolateral fusion above and below the unstable motion segment. In the absence of cord compromise and neurological deficit, no posterior decompression is required (A and E are incorrect). A TLSO brace would not provide enough stability in an unstable three-column injury and the patient's mechanical instability and risk for neurologic injury would persist with weight-bearing. Antibiologics are effective in preventing disease progression but would not help a pre-existing fracture heal, making B incorrect.

▸▸ Answer 18

Correct answer is E

Several radiographic features have been suggested to be predictive of postoperative stability with lumbar laminectomy without fusion. Certain findings associated with lumbar spondylosis, including degenerative disc disease with disc space narrowing, and end plate sclerosis with bridging osteophytes may act to stabilize the motion segment following posterior decompression. Facets that are more coronally oriented have greater ability to counteract shear forces that may lead to spondylolisthesis following posterior decompression. However, advanced facet arthropathy with gapping in the joint suggests joint laxity that may increase postoperative instability, making E the correct answer.

▸▸ Answer 19

Correct answer is B

Understanding the clinical presentation of mechanical low back pain is essential during the consideration of lumbar fusion surgery. Mechanical axial spine pain is characterized by (1) deep and agonizing pain that is (2) worsened with axial loading (making E incorrect) and is improved with unloading, meaning that the patient should find a comfortable position, such as sitting or lying down. This patient states that he is unable to find a comfortable position, and his back pain is also present when he is in a resting position in the absence of axial loading, calling into question the mechanical nature of his back pain. This is a negative predictor in response to fusion surgery. Decompression and fusion procedures are common for concurrent radicular symptoms and mechanical low back pain (making A incorrect). Deep and agonizing low back pain by itself is not enough to include or exclude mechanical low back pain and must be further characterized to differentiate from other back pain etiologies (making D incorrect). If a patient has clinical findings of mechanical axial back pain in the setting of previous spine surgery with radiographic findings consistent with adjacent segment disease, this is not a negative predictor in outcome (making C incorrect).

▸▸ Answer 20

Correct answer is C

The patient's worsening neurologic symptoms in the setting of multiple herniated discs warrant surgical intervention. Three levels of significant ventral compression in the setting of a kyphotic deformity would best be treated with a ventral approach for both direct decompression and correction of the kyphotic deformity. A three-level anterior cervical discectomy and fusion would be the best treatment strategy, with consideration of posterior fusion if concerns for pseudoarthrosis arise. Artificial disc replacement has only been approved for two levels, making D incorrect.[5] Additionally, artificial disc replacement would not be expected to adequately restore cervical lordosis in the setting of a kyphotic deformity. Posterior approaches are popular for compression greater than two motion segments; however, in the presence of significant kyphotic deformity, the ventral portion of the spinal cord may be draped over the posterior vertebral bodies and disc herniations, leading to residual compression (B is incorrect). Cervical laminoplasties are contraindicated in the setting of cervical kyphosis (A is incorrect)

Key Principles

- Degenerative disease of the spine begins with degenerative disc disease from repetitive axial loading and unloading, and eventually undergoes spinal restabilization through reactive end plate changes and eventual osteophyte formation across the motion segment.
- Inflammatory spinal arthropathies are complex disease processes that have significant implications on spinal stability and require unique treatment considerations compared with degenerative disease.
- Ankylosing spondylitis and DISH may become highly unstable in the setting of trauma given the long moment arms formed by autofusion.
- In the cervical spine, ventral compression is best corrected from a ventral approach, whereas dorsal compression is best decompressed from a dorsal approach. Associated deformities including cervical kyphosis should be taken into consideration during surgical planning.
- The various etiologies of axial spine pain have different forms of management and should be carefully differentiated from each other.

References

[1] Goel A. Indicators of atlantoaxial instability. J Craniovertebr Junction Spine 2021;12(2):103–106

[2] Goel A. Treatment of basilar invagination by atlantoaxial joint distraction and direct lateral mass fixation. J Neurosurg Spine 2004;1(3):281–286

[3] Fiani B, Houston R, Siddiqi I, et al. Retro-odontoid pseudotumor formation in the context of various acquired and congenital pathologies of the craniovertebral junction and surgical techniques. Neurospine 2021;18(1):67–78

[4] Laouissat F, Sebaaly A, Gehrchen M, et al. Classification of normal sagittal spine alignment: refounding the Roussouly classification. Eur Spine J 2018;27(8):2002–2011

[5] Roberts T, Filler RJ, Savage JW, et al. Cervical total disk arthroplasty. Clinical Spine Surg 2018;31(1):6–13

6 Trauma, Tumor, and Infection

Shawn W. Adams, Brian J. Williams

A common descriptive language identifying and describing spine fractures is essential for professional communication. Radiographic identification of spine fractures alone provides only some of the information needed to guide clinical decision making and treatment algorithms. Often, the assessment of fracture stability is important in dictating management. Understanding the biomechanical forces and mechanisms that cause injury patterns will provide further information about mechanical integrity, stability, ligamentous damage, and associated injuries. Proper identification of fractures or classification additionally allows for better data with which to study treatments and outcomes.

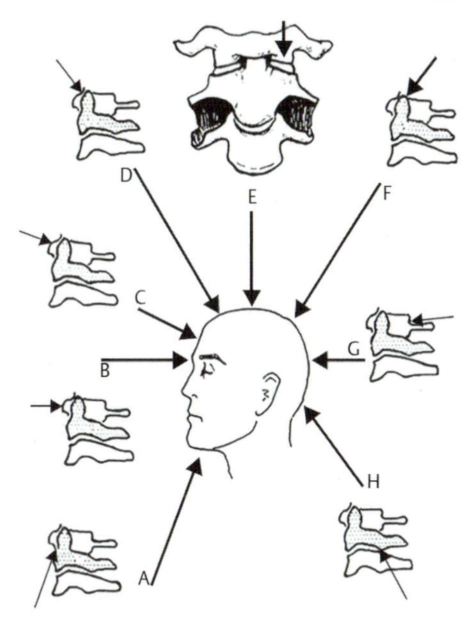

Fig. 6.1 The mechanism of injury (orientation of injury force vector) partly dictates the type of injury incurred. Sagittal plane injury. (Source: Biomechanics of Spine Stabilization: Third Edition, © 2015 Thieme Medical Publishers, Inc.)

Learning Objectives

- Understand how local, regional, and global spine anatomy affects the response to force, particularly traumatic forces.
- Learn which injury patterns are associated with which mechanisms or force vectors.
- Review a common descriptive nomenclature for identifying specific fracture patterns.
- Apply biomechanical principles with anatomic knowledge and fracture identification to help guide treatment.
- Tumor and infection can alter the structural integrity such that injury common to high forces may be seen after seemingly nontraumatic events.

Questions

▸▸ Question 1

Which letter in ▶ Fig. 6.1 corresponds to the force vector most likely to be associated with a C1 burst fracture (Jefferson fracture)?

- A. A
- B. B
- C. C
- D. D
- E. E

▸▸ Question 2

According to the Anderson and Montesano classification, an extension of a basilar skull fracture results in which type of occipital condyle fracture?

- A. Type I
- B. Type II
- C. Type III
- D. Type IV
- E. Atypical

▸▸ Question 3

Which letter in ▶ Fig. 6.2 corresponds to the force vector associated with a traumatic spondylolisthesis of the axis (hangman's fracture)?

- A. F
- B. B
- C. G
- D. D
- E. E

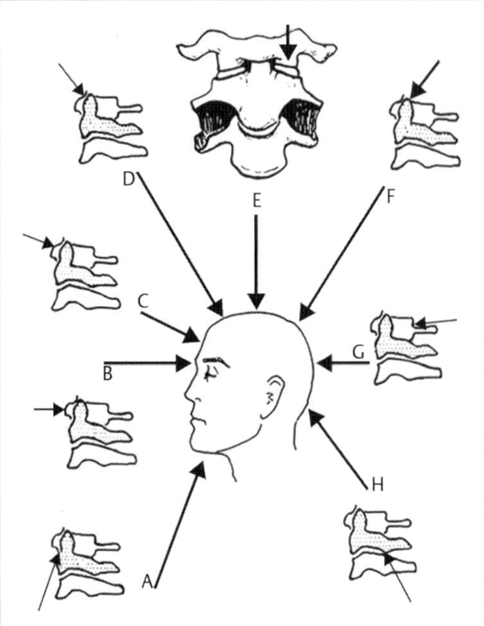

Fig. 6.2 The mechanism of injury (orientation of injury force vector) partly dictates the type of injury incurred. Sagittal plane injury. (Source: Biomechanics of Spine Stabilization: Third Edition, © 2015 Thieme Medical Publishers, Inc.)

▸▸ Question 4

Which of the following injuries is NOT typically caused by an axial loading mechanism?

- A. C1 burst fracture (Jefferson fracture)
- B. Type I occipital condyle
- C. Type II occipital condyle
- D. Vertical, sagittal-oriented C2 burst-pedicle fracture (type II C2 body fracture)
- E. Horizontal C1 fracture

▸▸ Question 5

Nonunion is a common complication of nonoperative management when following which type(s) of odontoid fracture as classified by Anderson and D'Alonzo?

- A. Type I
- B. Type II
- C. Type III
- D. Type I and III
- E. All types

▸▸ Question 6

A type III occipital condyle injury of the Anderson and Montesano classification is associated with an avulsion of bony fragment from the occipital condyle by which structure?

- A. Transverse ligament
- B. Tectorial membrane
- C. Alar ligament
- D. Apical ligament
- E. Ligamentum flava

▸▸ Question 7

An injury-causing force that is the product of an axial load and ventrally oriented bending moment (to failure)—that is, the axial load is eccentrically placed—is most likely to produce which type of injury pattern?

- A. Wedge compression fracture
- B. Burst fracture
- C. Lateral wedge compression fracture
- D. Flexion–distraction (Chance) fracture
- E. Hyperextension subluxation

▸▸ Question 8

In Benzel's biomechanical model, a true axial load (to failure) if applied to the subaxial spine symmetrically results in which type of injury pattern, regardless of retropulsion of body fragments into the spinal canal?

- A. Wedge compression fracture
- B. Burst fracture
- C. Lateral wedge compression fracture
- D. Flexion–distraction (Chance) fracture
- E. Fracture dislocation

▸▸ Question 9

A Chance-type fracture is caused by which mechanism?

- A. Axial loading force through the IAR
- B. Axial loading force lateral to the IAR
- C. Axial loading force anterior to the IAR
- D. Distraction force with flexion bending moment
- E. Distraction force

▸▸ Question 10

Most upper cervical spine injuries result from___________.

- A. Blunt trauma to the neck
- B. Projectile injury to the neck
- C. Metastatic or primary tumor of the segment
- D. Osteomyelitis of the segment
- E. Blunt trauma to the head

▸▸ Question 11

When assessing the stability of a C1 burst fracture (see ▸ Fig. 6.3), which value is the cutoff, such that the sum of a and b greater than this is associated with rupture of the transverse ligament?

- A. 3 mm
- B. 5 mm
- C. 7 mm
- D. 9 mm
- E. 13 mm

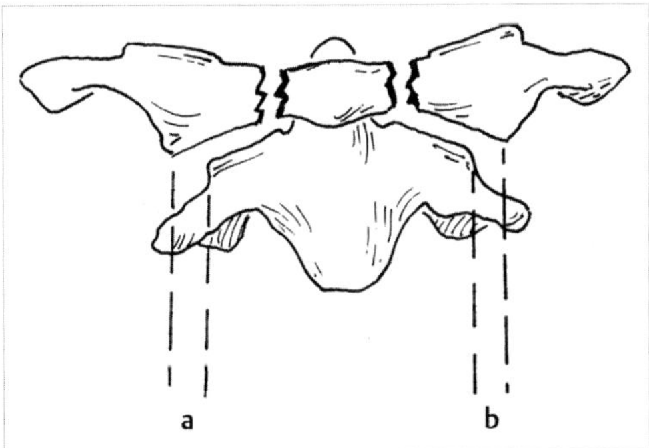

Fig. 6.3 A lateral displacement of the C1 facet on the C2 facet of more than 7mm, adding together the **(a)** right and **(b)** left displacements, implies disruption of the transverse ligament of the atlas and significant instability. (Source: Biomechanics of Spine Stabilization: Third Edition, © 2015 Thieme Medical Publishers, Inc.)

▸▸ Question 12

In the Effendi classification of traumatic spondylolisthesis of the axis (hangman's fracture), which type(s) is/are generally considered unstable and in need of surgical stabilization?

- A. Type I
- B. Type II
- C. Type III
- D. All
- E. None

▸▸ Question 13

In a C1 arch fracture, as depicted in ▸ Fig. 6.4, the typical point of fracture is closely associated with what anatomical structure?

- A. C1 pedicle
- B. Atlanto-occipital membrane
- C. Insertion of the ligament of flavum
- D. Vertebral artery
- E. C2 nerve root

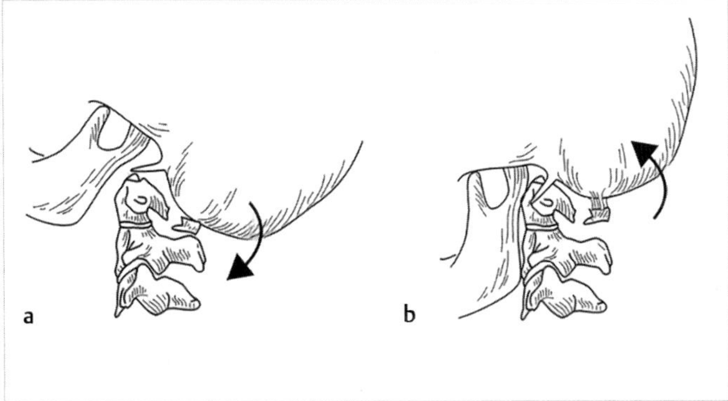

Fig. 6.4 **(a)** Hyperextension of the calvaria (*curved arrow*) can cause a fracture of the posterior arch of C1 by impingement on the dorsal arch of C1 via the occiput or the lamina of C2. **(b)** Hyperflexion (*curved arrow*) can cause a similar injury via ligamentous attachments. The latter two injuries do not usually degrade spinal stability, as can the C1 burst fracture. (Source: Biomechanics of Spine Stabilization: Third Edition, © 2015 Thieme Medical Publishers, Inc.)

▸▸ **Question 14**

If a force vector passes precisely through the IAR of a vertebral body, the moment arm of this force vector is________.

- A. 0
- B. Parallel
- C. Maximal
- D. Proportional
- E. Equal but opposite

▸▸ **Question 15**

What scenario/mechanism is commonly associated with Chance fractures?

- A. Fall forward striking face
- B. Fall backward landing on back
- C. Fall from height landing on feet
- D. Restrained motorist
- E. Dive into shallow pool

▸▸ **Question 16**

Due to regional anatomical differences, which area of the spine is more likely to suffer lamina and/or pars interarticularis injuries from hyperextension?

- A. Subaxial cervical spine
- B. Cervical–thoracic junction
- C. Thoracic spine
- D. Thoracolumbar junction
- E. Lumbar spine

▸▸ **Question 17**

Excessive shear and rotational force vectors applied to the spine can result in which injury pattern?

- A. Wedge compression fracture
- B. Burst fracture
- C. Lateral wedge compression fracture
- D. Flexion–distraction (Chance) fracture
- E. Fracture dislocation

▸▸ **Question 18**

In the cervical spine, isolated (without fracture) ligamentous injuries are common. Ligament injuries are evidenced by the high incidence of positive magnetic resonance imaging (MRI) finding in cervical soft tissue in the face of negative radiographs or computed tomography (CT) scans after cervical spine trauma. These findings can be evidence of what?

- A. Spinal cord injury without radiological evidence
- B. Cervicalgia
- C. Whiplash
- D. Torticollis
- E. Fibromyalgia

▸▸ **Question 19**

Regarding sacral fractures, what is a vertical fracture that involves the ventral neuroforamina best classified as?

- A. Zone 1 fracture
- B. Zone 2 fracture
- C. Zone 3 fracture
- D. Zone 4 fracture
- E. H type

▸▸ **Question 20**

What is the predominant factor dictating the type of cervical spine injury?

- A. Age of the person
- B. The orientation of the force vector applied
- C. Tumor biology
- D. Identity of infectious agent
- E. Bone density

Answers

▸▸ **Answer 1**

Correct answer is E

Axial loads applied to the vertex of the calvaria (injury mechanism E) can cause several types of injury. The most common of these is the C1 burst fracture (Jefferson fracture). The other vectors are not pure axial loads, although one could imagine intermediate vectors with a significant axial load component that could be sufficient to cause the mechanical failure of the C1 ring seen in a Jefferson fracture.

▸▸ **Answer 2**

Correct answer is B

There are three types of occipital condyle fractures in the Anderson and Montesano system. "Types I and II usually are incurred via an axially applied load. A type I fracture is a medial disruption of the condyle (impacted occipital condyle) ... The type II occipital condyle fracture (an extension of a basilar skull fracture) most likely also results from an axially applied load."[1]

▸▸ **Answer 3**

Correct answer is B

"The sudden hyperextension of the head, without an associated distraction component, causes the commonly observed hangman's fracture (traumatic spondylolisthesis of the axis)."[2] This is typically seen with a blow to the face, particularly in an elderly person who sustains a forward fall with significant face trauma causing cervical hyperextension. Vector A is associated with the "judicial hangman's" injury; this is not a choice. The other vectors depicted are not associated with the bilateral pars interarticularis fracture of a hangman's type injury.

▸▸ **Answer 4**

Correct answer is E

A horizontal split of the ventral C1 arch results from violent distraction and extension. The longus coli muscle attaches to the anterior tubercle of C1 and likely applies the force that results in the avulsion or separation between the rostral and caudal portions of the ventral C1 ring. All the other fractures listed are typically associated with an axial loading force.

▸▸ **Answer 5**

Correct answer is B

Nonunion is common with type II fractures. Advancing age portends an increasingly poor prognosis regarding fracture healing. Displacement, less cancellous bone, poor blood supply, inadequate immobilization—all seem to be implicated in the development of a nonunion.

▸▸ **Answer 6**

Correct answer is C

A lateral blow to the head uncommonly results in a medial avulsion of the occipital condyle. This is termed a *type III occipital condyle fracture*. It is an avulsion injury caused by shearing forces that put tension on the occipital condyle via the alar and capsular ligaments.

▸▸ **Answer 7**

Correct answer is A

Ventral wedge compression fractures are the product of an axial load and ventrally oriented bending moment (to failure), that is, the axial load is eccentrically placed ventral to the instantaneous axis of rotation (IAR). Burst fractures result from symmetric compression with the load near or over the IAR. Lateral wedge compression fractures also have an axial load eccentric to the IAR, but it would be lateral not ventral. Flexion–distraction (Chance) fracture, by definition, has a distracting force component, not axial loading.

▸▸ **Answer 8**

Correct answer is B

If a true axial load (to failure) is applied to the subaxial spine, a symmetric compression of the vertebral body results—a burst fracture.

▸▸ **Answer 9**

Correct answer is D

The injury pattern described by Chance and known as a Chance fracture is caused by a flexion-distraction mechanism. Axial loading force through the IAR causes burst fractures. Axial loading force lateral to the IAR causes lateral wedge compression fractures. Axial loading force anterior to the IAR causes ventral wedge compression fractures.

▸▸ **Answer 10**

Correct answer is E

Most upper cervical spine injuries result from blows to the head. This is due to (1) the unique

- B. Evaluation of cervical distraction versus traction weight can be done via fraction = $K_{neck}Sx$, where K_{neck} (spring constant) is same for bilateral and unilateral cervical spine dislocation
- C. For height reduction of a spinal bony component, the applied load must be perpendicular with the instantaneous axis of rotation (IAR)
- D. True axial load application to the spine along an axially oriented axis can result in the failure of a spinal segment component resulting in loss of height of that component (bone and soft tissue)
- E. An isolated axial load with applied bending movement will result in loss of vertebral height of spinal segments

▸▸ Question 10

Most spinal deformities are manifestations of more than one type of deformation. All are examples of combination deformation, except__________.

- A. Wedge compression fracture
- B. Type I C2 body fracture
- C. Chance fracture
- D. Burst fracture
- E. Post traumatic kyphosis.

▸▸ Question 11

Spinal dislocation or listhesis involves a__________.

- A. Combination deformation with flexion–distraction of the spine
- B. Translation and shearing of the spinal elements along coronal and sagittal axis of the spine resulting from application of parallel noncoincident force vector in opposite direction
- C. Combination deformation with translation along the axis of the spine
- D. Translation deformation force vector applied along the longitudinal axis of the spine
- E. Rotation deformation combined with flexion

▸▸ Question 12

For deformation progression to occur, at least one unstable spinal segment must be present. This instability may be either acute or chronic. Instability as an isolated entity, however, is not sufficient to create a deformation or to cause it to progress.

All of the below are contributing factors to deformity progression, except__________.

- A. Application of pathological (excessive) stress on spine
- B. Nutrient and metabolic level change in affected disc
- C. Sagittal imbalance of spine
- D. Symmetrical loading of disc
- E. Application of nonpathological stresses to an already deformed spine

▸▸ Question 13

Spinal balance is an important consideration with all deformities. If the head cannot be naturally maintained above the hips, excessive strain is placed on the spine, thus predisposing the spine to further deformation. In addition, excessive strain may be applied to the spine, leading to a pain syndrome. Such a situation exists with the flat back syndrome characterized by a mechanical pain that extends into the buttocks and dorsal thigh region. A patient so affected cannot stand erect without bending his or her knees and hips. Understanding the concept of sagittal spinal balance and compensatory mechanisms is essential to planning the surgical treatment of sagittal spinal deformity. Which of the following spinopelvic parameters is the most important initiating factor for flat back syndrome and is the main aim for restoration during deformity correction surgery in patient with flat back syndrome?

- A. High pelvic incidence (PI)
- B. High lumbar lordosis (LL)
- C. Low LL
- D. Low sacral slope (SS)
- E. High PI

▸▸ Question 14

Excessive angular deformity or posture can result in a translational deformity. Such a situation may exist at the lumbosacral junction. In this circumstance, subluxation and/or degenerative changes may occur. The shear strain associated with pathologic lumbar angles and other pelvic parameters is a strong predictor of progressive anterolisthesis at the L5–S1 junction. Which of the following spinopelvic parameters are strongly associated with spondylolisthesis at L5–S1 level?

- A. Low PI
- B. Less LL
- C. High PI
- D. Low SS
- E. Low pelvic tilt

Answers

▸▸ Answer 1

Correct answer is C

Translation and rotation can occur along and about each of the three axes of the Cartesian coordinate system, leading to a potential of six fundamental movements. The six fundamental types of spinal deformation are (1) rotation about the long axis of the spine, (2) rotation about the coronal axis of the spine, (3) rotation about the sagittal axis of the spine, (4) translation along the long axis of the spine, (5) translation along the coronal axis of the spine, and (6) translation along the sagittal axis of the spine. Each of these movements or deformations can occur in either of two directions (see ▸ Fig. 7.1).

Posttraumatic kyphosis occurs due to rotation deformation about an axially oriented axis (coronal or sagittal) that occurs at the level of the vertebral body along with an asymmetric load application (see ▸ Fig. 7.2). Answer C is correct.

▸▸ Answer 2

Correct answer is B

Biomechanical coupling is a 3D process occurring within six degrees of freedom in which the vertebrae can translate along or rotate about each orthogonal axis. The 3D motions in human vertebral segments correspond to flexion–extension, rotation, and side-bending (lateral flexion) forces. Coupling, essentially, is the obligatory secondary motion to an applied force—e.g., rotation in response to side-bending. It occurs due to orientation of facet joints and the presence or absence of uncovertebral joints.

This coupling behavior is dependent on the first motion of initiation (i.e., side-bending), the posture of the spine, and the pathology of the segment (option A is incorrect). It plays roles in both the prevention of spinal deformation by contributing to movement restriction and the exaggeration of complexity of the deformation itself when a deformity indeed occurs (options C and E are incorrect).

Because the movements are 3D, measurement should incorporate appropriate devices that address the multidimensional nature of movement (option D is incorrect). Failure to use an appropriate measurement device may lead to errors and inaccuracies associated with coupling biomechanics.[1]

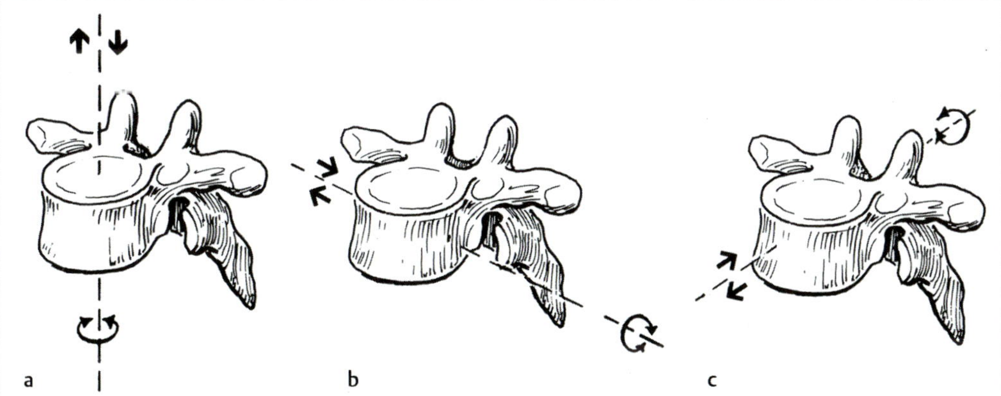

Fig. 7.1 The six fundamental segmental movements, or types of deformation, of the spine along (straight arrows) or about (curved arrows) the instantaneous axis of rotation are the following: (1) rotation or translation about the long axis of the spine **(a)**; (2) rotation or translation about the coronal axis of the spine **(b)**; (3) rotation or translation about the sagittal axis of the spine **(C)**; (4) translation along the long axis of the spine **(a)**; (5) translation along the coronal axis of the spine **(b)**; and (6) translation along the sagittal axis of the spine **(c)**. (Source: Biomechanics of Spine Stabilization: Third Edition, © 2015 Thieme Medical Publishers, Inc.)

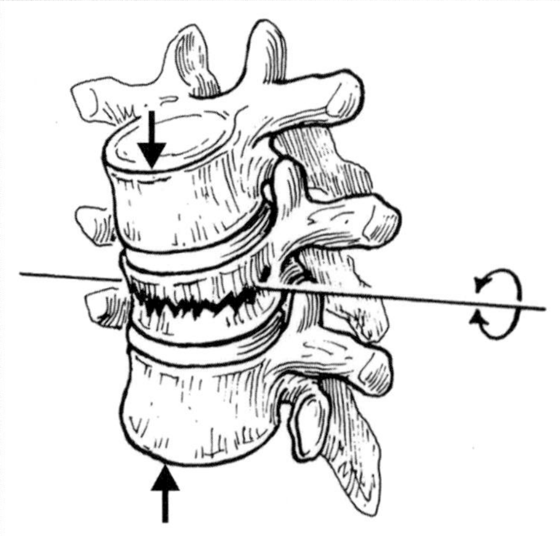

Fig. 7.2 A depiction of the forces and the resultant rotation deformation about a coronally oriented axis of the spine, resulting in a wedgelike deformation. Curved arrow depict bending moments. Straight arrows depict applied forces. (Source: Biomechanics of Spine Stabilization: Third Edition, © 2015 Thieme Medical Publishers, Inc.)

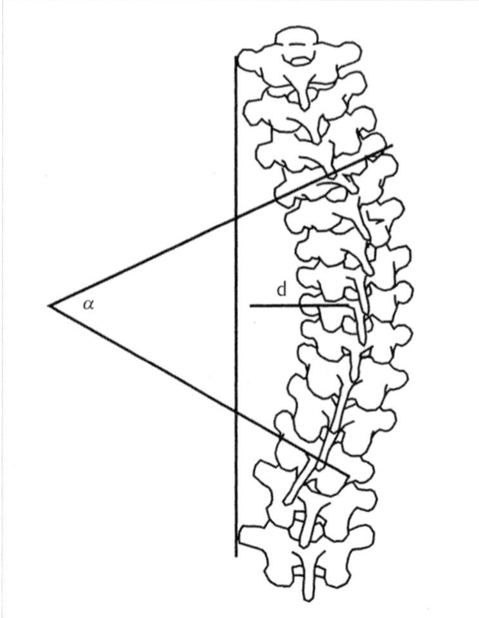

Fig. 7.3 Deformity begets deformity by increasing the length of the moment arm (*d*). Determination of the Cobb angle (α) in a spine with a moderate scoliotic deformity is depicted. The Cobb angle is measured from end vertebra to end vertebra. (Source: Biomechanics of Spine Stabilization: Third Edition, © 2015 Thieme Medical Publishers, Inc.)

▸▸ Answer 3

Correct answer is C

In a traumatic permanent deformation, ligamentous and bony elements (e.g., facet joints) are often disrupted. Classic examples of such acute injuries are the unilateral cervical locked facet due to rotation combined with flexion movement (option C is correct).

Rotation deformation with fracture dislocation is the mechanism leading to posttraumatic fracture dislocation (option A is incorrect). Extension combined with rotation deformation leads to a lordotic deformity (option B is incorrect). Translation along the long axis with flexion leads to a wedge compression (option D is incorrect), and translation along the long axis with extension leads to a distraction injury (option E is incorrect).

▸▸ Answer 4

Correct answer is A

A classic rotation deformation about the sagittal or coronal axis resulting from asymmetric load application leads to a wedge compression fracture. Rotation can take the form of kyphosis with flexion rotation deformation (option B is incorrect), lordosis with extension rotation deformation (option C is incorrect), scoliosis with lateral bending rotation deformation (option D is incorrect), or a combination of these.

▸▸ Answer 5

Correct answer is A

The Cobb angle is measured from end vertebra to end vertebra (see ▸ Fig. 7.3). Determination of the Cobb angle (α) in a spine with a moderate scoliotic deformity is depicted. The Cobb angle is measured from the superior end plate of the superior end vertebra to the inferior end plate of the inferior end vertebra.

▸▸ Answer 6

Correct answer is C

The Cobb angle is more appropriately used to quantitate multilevel curves as opposed to a short-segment curve (option C is correct).

The Cobb angle can be deceptive even when used in multilevel curves. Its utility in the cervical spine has also been questioned (options A and B are incorrect).

The radii of curvature of two spinal deformities may be widely disparate despite their having the same Cobb angle (option D is incorrect).

A lesser radius of curvature is observed at the injured segment in a situation in which an acute segmental angulation occurs, compared with less acute multisegmental angulations (option E is incorrect) (see ▸ Fig. 7.4). Deformity begets deformity by increasing the length of the moment arm (d). **(a)** Determination of the Cobb angle (α) in a spine with a moderate scoliotic deformity is depicted. The Cobb angle is measured from end vertebra to end vertebra. **(b)** The end vertebrae are located between curves that are concave toward opposite directions, as depicted in the Cobb angle β. The radii of curvature of two spinal deformities may be widely disparate despite their having the same Cobb angle. **(c)** A lesser radius of curvature is observed at the injured segment in a situation in which an acute segmental angulation occurs, as in the Cobb angle Δ, compared with (b) less acute multisegmental angulations. Note that each spine has the same Cobb angle (α = β = Δ).

▸▸ Answer 7

Correct answer is D

Translational deformation of the spine occurs along an axis defined by the direction of the deformation-creating force vector (option D is correct).

Translational deformation differs from rotational deformation, which is created by a bending moment caused by the application of a force vector at some distance from the axis of deformation (option E is incorrect). Translational deformation can occur in any plane and can be acute or chronic (option A is incorrect). In burst fractures, the

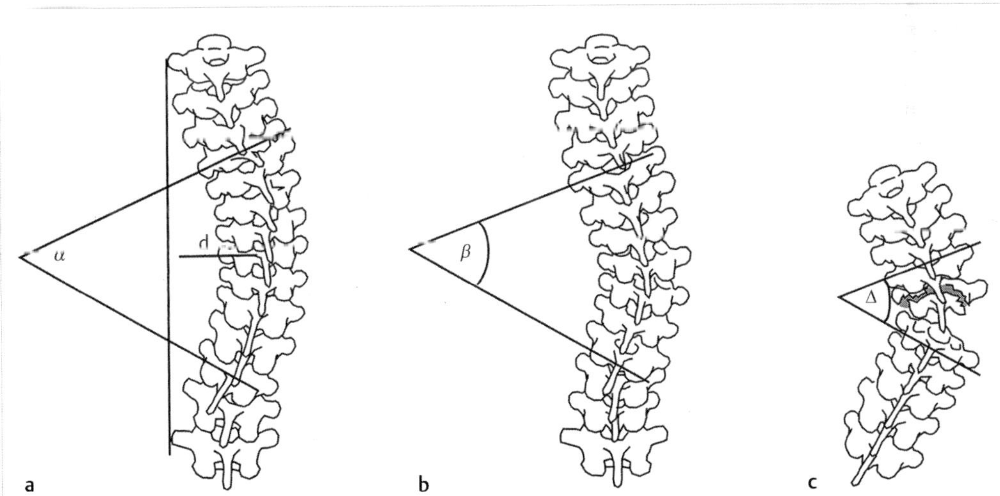

Fig. 7.4 Deformity begets deformity by increasing the length of the moment arm (*d*). **(a)** Determination of the Cobb angle (α) in a spine with a moderate scoliotic deformity is depicted. The Cobb angle is measured from neutral vertebra to neutral vertebra. **(b)** The neutral vertebrae are located between curves that are concave toward opposite directions, as depicted in Cobb angle β. The radii of curvature of two spinal deformities may be widely disparate despite their having the same Cobb angle. **(c)** A lesser radius of curvature is observed at the injured segment in a situation in which an acute segmental angulation occurs, as in Cobb angle Δ, compared with (B) less acute multisegmental angulations. Note that each spine has the same Cobb angle (α = β = Δ). (Source: Biomechanics of Spine Stabilization: Third Edition, © 2015 Thieme Medical Publishers, Inc.)

deforming force vector is applied along the longitudinal axis of the spine, not along one of the axially oriented axes of the spine, which leads to fracture-dislocation deformation (option B is incorrect).

In spondylolistheses, the deforming force vector is applied along one of the axially oriented axes of the spine, not along the long axis of spine (option C is incorrect). ▶ Fig. 7.5 shows depiction of forces.

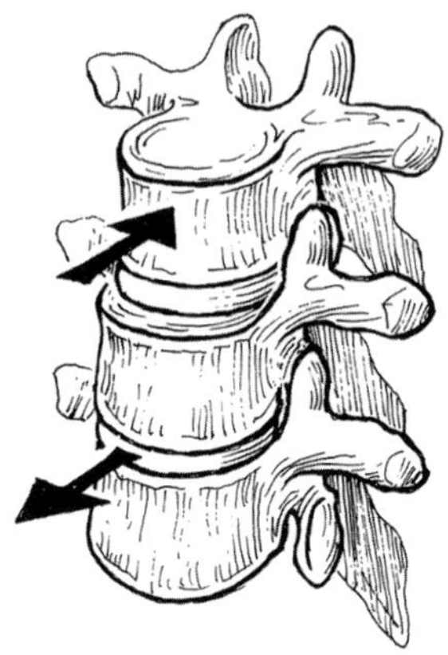

Fig. 7.5 A burst fracture results from translation of the upper and lower endplates of a vertebral body toward each other along the long axis of the spine. (*Arrows*) Axially oriented translational deformation, resulting in a fracture–dislocation, occurs via two parallel but non-coincident opposed force vectors. (Source: Biomechanics of Spine Stabilization: Third Edition, © 2015 Thieme Medical Publishers, Inc.)

▸▸ Answer 8

Correct answer is C

Translational deformation of the spine occurs along an axis defined by the direction of the deformation-creating force vector resulting in shearing, compression, and distraction of the spinal elements.

Distraction deformation of the spine is uncommon, particularly in a chronic form (option B is incorrect). This is so because assumption of the upright posture induces axial (compression) loading (option A is incorrect).

Because axial loads are borne by the spine during the activities of daily living, compression of the spine is common (option C is correct).

Type I C2 body fractures resulting from flexion–distraction and Chance fractures due to flexion–distraction are examples of combination deformations (options D and E are incorrect).

Flexion–distraction of the spine, (See ▶ Fig. 7.6), can result in (**a**) a type I C2 body fracture in the cervical region or (**b**) a Chance fracture in the thoracic or lumbar region.

▸▸ Answer 9

Correct answer is D

Translational deformation along the long axis of the spine occurs via the application of two *coincident* forces along the neutral axis of the spine (option A is incorrect).

Evaluation of cervical distraction versus traction weight indicates that $F_{traction} = K_{neck}$ delta x, where

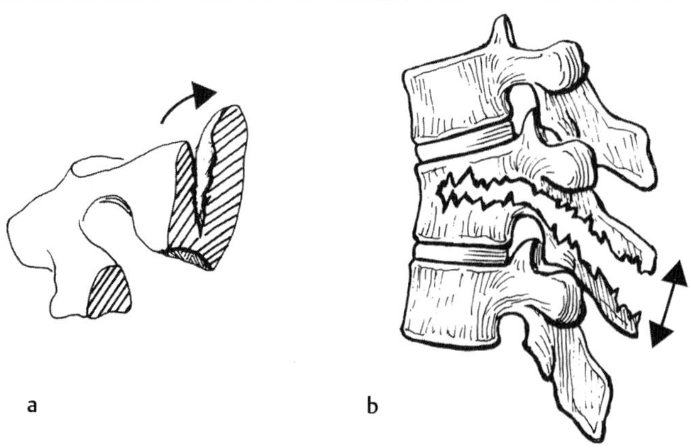

Fig. 7.6 (**a**) Flexion–distraction of the spine can result in a type I C2 body fracture in the cervical region or (**b**) a Chance fracture in the thoracic or lumbar region. (Source: Biomechanics of Spine Stabilization: Third Edition, © 2015 Thieme Medical Publishers, Inc.)

F = traction weight and x = distraction at the injured level. The constant, K_{neck}, is different for bilateral and unilateral dislocations ($p < 0.001$) and is a function of magnitude of injury and neck morphology (option B is incorrect).[2]

The application of true axial loads to the spine along an axially oriented axis can result in the failure of a component of a spinal segment (bone or soft tissue), with a resultant loss of height of that component (option D is correct). For this to occur, the force vector of the applied load must be in line with the IAR along the neutral axis of the spine (option C is incorrect). Applying an isolated axial load with no applied bending moment along the neutral axis of spine results in loss of vertebral height of a spinal segment (option E is incorrect).

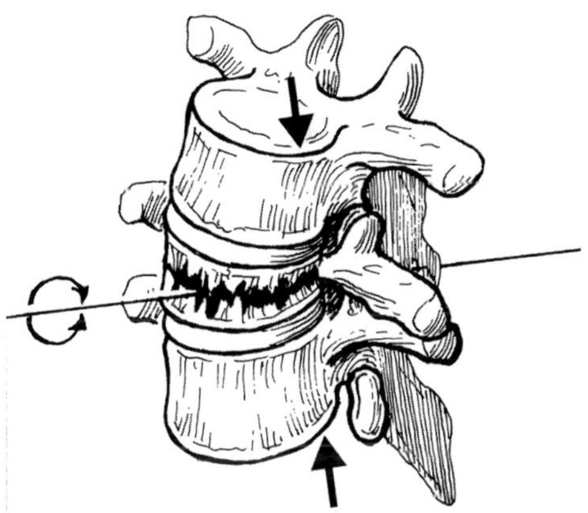

Fig. 7.7 Rotation deformation can occur about the coronal axis of the spine (ventral wedge compression fracture and about the sagittal axis (lateral wedge compression fracture, as shown here). Curved arrow depicts bending moment. Straight arrows depict applied forces. (Source: Biomechanics of Spine Stabilization: Third Edition, © 2015 Thieme Medical Publishers, Inc.)

▸▸ **Answer 10**

Correct answer is D

Most spinal deformities are manifestations of more than one type of deformation—for example, a wedge compression deformation resulting from translational deformation along the axis of the spine with an associated bending movement or flexion (see ▶ Fig. 7.7). Rotation deformation can occur about the coronal axis of the spine (ventral wedge compression fracture and about the sagittal axis (lateral wedge compression fracture, as shown here). Curved arrow depicts bending moment. Straight arrows depict applied forces. Type I C2 body fractures (flexion–distraction) and Chance fractures (flexion–distraction) are other examples of combination deformations (see ▶ Fig. 7.8).

▸▸ **Answer 11**

Correct answer is B

Translation and shearing of the spinal elements along the coronal or sagittal axis of the spine result in spinal dislocations or listhesis. This outcome is a result of the application of parallel but not aligned force vectors in opposite directions (option B is correct).

Combination deformation with flexion–distraction of spine results in type I C2 body fracture and chance fracture (option A is incorrect).

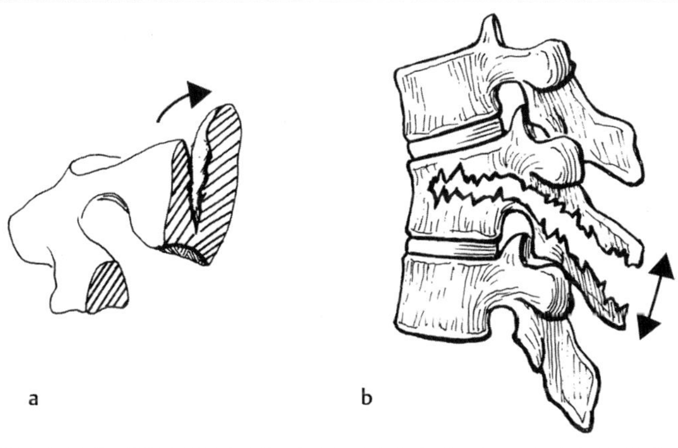

Fig. 7.8 (a) Flexion–distraction of the spine can result in a type I C2 body fracture in the cervical region or (b) a Chance fracture in the thoracic or lumbar region. (Source: Biomechanics of Spine Stabilization: Third Edition, © 2015 Thieme Medical Publishers, Inc.)

Combination deformation with translation along axis of the spine is biomechanics of compression deformation (option C is incorrect).

Translation deformation force vector applied along the longitudinal axis of the spine results in a burst fracture of a spine segment (option D is incorrect). Rotation deformation combined with flexion results in unilateral cervical locked facet (option E is incorrect).

▸▸ Answer 12

Correct answer is D

For deformation progression to occur, at least one unstable spinal segment must be present. This instability may be either acute or chronic. Instability as an isolated entity, however, is not sufficient to create a deformation or to cause it to progress.

Deformation creation or progression requires the application of pathologic (excessive) stresses to the spine and/or the application of nonpathological stresses to an already deformed spine (options A and E).

Spine deformation is associated with changes in nutrient and metabolite levels in affected discs. This can result in premature cell death and has a deleterious effect on disc function, thus contributing to the progressive nature of the deformation. Sagittal imbalance and spine deformity are significant contributing factors to excessive disc loading, which in turn lead to the aforementioned metabolic derangements and subsequent excessive degeneration and instability (options B and C).

Asymmetrical loading of the disc (rather than symmetrical loading) is associated with deformity progression (option D is incorrect).

▸▸ Answer 13

Correct answer is C

Understanding the concept of sagittal spinal balance and compensatory mechanism is essential to planning surgical treatment of sagittal spinal deformity. Sagittal imbalance can be caused by decreased LL and increased thoracic kyphosis and can furthermore be influenced by the PI and flexion contracture of the hip and knee joints. Compensation usually occurs at more rostral levels. Basically, flat back deformity occurs as a result of decrease in LL, and thus restoration of LL to the normal state is the main target of surgery.

The flat back syndrome is anatomically characterized by a loss of LL (option C is correct).

▸▸ Answer 14

Correct answer is C

The shear strain associated with pathologic lumbar angles and other pelvic parameters is a strong predictor of progressive anterolisthesis at the L5–S1 junction.

An excessive LL, with a vertically oriented L5–S1 disc interspace, places significant translational loads at the lumbosacral junction. This may result in spondylolisthesis if the L5–S1 facet joint is incompetent or, in accelerated degenerative changes, if it is competent (option C is correct).

Key Principles

- There are six fundamental segmental movements along and about each of the three axes of the Cartesian coordinate system, which lead to six fundamental types of spinal deformation.
- Coupling phenomenon is 3D and takes place within six degrees of freedom. It plays a role in the prevention of spinal deformation by contributing to movement restriction and in the exaggeration of the complexity of the deformation itself.
- Two parallel and coincident opposed force vectors lead to a burst fracture, while two parallel noncoincident opposed force create a fracture-dislocation deformation of the spine.
- At least one unstable spinal segment must be present for spinal deformation progression and even nonpathological stresses can cause deformity progression in an already deformed spine.
- Knowledge of the approximate location of the IAR and the neutral axis is very useful in the consideration of operative indications and construct design.
- A stable deformation is characterized by the absence of radiographic evidence of deformity progression and the accompanying absence of progressive neurological deficit and pains related to instability.

References

[1] Panjabi M, Yamamoto I, Oxland T, Crisco J. How does posture affect coupling in the lumbar spine? Spine 1989;14:1002–1011

[2] Miller LS, Cotler HB, De Lucia FA, Cotler JM, Hume EL. Biomechanical analysis of cervical distraction. Spine 1987;12:831–837

8 Neural Element Injury

Karl Janich, Marjorie C. Wang

Learning Objectives

- Understand the mechanisms of neural injury at the cellular level.
- Characterize injuries to the neural elements based on fundamental mechanisms.
- Identify mechanisms by which surgical intervention can cause neural element injury.
- Understand spinal cord injury syndromes and anatomy.

Questions

▸▸ Question 1

What is the most common cause of neurologic dysfunction in the setting of degenerative disease or trauma?

- A. Extrinsic compression
- B. Distraction
- C. Sagittal bowstring
- D. Coronal bowstring
- E. Neural element avulsion

▸▸ Question 2

Which of the following mechanisms of neural injury typically results directly in cell death?

- A. Cell disruption
- B. Cell distortion
- C. Cell metabolic derangements
- D. Cell osmotic shifts
- E. Aerobic metabolism

▸▸ Question 3

Which of the following treatments can help relieve injury due to the three mechanisms of cellular injury?

- A. Administration of intravenous steroids
- B. Early parenteral nutrition
- C. Induced hypotension
- D. Hypertonic intravenous solution
- E. Surgical decompression

▸▸ Question 4

Early surgical treatment to relieve mechanisms of injury related to persistent neural element distortion should address which of the following?

- A. Compression and adhesions
- B. Compression, distraction, and tethering
- C. Compression and ligamentous injury
- D. Distraction and adhesions
- E. Restoration of normal spinal alignment

▸▸ Question 5

The radiculomedullary artery of Adamkiewicz typically arises from which level of the spine?

- A. C1–C2
- B. C7–T4
- C. T8–L1
- D. L3–S1
- E. L5–S5

▸▸ Question 6

Simple distraction of a neural element may result in which of the following?

- A. Hyperemia
- B. Reduction of retropulsed fragments
- C. Increased tissue perfusion pressure
- D. Neuronal distortion and impediment of the blood supply
- E. Neutrophilic infiltration

▸▸ Question 7

Tethering of the spinal cord over ventral structures in the sagittal plane may be exacerbated by which of the following?

- A. Dorsal decompression without fusion
- B. Lumbar puncture
- C. Medical management
- D. Anterior decompression with fusion
- E. Correction of kyphosis

▸▸ Question 8

What structure must be intact to allow ligamentotaxis to reduce a compressive lesion, such as a burst fracture?
- A. Anterior longitudinal ligament
- B. Annulus fibrosus
- C. Posterior longitudinal ligament
- D. Ligamentum flavum
- E. Interspinous ligament

▸▸ Question 9

Which of the following may lead to decline in neurological function after attempted ligamentotaxis?
- A. Compression-type injury
- B. Intact anterior longitudinal ligament
- C. Intact posterior longitudinal ligament
- D. Osteoporosis
- E. Spinal cord tethered over bony fragments

▸▸ Question 10

Why may a dorsal decompression procedure fail to reduce spinal cord distortion?
- A. Coronal tethering/ventral compression of the spinal cord
- B. Distraction-type injury pattern
- C. Increased risk of durotomy
- D. Intact posterior longitudinal ligament
- E. Presence of laminar fractures

▸▸ Question 11

Allodynia, or central pain, after nerve root injuries is thought to arise from central sensitization through what process?
- A. Activation of immune mediators
- B. Hypervascularity
- C. Lymphocytic infiltration
- D. Macrophage sequestration outside the blood-brain barrier
- E. Upregulation of mu receptors

▸▸ Question 12

C5 palsy following cervical spine decompression procedures is thought to be caused by which of the following mechanisms?
- A. Direct crush injury
- B. Infarction
- C. Infection
- D. Inflammation
- E. Stretching

▸▸ Question 13

Visualization of which of the following is the most appropriate landmark to use to assess for adequate decompression of the spinal canal after laminectomy?
- A. Lateral dorsal ganglion
- B. Lateral dural sac
- C. Midline dural sac
- D. Transverse process
- E. Vertebral body

▸▸ Question 14

Multilevel cervical laminectomies that extend into the thoracic spine may result in which of the following?
- A. Cerebrospinal fluid leak
- B. Infection
- C. Development of kyphosis
- D. Spinal cord herniation
- E. Development of spondylolisthesis

▸▸ Question 15

Multilevel laminectomies that do not extend rostrally and caudally beyond an extrinsic mass, ventral to the spinal cord, may result in which of the following?
- A. Arachnoiditis
- B. Development of a Chiari 1 malformation
- C. Dorsal kinking of the spinal cord
- D. Hydrocephalus
- E. Instability

▸▸ **Question 16**

A surgeon should have heightened awareness of aberrant anatomy such as a conjoined nerve root because this may result in which of the following findings in surgery?

- A. Iatrogenic instability after decompression
- B. Tethering of the nerve root during decompression
- C. Vascular injury
- D. Wrong level surgery
- E. Unintended durotomy

▸▸ **Question 17**

Injury to the ventral spinal cord typically presents with deficits of which of the following?

- A. Gross touch
- B. Joint position sense
- C. Pain and temperature
- D. Two-point discrimination
- E. Vibration

▸▸ **Question 18**

Hemisection of the spinal cord typically presents with deficits of which of the following?

- A. Bilateral motor function
- B. Contralateral motor function
- C. Contralateral pain and temperature function
- D. Ipsilateral pain and temperature function
- E. Bilateral vibration sense

▸▸ **Question 19**

In the dorsal spinal cord, which part of the spine has traditionally thought to be represented most medially?

- A. Cervical
- B. Thoracic
- C. Lumbar
- D. Sacral
- E. Coccygeal

▸▸ **Question 20**

The clinical scenario of loss of motor and sensory function in the upper extremities greater than loss in the lower extremities is described as what type of neurological injury?

- A. Anterior spinal injury
- B. Brown-Séquard injury
- C. Central cord injury
- D. Cord transection
- E. Nerve root injury

Answers

▸▸ **Answer 1**

Correct answer is A

Extrinsic compression is the most common cause of neurologic dysfunction in these settings. Compression from extrinsic structures, such as ligamentum flavum, facet hypertrophy, traumatic listhesis, and disc osteophytes, can cause dysfunction.

▸▸ **Answer 2**

Correct answer is A

Cell disruption typically results directly in cell death. Cell distortion and metabolic derangements can result in cell disruption, which then can lead to cell death. Cell death may result in spinal cord atrophy, but atrophy does not cause cell death.

▸▸ **Answer 3**

Correct answer is E

Surgical decompression of a compressive lesion can help relieve cell distortion. Maintenance or increased tissue perfusion pressure, not induced hypotension, may help decrease metabolic derangements.

▸▸ **Answer 4**

Correct answer is B

There are four mechanisms of neural element distortion–related injury (see ▸ Fig. 8.1) neural element compression, simple distraction, and tethering in the sagittal or coronal planes. In surgical planning, each of these mechanisms of injury should be considered. Adhesions would not typically be a consideration in early surgery. Osmotic shifts would not be directly addressed in surgical planning. Normal spinal alignment is not absolutely necessary; however, restoration of a nonpathologic relationship between the neural elements and structural elements (e.g., bone and soft tissue) is the goal of surgery.[1]

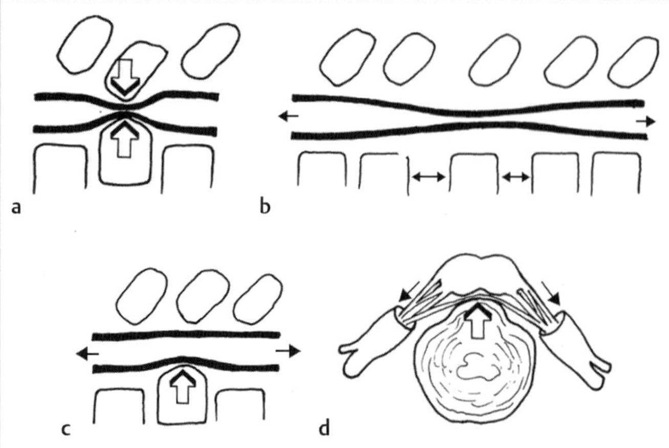

Fig. 8.1 The four mechanisms of neural element distortion-related injury: **(a)** neural element compression, **(b)** simple distraction resulting in spinal cord stretching and narrowing, **(c)** tethering over an extrinsic mass in the sagittal plane ("sagittal bowstring" effect), and **(d)** tethering of neural elements over an extrinsic mass in the coronal plane ("coronal bowstring" effect). Solid arrows depict "distractive" forces; hollow arrows depict forces applied directly to the dural sac. (Source: Biomechanics of Spine Stabilization: Third Edition, © 2015 Thieme Medical Publishers, Inc.)

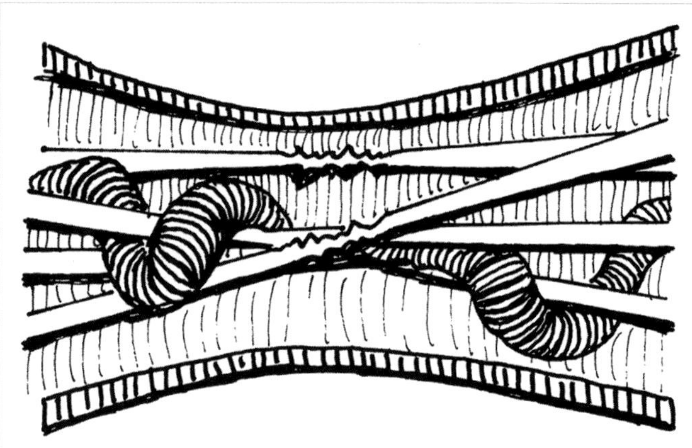

Fig. 8.2 Spinal cord distraction can distort and disrupt both neurons and the blood supply to the spinal cord. (Source: Biomechanics of Spine Stabilization: Third Edition, © 2015 Thieme Medical Publishers, Inc.)

▸▸ Answer 5

Correct answer is C

The radiculomedullary artery of Adamkiewicz, if it is present (87%), typically arises from the left (77%) and at T8–L1 (89%) but can arise from elsewhere.[2] Procedures where localization of the artery is necessary must involve full spinal angiography to characterize the spinal cord vasculature with the high incidence of variants.

▸▸ Answer 6

Correct answer is D

While mechanisms of neural injury continue to be studied, distraction is postulated to cause two potentially harmful effects (see ▶ Fig. 8.2) neuronal distortion and impediment of the blood supply. Ischemia is more likely a contributor to injury, but neutrophilic infiltration has not been described.

▸▸ Answer 7

Correct answer is A

The sagittal "bowstring" effect, or tethering of the spinal cord over ventral extrinsic structures, may be worsened by cervical flexion or focal kyphosis and by dorsal decompression procedures without fusion if they allow for worsening kyphosis or exaggerated flexion. This may be related to vascular compression. A decompression with fusion may prevent worsening kyphosis or exaggerated flexion in this case.

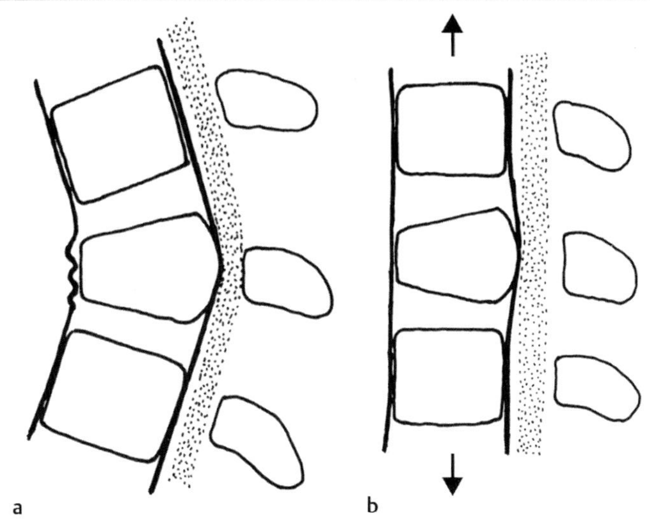

Fig. 8.3 (a) Spinal distraction can be used as a mechanism of reducing (relocating) ventral retropulsed bone and/or disc fragments. This is termed *ligamentotaxis* (*annulotaxis*). (b) Both an intact posterior longitudinal ligament and an anterior longitudinal ligament that does not effectively impede distraction are required for this technique to be anatomically effective. (Source: Biomechanics of Spine Stabilization: Third Edition, © 2015 Thieme Medical Publishers, Inc.)

▸▸ Answer 8

Correct answer is C

Ligamentotaxis, or annulotaxis (see ▶ Fig. 8.3), requires an intact posterior longitudinal ligament and mobile bone and disc fragments. The strength of an anterior longitudinal ligament will potentially prevent effective ligamentotaxis. The annulus fibrosus interruption often is the inciting factor for nucleus pulposus herniation. Ligamentum flavum and interspinous ligament do not contribute to reduction of fragments.

▸▸ Answer 9

Correct answer is E

Tethering of the spinal cord over bony fragments may lead to neurological decline after attempted ligamentotaxis. Ligamentotaxis may fail to reduce bony fracture fragments in the presence of an intact anterior longitudinal ligament, which may also be associated with a compression injury. Osteoporosis is a consideration for surgical planning. An intact posterior longitudinal ligament is required for ligamentotaxis.[4]

▸▸ Answer 10

Correct answer is A

Unrecognized coronal tethering of the spinal cord may result in continued spinal cord distortion after a dorsal decompression procedure (see ▶ Fig. 8.4). The other answer options should not result in continued distortion. Laminar fracture fragments would be removed in the dorsal decompression procedure.

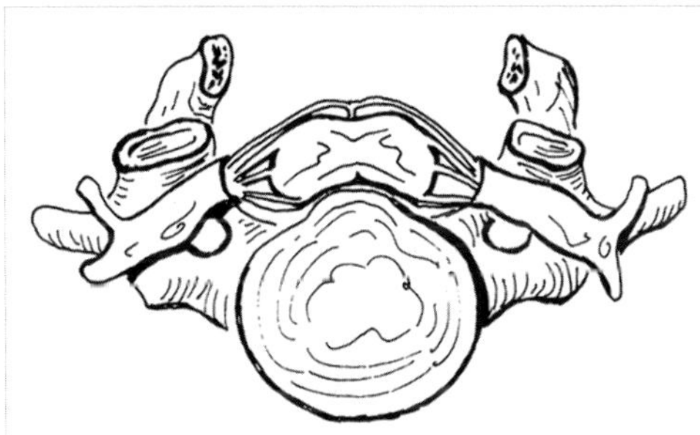

Fig. 8.4 Coronal plane tethering ("coronal bowstring" effect). Laminectomy may not relieve the distortion. (Source: Biomechanics of Spine Stabilization: Third Edition, © 2015 Thieme Medical Publishers, Inc.)

▸▸ Answer 11

Correct answer is A

Allodynia is thought to be related to activation of immune mediators and macrophage traffic across the blood–brain barrier, rather than sequestration. Hypervascularity, lymphocytic infiltration, and upregulation of mu receptors are not considered to be etiologies.

▸▸ Question 8

Which of the following is not a structural cause for neural element compression or distortion?
- A. Herniated intervertebral disc
- B. Spinal stenosis
- C. Compression by extrinsic space-occupying lesions
- D. Traumatic distortion of neural elements
- E. Spinal infarct

▸▸ Question 9

A patient with significant intervertebral disc degeneration comes to the clinic with dysfunctional segmental motion. How does such instability affect the stress–strain curve (see ▸ Fig. 9.2)?
- A. Narrowing of the neutral zone
- B. Rightward shift of the stress–strain curve
- C. Widening of the plastic zone
- D. Leftward shift of the elastic zone
- E. Leftward shift of the stress–strain curve

▸▸ Question 10

What is the most common indication for lumbar total disc arthroplasty?
- A. Degenerative disc disease with corresponding low back pain
- B. Myelopathy
- C. Radiculopathy
- D. Neck pain
- E. Trauma

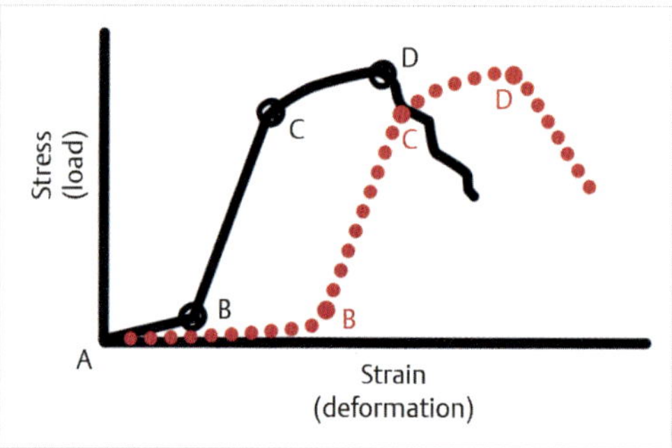

Fig. 9.2 The stress–strain curve. The dashed curve is the curve associated with a dysfunctional motion segment. Note the widening of he neutral zone, with a shift to the right of the elastic (*BC*) and plastic *CD*) zones. (Source: Biomechanics of Spine Stabilization: Third Edition, © 2015 Thieme Medical Publishers, Inc.)

▸▸ Question 11

For artificial disc applications in the cervical spine, which of the following clinical presentations would have the least correlation with imaging findings?
- A. Motor deficit
- B. Myelopathy
- C. Radicular pain
- D. Chronic neck pain
- E. Cervicalgia

▸▸ Question 12

If both spinal stabilization and artificial disc replacement are effective in surgeries for mechanical back pain, in which phase of the pathology would artificial disc surgery likely be more efficacious?
- A. Late phase
- B. Middle phase
- C. Early phase
- D. No specific phase of the disease process
- E. Disease progression with neurologic symptoms

▸▸ Question 13

The sagittal computed tomography (CT) reconstruction shown below (see ▸ Fig. 9.3) demonstrates which type of instability?
- A. Overt
- B. Traumatic
- C. Neoplastic

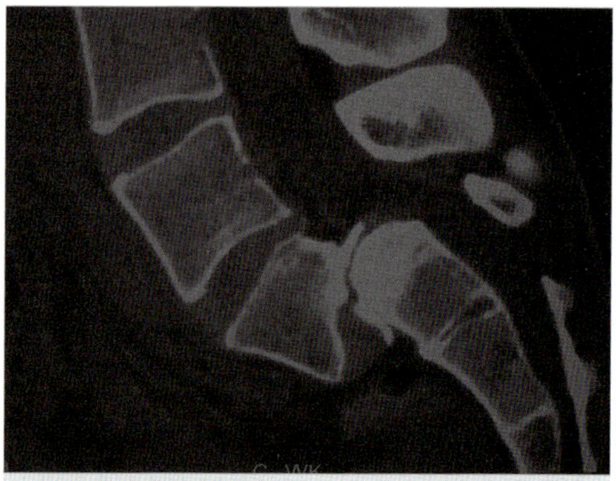

Fig. 9.3 A sagittal computed tomographic reconstruction of a patient with an isthmic spondylolisthesis. This case is illustrative of glacial instability. (Source: Biomechanics of Spine Stabilization: Third Edition, © 2015 Thieme Medical Publishers, Inc.)

- D. Glacial
- E. Dysfunctional segmental motion

▸▸ Question 14

Which of the following stages or points does not comprise a stress–strain curve?

- A. Upper yield point
- B. Elastic zone
- C. Plastic zone
- D. Recovery zone
- E. Strain hardening

▸▸ Question 15

What kind of clinical symptoms may result from a mechanical instability reflected by a rightward shift in the neutral zone of the stress–strain curve?

- A. Unilateral radiculopathy improved by sitting
- B. Deep mechanical back pain worsened by spinal loading and improved by unloading
- C. Bilateral paresthesias in multiple dermatomes
- D. Deep mechanical back pain worsened by spinal unloading and improved by loading
- E. Gait instability due to myelopathy

▸▸ Question 16

Which type of spondylolisthesis is associated with glacial instability?

- A. Isthmic
- B. Traumatic
- C. Congenital
- D. Pathological
- E. Postsurgical

▸▸ Question 17

Which type of spondylolisthesis is associated with dysfunctional segmental motion?

- A. Isthmic
- B. Traumatic
- C. Congenital
- D. Pathological
- E. Degenerative

▸▸ Question 18

Which of these pathologies is not considered a cause of acute instability of the spine?

- A. Trauma
- B. Pathologic fracture from metastatic disease
- C. Osteomyelitis
- D. Isthmic spondylolisthesis
- E. Primary spinal tumor

▸▸ Question 19

What is the index treatment in cervical total disc arthroplasty?

- A. The placement of a strut
- B. Neural decompression with discectomy
- C. Deployment of an artificial disc
- D. Provision of an intervertebral spacer
- E. Motion preservation

▸▸ Question 20

A patient presents with bilateral C6–C7 perched facets after a motorcycle accident. What type of instability does this pathology represent?

- A. Glacial
- B. Chronic
- C. Overt
- D. Limited
- E. Dysfunctional segmental motion

▸▸ Question 21

A patient presents with a nondisplaced unilateral C6–C7 facet fracture after a motorcycle accident. What type of instability does this pathology represent?

- A. Glacial
- B. Chronic
- C. Overt
- D. Limited
- E. Dysfunctional segmental motion

Answers

▸▸ Answer 1

Correct answer is C

The causes of neural element compression and distortion are numerous, including herniated intervertebral discs, spinal stenosis, foraminal stenosis, or extrinsic space-occupying lesions such as extramedullary tumors, hematomas, phlegmon, intrinsic lesions such as intramedullary tumors, or infection. Patients with these anatomical/radiologic findings may have various levels of clinical symptoms and neurologic deficits. The strongest indication for surgery would be significant anatomical findings that correlate with progressive neurologic deficits.

▸▸ Answer 2

Correct answer is B

The decision process is simple when a patient presents with a normal anatomy despite significant clinical symptoms without any neurologic deficits. The patient should be aggressively counseled for the use of nonoperative strategies. Longitudinal studies in such patients demonstrated that the outcomes of surgically treated and nonoperatively managed patients are equivalent. Thus, the rationale for surgery is lacking.

▸▸ Answer 3

Correct answer is E

Many factors should be considered in ambiguous cases in which patients present with anatomically relevant pathologies with no or medically manageable symptoms without neurologic deficits. Armed with the surgeon's knowledge of surgical risks for catastrophic or less impactful complications and individual patient's estimated risk profile for progression of spinal pathology best informed by the current literature, the surgeon and patient can develop reasonable plans to address both the pathology at hand and the patient's clinical, functional, and personal needs.

▸▸ Answer 4

Correct answer is A

Dysfunctional segmental motion may result when significant intervertebral disc degeneration has occurred, leading to a loosening or destabilization of the spine that in turn may lead to mechanical pain. Overt or limited instability is considered acute and can have causes such as trauma, infection, or neoplastic processes. In these cases, there may be clearer correlation between anatomic abnormality and neurologic symptoms due to compression or distortion of neural elements.

▸▸ Answer 5

Correct answer is E

There is no strong literature supporting the idea that spinal fusion and instrumentation always improves chronic pain associated with chronic instability. The extent of degeneration identified on radiologic studies often does not reflect the extent of instability or the characteristics of chronic pain. In chronic instability with a dysfunctional segmental motion after significant intervertebral disc degeneration, mechanical axial pain often improves with spinal unloading. In dysfunctional segmental motion, the pathology pushes the stress–strain curve to the right and widens the neutral zone (AB). Although spinal fusion and instrumentation may improve the rightward push of the stress–strain curve and widening of the neutral zone, there are no strong data to correlate the widening of the neutral zone with worsening of pain.

▸▸ Answer 6

Correct answer is D

The indications for total disc arthroplasty are very dissimilar in the cervical and lumbar spine. In the lumbar spine, artificial disc replacement is often applied to relieve chronic pain whose imaging findings may be very similar to those where spinal stabilization surgeries may be indicated. In the cervical spine, there is little correlation between imaging findings and clinical symptoms that indicate artificial disc applications beyond radiculopathy, motor deficits, or myelopathy. Moreover, in the cervical spine, the artificial disc deployment is often a secondary treatment as an intervertebral spacer that permits motion after a discectomy to treat myelopathy, radiculopathy, or chronic pain. Although, in theory, artificial disc replacement may provide benefit in earlier phases of disease and spinal stabilization in the latter phases, the correlation between anatomical considerations and clinical symptoms remains poor in both artificial disc replacement and spinal stabilization in management of mechanical back pain.

▸▸ Answer 7

Correct answer is C

There are three fundamental and fairly discrete categories of surgery for spinal pathologies. These are surgery for neural element compression or distortion, surgery for spine stabilization through fusion with or without instrumentation, and surgery to preserve motion or to establish nonpathologic motion. To determine whether a treatment plan is indicated for a specific spine pathology at hand, it is critical to consider the association between anatomy/radiologic findings with individual patient's clinical and neurologic status.

▸▸ Answer 8

Correct answer is E

Structural causes of neural element distortion or compression can provide clear correlations between anatomy/radiologic findings with clinical considerations. Herniated intervertebral discs, spinal or neuroforaminal stenosis, compression of neural elements by extrinsic masses such as tumors, phlegmon, hematomas or intrinsic lesions such as intramedullary tumors, and traumatic injuries that distort or compress neural elements are indications for surgery to address neural element compression or distortion.

▸▸ Answer 9

Correct answer is B

This patient may present with dysfunctional segmental motion, which is a type of chronic instability where the spine is destabilized or loosened. Such instability is associated with a rightward shift of the stress–strain curve including the elastic and plastic zones.

▸▸ Answer 10

Correct answer is A

In the lumbar spine, the management of degenerative disc disease with corresponding low back pain is often the common indication for total disc arthroplasty. Compared with the cervical spine, the artificial disc is employed with the intent of providing the index portion of the procedure—the management of degenerative disc disease and low back pain. In the cervical spine, the artificial disc functions as a spacer that maintains disc interspace height.

▸▸ Answer 11

Correct answer is D

For artificial disc application in the cervical spine, the strongest correlations between imaging/anatomical findings with clinical symptoms are radicular pain, myelopathy, and motor deficit. The artificial disc acts as a spacer following an anterior cervical discectomy and is really a secondary treatment following the neural decompression.

▸▸ Answer 12

Correct answer is C

There are no substantive data to support that either spinal stabilization or artificial disc replacement is superior in the management of chronic back pain. However, in theory, if both spine stabilization and artificial disc replacement surgeries are considered efficacious, then artificial disc replacement may be more effective if employed in the early phases of the degenerative processes before the development of advanced spondylosis. Fusion surgery, conversely, would be more effective in addressing more advanced degeneration and if instability is present.

▸▸ Answer 13

Correct answer is D

The CT reconstruction demonstrates an isthmic spondylolisthesis at L5–S1, which is consistent with a glacial instability. Glacial instability describes a gradual deformation or slippage of one spine component over another. Dynamic studies such as flexion/extension radiographs will further distinguish glacial instability from dysfunctional segmental motion. Unlike in acute instability of the spine, chronic instability often presents with more nebulous correlation between anatomical findings and clinical symptoms. This aspect is reflected in the high rates of failure in managing chronic back pain with spinal fusion and instrumentation procedure.

▸▸ **Answer 14**

Correct answer is D

A stress–strain curve (see ▶ Fig. 9.4) reflects the relationship between stress and strain. It is obtained by gradually applying load to a test subject and measuring the deformation, from which the stress and strain can be determined. In a stress–strain curve, there are several stages that suggest differential mechanical properties of a particular material or construct. The first phase is the linear elastic region where the stress is proportional to the strain in accordance with the general Hooke's law and from which Young's modulus can be determined from the slope of this phase. The end of the elastic stage is also the beginning of the plastic zone. The stress component at this point is the upper yield point or yield strength. The next stage is the strain hardening region, in which the stress rises beyond the upper yield point and reaches the maximum at the upper tensile strength. The material undergoes a plastic deformation until the following stage—necking—is reached after the stress meets the upper tensile strength and fractures at the fracture point.

▸▸ **Answer 15**

Correct answer is B

In patients with glacial instability, a gradual deformation occurs in elements of spinal components that results in slippage or possibly dysfunctional segmental motion. Such loosening or destabilization of the spine is associated with a shift to the right of the stress–strain curve and a widening of the neutral zone. This kind of instability is associated with deep mechanical back pain that is worsened with spinal loading and improved by unloading.

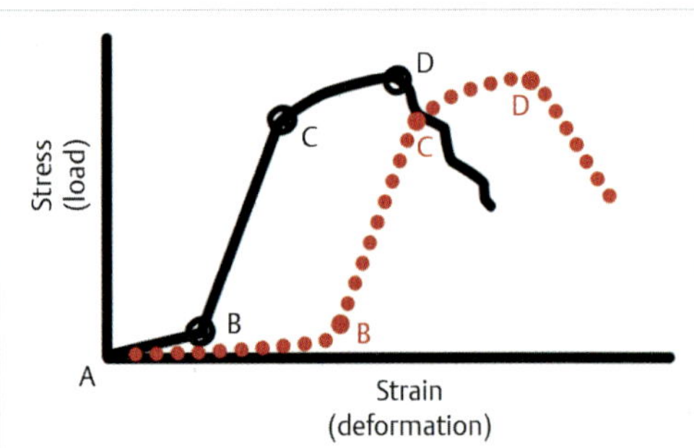

Fig. 9.4 The stress–strain curve. The dashed curve is the curve associated with a dysfunctional motion segment. Note the widening of he neutral zone, with a shift to the right of the elastic (*BC*) and plastic *CD*) zones. (Source: Biomechanics of Spine Stabilization: Third Edition, © 2015 Thieme Medical Publishers, Inc.)

▸▸ **Answer 16**

Correct answer is A

Isthmic spondylolisthesis is associated glacial instability. Defects in the pars interarticularis result in a gradual deformation or slippage of one vertebral body over another, with a progression of the slip over time.

▸▸ **Answer 17**

Correct answer is E

Degenerative spondylolisthesis is a form of chronic instability that results in dysfunctional segmental motion. Significant intervertebral disc space degeneration and/or degeneration of the facet joint complex may result in a loosening or destabilization of the spine. This instability is associated with the widening of the neutral zone and a rightward shift of the stress–strain curve.

▸▸ **Answer 18**

Correct answer is D

Overt instability is a common indication for spinal stabilization surgery. These pathologies arise when the integrity of the spine is compromised by traumatic injury, infectious insults, or neoplastic processes. They often present a strong correlation between anatomy and clinical indications for surgery. In fact, the anatomical findings from imaging studies are usually employed as primary indicators for surgery.

▸▸ **Answer 19**

Correct answer is B

Unlike in the lumbar spine, cervical total disc arthroplasty is applied to treat cervical radiculopathy, myelopathy, or occasionally chronic neck pain, where there is a correlation between clinical symptoms and imaging findings. For the cervical spine, the index treatment is discectomy. The artificial disc is used as a spacer between two vertebrae as a secondary treatment.

▸▸ **Answer 20**

Correct answer is C

Traumatic injuries to the spine represent a common etiology for acute instability. Imaging findings such as bilateral perched facets demonstrate overt instability. The presence of neural element compression or compromise in addition to the overt instability provides further indication for surgical stabilization of the fractures.

▸▸ **Answer 21**

Correct answer is D

Trauma is a common cause of acute instability, but the extent of injury may not be as extensive as in overt instability and suggests limited instability. Although the presence of neural element compression or compromise may provide further indications for surgery, limited instability alone may not be the primary indicator for surgery.

Key Principles

- There are three major types of spine surgery: (1) surgery for neural element compression or distortion; (2) surgery for spine stabilization via fusion, with or without instrumentation; and (3) surgery for preservation of motion or establishment of nonpathological motion.
- In cases with significant anatomical or radiographical findings without impressive clinical symptoms, the surgical risk data for the age-matched general population—e.g., risks for worsened neurologic deficits, a lack of efficacy, surgical site infections, anesthetic complications—must be weighed and discussed with patients to arrive at shared decision-making to best address spinal pathologies.
- In chronic instability, the data are lacking to establish any strong correlation between the extent of degeneration and the extent of instability or qualitative character of chronic back pain.
- The artificial disc is used in the cervical spine as a secondary treatment to maintain disc interspace height and permit motion after decompression of neural elements.
- The clinical/radiographical correlation and indications for lumbar artificial disc application are not dissimilar to those with lumbar spine stabilization/fusion surgery for chronic back pain.

Part III

Spine Surgery

III

10 Surgical Approaches to the Subaxial Spine

Luis M. Tumialán

Understanding the various approaches to the spine will enable the surgeon to select the most appropriate corridor to address the compression of the neural elements and/or provide stability to spine. Selection of the surgical corridor is determined by the nature of the compression of the neural elements at hand in a manner that will provide a safe corridor for a comprehensive decompression.

Learning Objectives

- Understand the ventral and lateral approaches to the cervical and upper thoracic spine.
- Understand the ventrolateral and extrapleural thoracotomy approaches.
- Understand the ventrolateral extraperitoneal approach to the upper and midlumbar spine.
- Understand the lateral extracavitary approach to the thoracic and lumbar spine.

Questions

►► Question 1

To decrease the incidence of recurrent laryngeal nerve palsy in anterior cervical approaches, which of the following is a reliable surgical technique to remember?

- A. Completely expose and mobilize the recurrent laryngeal nerve, making it less prone to traction injury when the retractors are in position
- B. Revision anterior cervical approaches carry less risk because the recurrent laryngeal nerve is enveloped in scar tissue
- C. A left-sided approach will prevent the neuropraxia of the laryngeal nerve commonly seen in right-sided approaches
- D. Request the anesthesiologist employ a fiber optic technique to secure the airway
- E. Lower endotracheal cuff pressures after exposure of the anatomy and placement of the retractors

►► Question 2

Which of the following statements is true when considering a ventrolateral transthoracic approach to the thoracic spine?

- A. A ventrolateral exposure is ideal for exposure from the second thoracic vertebra to the fifth thoracic vertebra
- B. Exposure from the left is limited by the aorta and from the right by the vena cava
- C. Decompression of the spinal cord is readily achievable without removing all ventral structures
- D. Mobilization and retraction of the endothoracic fascia are essential to prevent disruption of the parietal pleura
- E. The exposure allows for a symmetrical view and, thereby, symmetrical decompression of the central canal

►► Question 3

The main advantage of the transperitoneal approach to the lumbar spine is ________.

- A. There is essentially no risk to the ureters when traversing the peritoneum into the retroperitoneum
- B. The sigmoid colon will not need to be retracted because of the transperitoneal nature of the approach
- C. The sacral promontory is readily identifiable and facilitates localization and exposure
- D. The need to repair the ventral and dorsal peritoneum upon completion of the spinal component of the procedure
- E. It allows for a vertical midline abdominal incision that will have a minimal effect on stability

►► Question 4

Which of the following would not be an accurate anatomic description of the lateral extracavitary approach to the thoracic and lumbar spine?

- A. The lack of intrathoracic, intrapelvic dissection or the need for a diaphragm incision
- B. The ability to extend the dissection farther laterally than would be possible with a wide foraminotomy approach
- C. Provides a line of sight for exposure of the ventral spinal cord to achieve decompression
- D. The minimal effect on muscle dissection of the paraspinal muscles
- E. The ability to simultaneously decompress and instrument the spine from a single position

►► Question 5

When considering approaches to intradural pathologies, which of the following accurately describes a sound anatomical basis for approaching the lesion?

- A. Ventral approaches to intradural lesions are advantageous for the closure of the dura
- B. The malignant nerve sheath lesions are the most common intradural pathology, requiring extensive exposure
- C. Most intradural and ventral lesions may be approached via a dorsal exposure
- D. Cerebrospinal fluid leakage is a more common issue in posterior approaches to the thoracic spine than in ventral approaches
- E. Limited exposures through the vertebral bodies are the main limitation of dorsal exposure

►► Question 6

What is the most important component to keep in mind when selecting the most appropriate surgical approach?

- A. Consider the view of the spine needed to access the pathology
- B. The angle of exposure is relevant only in ventral exposures
- C. The role of minimally invasive techniques is less applicable in cases of thoracic spinal cord compression
- D. The nature and location of spinal cord compression are less relevant for ventral approaches because of the angle of exposure

►► Question 7

The best surgical approach to the thoracic disc in ► Fig. 10.1 would be _______.

- A. Dorsal approach
- B. Dorsolateral approach
- C. Either a dorsal or dorsolateral approach would be anatomically feasible
- D. Lateral approach
- E. Ventral approach

►► Question 8

► Fig. 10.2 illustrates which approach to the spine?

- A. Translaminar approach
- B. Interlaminar approach
- C. Transpedicular approach
- D. Costotransversectomy approach
- E. Lateral extracavitary approach

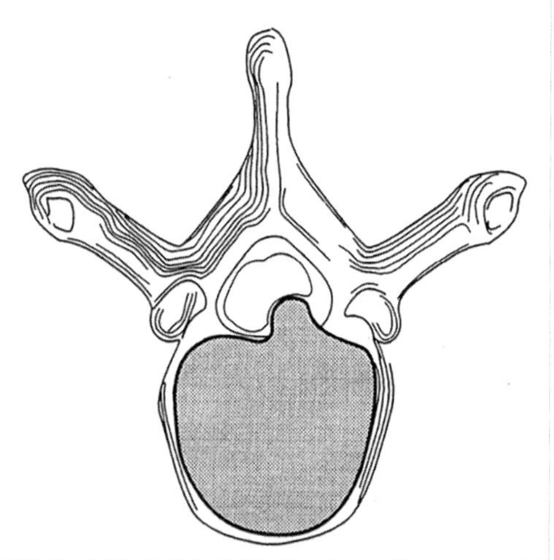

Fig. 10.1 The relationship of a thoracic herniated disc fragment to the dural sac affects the orientation of the surgical exposure. A more medially situated herniation can be approached laterally. The latter is appropriate only if the dural sac does not "sag" over the lateral aspect of the herniation. (Source: Biomechanics of Spine Stabilization: Third Edition, © 2015 Thieme Medical Publishers, Inc.)

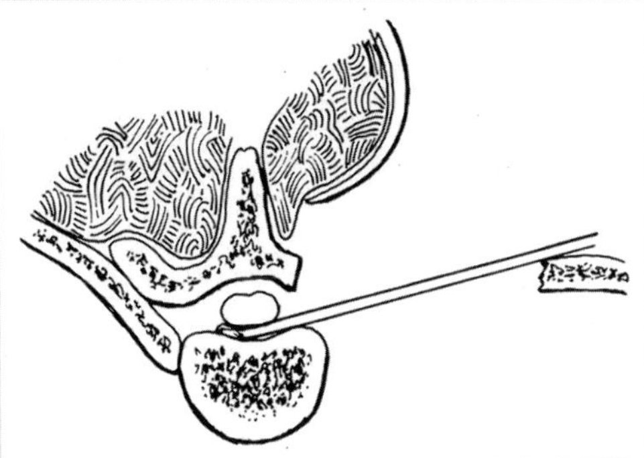

Fig. 10.2 The potential ventral dural sac decompression achieved with a reversed-angle curet through the dorsal surgical exposures, seen in axial views. Lateral extracavitary approach (for comparison). Note that the main difference between the costotransversectomy approach and the lateral extracavitary approach is the direction of the resection of the erector spinae muscle (medial for the lateral extracavitary, lateral for the costotransversectomy). Also note that an approximately 20- to 40-degree "angle of view" advantage for ventral dural sac decompression is realized with the lateral extracavitary approach versus the costotransversectomy approach. Resection of the erector spinae muscle eliminates much of this difference. (Source: Biomechanics of Spine Stabilization: Third Edition, © 2015 Thieme Medical Publishers, Inc.)

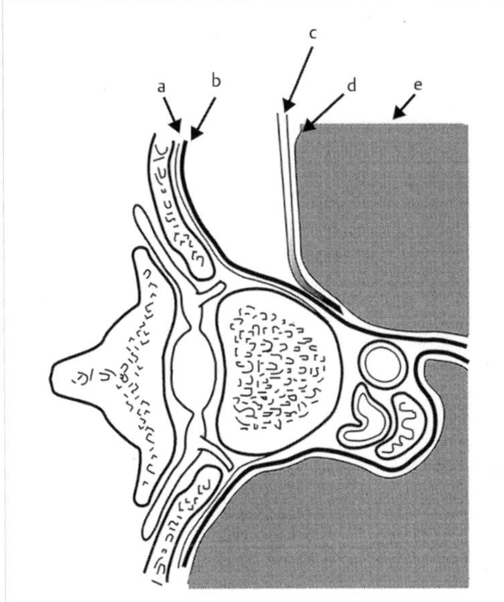

Fig. 10.3 The ventrolateral transthoracic approach to the spine, seen in an axial view. (A) The exposure gained is lateral to that gained in the cervical region with the ventral approach. Note the exposure between the parietal pleura and the visceral pleura. (Source: Biomechanics of Spine Stabilization: Third Edition, © 2015 Thieme Medical Publishers, Inc.)

►► **Question 9**

In the ventrolateral transthoracic approach to the spine, which letter represents the parietal pleura in ► Fig. 10.3?

- A. Endothoracic fascia
- B. Parietal pleura
- C. Retractor
- D. Visceral pleura
- E. Lung parenchyma

►► **Question 10**

In ventral approaches to the cervical spine, traction to the sympathetic chain may result in Horner's syndrome. In ► Fig. 10.4, which letter represents the sympathetic chain?

- A. Carotid artery
- B. Trachea
- C. Esophagus
- D. Jugular vein
- E. Sympathetic chain

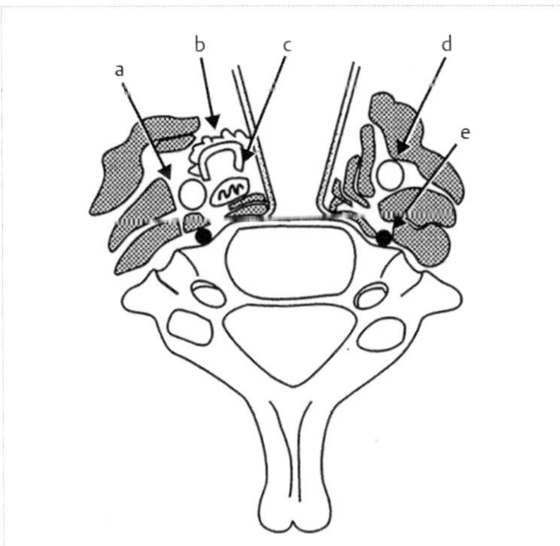

Fig. 10.4 The ventral and ventrolateral and lateral approaches to the subaxial cervical spine, seen in axial views. Note the subperiosteal dissection, placement of retractors, and exposures thus gained. Dots depict sympathetic chain and ganglia. (Source: Biomechanics of Spine Stabilization: Third Edition, © 2015 Thieme Medical Publishers, Inc.)

▸▸ Question 11

In an anterior approach to the cervical spine, which structure presents an avascular medial plane that allows safe passage onto the subaxial spine (see ▸ Fig. 10.5)?

- A. Sternohyoid muscle
- B. Thyrohyoid muscle
- C. Omohyoid muscle
- D. Common carotid artery
- E. Sternocleidomastoid muscle

▸▸ Question 12

A table-mounted anterior cervical retraction system allows for _______.

- A. Maintenance of lateral exposure of the cervical spine but not rostral–caudal exposure
- B. Maintenance of rostral–caudal exposure of the cervical spine but not lateral exposure
- C. Maintenance of both rostral–caudal and lateral exposure of the cervical spine
- D. Visualization, although a table-mounted retraction system causes asymmetric and, at times, excessive soft tissue pressure
- E. Less exposure of the cervical than a patient-mounted system but has less tissue trauma

▸▸ Question 13

The extrapleural thoracotomy approach to the thoracic spine _______.

- A. Has the disadvantage of an increased incidence of pulmonary complications
- B. Provides nearly the same exposure as the thoracotomy approach
- C. Is less advantageous at the thoracolumbar junction
- D. Requires the diaphragm to be incised instead of displaced forward
- E. The transdiaphragmatic approach is the preferred approach at the thoracolumbar junction

▸▸ Question 14

In the exposure of the upper thoracic spine, which structure may need to be secured for adequate exposure of the thoracic vertebral body (see ▸ Fig. 10.6)?

- A. Aortic arch
- B. Left brachiocephalic
- C. Sternocleidomastoid muscle
- D. Common carotid artery
- E. Thyrohyoid muscle

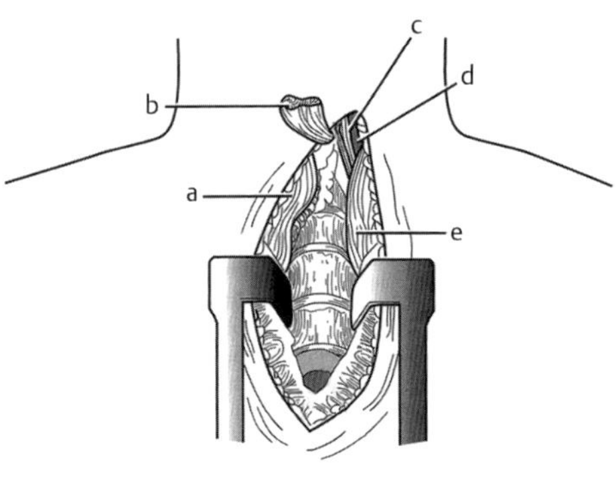

Fig. 10.5 The median sternotomy approach gains access to mediastinal structures and the upper thoracic spine. The innominate vein can be ligated, but the aorta still limits caudal exposure significantly. Therefore, resection of the manubrium and medial clavicle provides essentially the same exposure as does the median sternotomy approach. (Source: Biomechanics of Spine Stabilization: Third Edition, © 2015 Thieme Medical Publishers, Inc.)

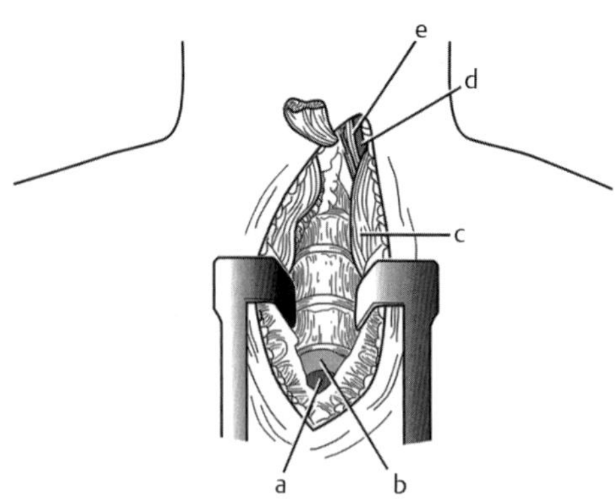

Fig. 10.6 The ventral and ventrolateral and lateral approaches to the subaxial cervical spine, seen in axial views. Note the subperiosteal dissection, placement of retractors, and exposures thus gained. Dots depict sympathetic chain and ganglia. (Source: Biomechanics of Spine Stabilization: Third Edition, © 2015 Thieme Medical Publishers, Inc.)

▸▸ Question 15

In a thin, poorly nourished, insensate patient, which of the following surgical strategies may be considered advantageous for dorsal exposure of the spine?

- A. A midline, intermuscular, and subperiosteal dissection
- B. A paramedian incision to optimize muscle coverage of the wound
- C. Refrain from the use of cautery to avoid devascularization of the tissue
- D. Preservation of the midline structures to prevent postoperative kyphosis
- E. The greater the lateral dissection of the paraspinal muscles, the less chance of paraspinal muscle denervation

▸▸ Question 16

What distinguishes a transpedicular approach in ▸ Fig. 10.7 from a costotransversectomy approach?

- A. The ability to achieve better ventral access with the transpedicular approach
- B. Preservation of the rib head in the transpedicular approach
- C. Increased risk to the parietal pleura in the transpedicular approach when compared with the costotransversectomy approach
- D. The preservation of the transverse process in the transpedicular approach
- E. Less disruption of the paraspinal muscles in the costotransversectomy approach

▸▸ Question 17

When considering a surgical decompression of a thoracic disc herniation in ▸ Fig. 10.8, which approach would offer the necessary exposure without risk to the neural elements?

- A. Dorsal approach
- B. Dorsolateral approach
- C. Either a dorsal or dorsolateral approach would be anatomically feasible
- D. Lateral approach
- E. Ventral approach

▸▸ Question 18

In a ventrolateral extraperitoneal approach to the upper lumbar spine, which statement best captures the anatomical circumstance of that corridor?

- A. It provides a disappointingly narrow longitudinal exposure

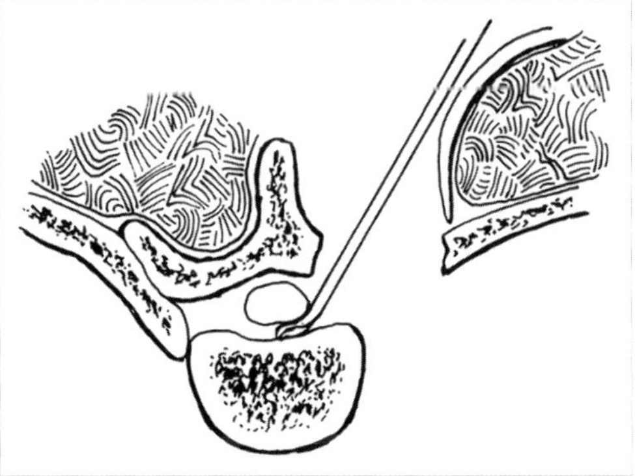

Fig. 10.7 The median sternotomy approach gains access to mediastinal structures and the upper thoracic spine. (Source: Biomechanics of Spine Stabilization: Third Edition, © 2015 Thieme Medical Publishers, Inc.)

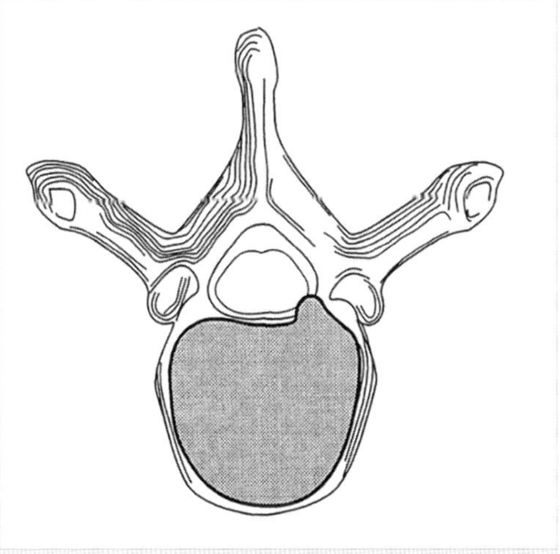

Fig. 10.8 The relationship of a thoracic herniated disc fragment to the dural sac affects the orientation of the surgical exposure. A lateral herniation can be approached dorsally. (Source: Biomechanics of Spine Stabilization: Third Edition, © 2015 Thieme Medical Publishers, Inc.)

with the assistance of a cardiothoracic surgeon prior to proceeding with surgery on the thoracic vertebral body. In the event of disruption control of bleeding and repair of the vessel is tenable.

▸▸ Answer 15

Correct answer is B

A paramedian incision may help avoid wound-healing problems by optimizing wound coverage with a muscle flap. In contrast, a midline intermuscular and subperiosteal dissection may be disadvantageous because of the compromised blood flow.

▸▸ Answer 16

Correct answer is B

Ventral access is superior with a costotransversectomy approach because of the increased angle of view. The rib and the rib head are preserved in the transpedicular approach, while both are removed in the costotransversectomy approach. Both approaches remove the transverse process. The costotransversectomy results in significantly more disruption of the paraspinal muscles.

▸▸ Answer 17

Correct answer is B

There is no contact with the spinal cord in this circumstance. Therefore, neither a lateral nor a ventral approach would be necessary. Given the lateral nature of the disc herniation, a dorsolateral approach would provide the necessary exposure.

▸▸ Answer 18

Correct answer is A

The major advantage of the ventrolateral extraperitoneal approach to the lumbar spine is the straightforward nature of the exposure for vascular and general surgeons. However, it provides a disappointingly narrow longitudinal exposure, limited by the crus of the diaphragm. The neuroforamina cannot be readily seen, and the exiting nerve roots remain at risk in the psoas muscle from this exposure.

▸▸ Answer 19

Correct answer is D

Preoperative imaging in the form of a magnetic resonance imaging (MRI) or even computed tomography angiography (CTA) will best define the access corridor onto the thoracic spine. The exposure is limited by vascular structures and best exposed by a cardiothoracic surgeon. Splitting the sternum is unnecessary in many cases and should be avoided if possible because of its associated morbidity.

▸▸ Answer 20

Correct answer is E

Ventral cervical spine exposure via the ventral approach does not result in significant deinnervation of muscles. Although the longus colli muscles are injured, they are injured symmetrically along the midline raphe. Furthermore, their importance in preventing spinal deformity is unknown but is likely minimal. There is not one factor that causes dysphagia; it is multifactorial. The incidence of recurrent laryngeal injury is higher in more extensive (multiple levels) and revision cases.

Key Principles

- Various approaches to the subaxial spine may be used, each with its unique advantages and disadvantages.
- Understanding the limitations of each posterior corridor of access—transpedicular versus costotransversectomy—will allow for safe and comprehensive decompression of the spinal cord.
- Understanding the anatomy of the vascular, muscular, and nervous systems is fundamental for avoiding complications with anterior approaches to the subaxial spine.
- Understanding the anatomy of the parietal and visceral pleura is essential for safely working within the transthoracic approach corridor.

References

[1] Apfelbaum RI, Kriskovich MD, Haller JR. On the incidence, cause, and prevention of recurrent laryngeal nerve palsies during anterior cervical spine surgery. Spine (Phila Pa 1976) 2000;25(22):2906–2912

[2] McCormick PC. Retropleural approach to the thoracic and thoracolumbar spine. Neurosurgery 1995;37(5):908–914

11 Destabilizing Effects of Spine Surgery

Kevin Hines, India Shelley, James S. Harrop

Spine operations have both intended and unintended impacts on spinal stability. Destabilization may occur through pathology, approach, decompression, and instrumentation techniques. Understanding how spine surgeons may iatrogenically destabilize the spine will allow for better operative planning and better patient outcomes.

Learning Objectives

- Understand methods and techniques by which a spine may be destabilized during surgery.
- Understand how ligamentous disruption may occur during ventral spine decompression.
- Understand how bony disruption may occur during ventral spine decompression.
- Understand how dorsal spine decompression may induce spinal instability.

Questions

▸▸ Question 1

What three structures provide substantial column support and may be compromised during ventral approaches?

- A. Ligamentum flavum, interspinous ligament, cruciate ligament
- B. Anterior longitudinal ligament, posterior longitudinal ligament, ligamentum flavum
- C. Anterior longitudinal ligament, posterior longitudinal ligament, annulus fibrosus
- D. Annulus fibrosis, facet capsule, interspinous ligament
- E. Ligamentum flavum, anterior longitudinal ligament, annulus fibrosis

▸▸ Question 2

Which structure is described as strong, wide, and unlikely to be significantly disrupted and affect stability during ventral spine surgery?

- A. Anterior longitudinal ligament
- B. Posterior longitudinal ligament
- C. Annulus fibrosis
- D. Interspinous ligament
- E. Intertransverse ligament

▸▸ Question 3

Which structure is described as providing weaker support, narrower than the dural sac, and likely to be disrupted during ventral spine surgery?

- A. Anterior longitudinal ligament
- B. Posterior longitudinal ligament
- C. Annulus fibrosis
- D. Interspinous ligament
- E. Intertransverse ligament

▸▸ Question 4

Ligamentous stability plays an important role in the function of strut graft stabilization. With insufficient de novo ligamentous stability, the interbody strut graft will not appropriately affix to the vertebral bodies above and below the strut graft. What may be used to supplement interbody fusion in the setting of ligamentous laxity?

- A. Early mobilization
- B. Spinal implant placed during distraction
- C. Anterior column release
- D. Cement augmentation
- E. Spinal implant placed during compression

▸▸ Question 5

Intervertebral disc disruption, unilateral or bilateral uncovertebral joint disruption, and posterior longitudinal ligament dysfunction all lead to spinal instability. Anterior cervical decompression decreases stability by disrupting these structures and primarily affecting which movement?

- A. Rotation and lateral bending
- B. Flexion and lateral bending
- C. Extension and lateral bending
- D. Flexion and extension
- E. Rotation and flexion

▸▸ Question 6

Bony disruption of the anterior column may significantly impact overall spinal stability and may be a source of iatrogenic destabilization.

Which configuration of bony removal during corpectomy will lead to the least iatrogenic destabilization?

- A. Resection of ventral coronal plane (anterior one-third)
- B. Resection of middle coronal plane
- C. Resection of dorsal coronal plane (posterior one-third)
- D. Resection of middle and dorsal coronal plane (posterior two-thirds)
- E. Resection of the middle axial plane

▸▸ Question 7

Iatrogenic spine destabilization from a dorsal approach can best be prevented by which of the following techniques?

- A. Addition of a stability augmentation procedure
- B. Addition of a stability augmentation procedure and limited disruption of spinal integrity
- C. Bracing
- D. Limited disruption of spinal integrity
- E. The creation of sharp angulation of the dural sac at the limits of laminectomy

▸▸ Question 8

Interspinous ligaments have a role in preventing iatrogenic destabilization and may be encountered during a dorsal approach. These interspinous ligaments are absent at which spinal level?

- A. L1–L2
- B. L1–L5
- C. L3–L5
- D. L4–L5
- E. L5–S1

▸▸ Question 9

Destabilization is a key consideration when addressing cervical spine compressive pathologies. Laminoplasty and laminectomy can both be considered as treatment options. Which of the following best describes the differences between laminoplasty and laminectomy when considering destabilization?

- A. Laminectomy allows for greater preservation of deep extensor muscle attachments when compared with laminoplasty
- B. Laminectomy better preserves facet joint complex integrity than laminoplasty
- C. Laminectomy minimizes bony and soft tissue disruption when compared with laminoplasty
- D. Laminoplasty allows for greater preservation of deep extensor muscle attachments when compared with laminectomy
- E. Laminoplasty results in greater disc interspace stress in the ventral annulus than laminectomy

▸▸ Question 10

The lumbar spine is especially predisposed to translational deformation. Which factor(s) contribute the most to this predisposition?

- A. The exaggerated lordotic posture of the lumbar spine only
- B. The horizontal orientation of the facet joint and an exaggerated lordotic posture
- C. The horizontal orientation of the facet joint only
- D. The vertical orientation of the facet joint and an exaggerated lordotic posture
- E. The vertical orientation of the facet joint only

▸▸ Question 11

The cervicothoracic junction is especially vulnerable to iatrogenic instability. What is the cause of this phenomenon?

- A. An abrupt change from immobility in the cervical spine to mobility in the thoracic spine
- B. An abrupt change from mobility in the cervical spine to immobility in the thoracic spine
- C. Lack of lateral masses in the thoracic spine
- D. Longer spinous processes in the thoracic spine
- E. Vertically aligned disc spaces

▸▸ Question 12

Laminectomy across the cervicothoracic junction should be supplemented with ___ to diminish destabilization.

- A. Disc arthroplasty
- B. Facet joint devices
- C. Instrumentation and fusion
- D. Spinous process tethering
- E. Vertebral corpectomy

▸▸ Question 13

A patient with a past medical history of prior cervical spine surgery, alcohol use disorder, prior lumbar decompression, and a 30-pack-year smoking history undergoes a laminectomy across the cervicothoracic junction. Supplemental instrumentation should be considered because she has which of the following two risk factors?

- A. A history of alcohol use and a history of tobacco use
- B. Prior cervical surgery and a history of alcohol use
- C. Prior cervical surgery and a history of tobacco use
- D. Prior lumbar decompression and a history of alcohol use
- E. Prior lumbar decompression and a history of tobacco use

▸▸ Question 14

Comorbid conditions can have significant effects on clinical outcomes. What two conditions are associated with decreased mobility following cervical laminectomy in patients with cervical myelopathy?

- A. Anxiety and hypertension
- B. Depression and alcohol use disorder
- C. Depression and anxiety
- D. Depression and hypertension
- E. Diabetes mellitus and hypertension

▸▸ Question 15

▸ Fig. 11.1 shows resections of different portions of the vertebral body. Which of the labeled resections affects stability the most?

- A. a
- B. b
- C. c
- D. d
- E. They all affect stability equally

▸▸ Question 16

The extent of ventral spinal decompression significantly affects spine stability. The fraction and portion of the vertebral body resected play an important role in the extent of destabilization. Which of the following variables has the greatest role in destabilization?

- A. The fraction of bone remaining in the ventral portion
- B. The fraction of bone remaining in the dorsal portion
- C. The fraction of bone remaining in the middle portion
- D. The fraction of bone remaining in the superior portion
- E. The fraction of bone remaining in the inferior portion

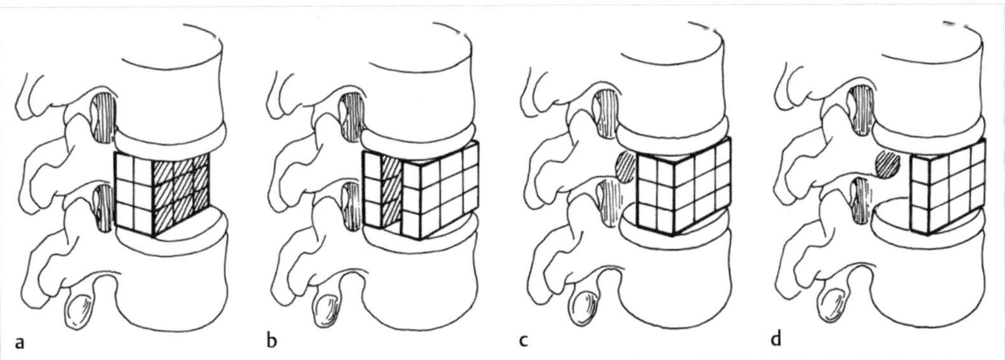

Fig. 11.1 Resections of portions of the "cubic" vertebral body depicted in Fig. 11.4. Partial vertebrectomy involving removal of the **(a)** ventral portion in the coronal plane of the vertebral body affects stability more than resection of the **(b)** middle or **(c)** dorsal portion of the vertebral body in the coronal plane. **(d)** In fact, resection of both the middle and dorsal thirds of the vertebral body (in the presence of an intact posterior column and an intact ventral third of the vertebral body) may not significantly disrupt spinal integrity. (Source: Biomechanics of Spine Stabilization: Third Edition, © 2015 Thieme Medical Publishers, Inc.)

▸▸ Question 17

What method of decompression is recommended to minimize iatrogenic destabilization while maximizing the decompression of neural elements in a ventral decompression?

- A. A narrow decompression both ventrally and dorsally
- B. A narrow decompression ventrally, with a wider decompression dorsally via an "Erlenmeyer flask" exposure
- C. A wide decompression both ventrally and dorsally
- D. A wide decompression ventrally, with a narrower decompression dorsally
- E. The width of decompression should not affect the amount of destabilization

▸▸ Question 18

The surgical technique of an individual surgeon can influence the amount of destabilization that occurs. When performing a decompression, surgeons should be aware of the natural tendency to ______.

- A. Excessively decompress the dural sac on the near side of the patient
- B. Excessively decompress the neural foramen on the side where they are standing
- C. Inadequately decompress the dural sac on the far side of the patient
- D. Inadequately decompress the dural sac on the near side of the patient
- E. Inadequately decompress the neural foramen on the side opposite where they are standing

▸▸ Question 19

Excessive facet joint disruption is a known contributor to instability. In the cervical spine, what amount of resection has been shown to be tolerable without causing extreme instability?

- A. One-third to one-half of the joint
- B. One-fourth to one-third
- C. One-half to three-fourths
- D. Less than one-fourth
- E. Any amount of resection causes extreme instability

Answers

▸▸ Answer 1

Correct answer is C

During ventral approaches to spinal pathology, the structures providing substantial support, such as the anterior longitudinal ligament, posterior longitudinal ligament, and annulus fibrosis, may be violated. Note ligamentum flavum and interspinous ligaments would not be part of an anterior approach.

▸▸ Answer 2

Correct answer is A

The anterior longitudinal ligament is a strong ligament that is wide enough that it will not be fully disrupted despite ventral exposure despite a small portion often being compromised with ventral approaches. As a result, the anterior longitudinal ligament contributes significantly to postoperative stability.

▸▸ Answer 3

Correct answer is B

The posterior longitudinal ligament is weaker than the anterior longitudinal ligament and narrower than the dural sac at the mid–vertebral body region at each spinal level. As a result, it is more likely to be disrupted, especially during vertebrectomy for decompression of the dural sac. This limits its ability to contribute to postoperative stability by limiting flexion and ligamentotaxis. Note some surgeons do not violate the posterior longitudinal ligament with decompression, but it provides less stability than the anterior longitudinal ligament.

▸▸ Answer 4

Correct answer is B

Spinal implants placed during distraction will maximize the "clamping down" of the end plates on the graft after distraction is released; this loading of the implant provides stability. Other options include bedrest and bracing to supplement the interbody in the absence of ligamentous integrity. The other choices here would only worsen the ligamentous laxity surrounding the graft and increase the failure rate of the construct.

▸▸ **Answer 5**

Correct answer is D

Chen et al[1] demonstrated that these structures' loss of integrity affected flexion and extension. Thus, an anterior cervical decompression destabilizes flexion and extension movements in the cervical spine.

▸▸ **Answer 6**

Correct answer is C

Partial vertebrectomies vary in destabilizing effects based on how much and which portion of the bony vertebral body is removed. By preserving the most ventral column of bone and the anterior longitudinal ligament, iatrogenic destabilization is minimized. It is even possible to resect the dorsal and middle coronal plane without inducing iatrogenic destabilization; however, by virtue of less remaining bony strut, it is less stable than dorsal resection alone.

▸▸ **Answer 7**

Correct answer is B

When using a dorsal approach, it has been shown that both the addition of a stability augmentation procedure and limited disruption of spinal integrity can help to prevent iatrogenic destabilization. Choices C and E have not been shown to prevent destabilization.

▸▸ **Answer 8**

Correct answer is E

The interspinous ligaments are absent at the level of L5–S1 and deficient at the level of L4–L5, thus providing minimal biomechanical support.

▸▸ **Answer 9**

Correct answer is D

Laminoplasty has been shown to better preserve the deep extensor muscle attachments when compared with laminectomy. Choices B and C are incorrect because laminoplasty better preserves facet joint complex integrity and minimizes bony and soft tissue disruption compared with laminectomy. Choice E is incorrect because laminectomy results in greater disc interspace stress in the ventral annulus compared with laminoplasty.

▸▸ **Answer 10**

Correct answer is D

The predisposition of the lumbar spine to translational deformation is primarily due to the vertical orientation of the facet joint and the exaggerated lordotic posture. The vertical orientation of the facet joints causes a shearing force on the spine when an axial force is applied.

▸▸ **Answer 11**

Correct answer is B

The cervical spine is highly mobile, while the thoracic spine has relatively limited mobility. The abrupt change between these two levels requires extra caution when operating at this junction.

▸▸ **Answer 12**

Correct answer is C

Steinmetz et al[2] determined that instrumentation and fusion should be used to supplement any laminectomy across the cervicothoracic junction. They determined that this helps decrease the risk of iatrogenic instability, a known possible outcome of operating at this junction.

▸▸ **Answer 13**

Correct answer is C

Prior cervical surgery, a history of tobacco use, or patients undergoing surgery for deformity correction are at increased risk of iatrogenic instability following laminectomy across the cervicothoracic junction. Surgeons should consider supplemental instrumentation in this population to decrease this risk.[2]

▸▸ **Answer 14**

Correct answer is C

Depression and anxiety scores are highly associated with decreased mobility postoperatively. Additionally, ambulatory dysfunction postoperatively could exacerbate depression and anxiety symptoms, which has been particularly demonstrated in patients with cervical spondylotic myelopathy.[3]

▸▸ **Answer 15**

Correct answer is A

A shows partial vertebrectomy removing the ventral portion in the coronal plane, which affects stability more than resection of the middle (B) and dorsal (C) portions of the vertebral body in the coronal plane. D shows resection of the middle and dorsal thirds of the vertebral body, which has not been shown to disrupt spinal integrity significantly.

▸▸ **Answer 16**

Correct answer is A

Preserving the amount of vertebral body remaining in the ventral section has a significant impact on the amount of stability that remains postoperatively. Surgical approaches should attempt to minimize the amount of ventral vertebral body resected to ensure maximum stability.

▸▸ **Answer 17**

Correct answer is B

An "Erlenmeyer flask" exposure involves a narrow decompression ventrally, with a wider decompression dorsally, as seen in ▸ Fig. 11.2. This minimizes multiple factors that contribute to destabilization, such as the amount of ventral vertebral body resected, ensuring a good view of the exposed spinal canal and a wide decompression of the dural sac.

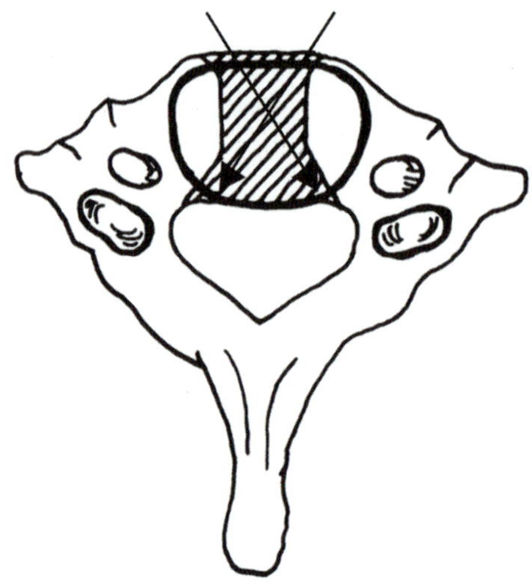

Fig. 11.2 The "Erlenmeyer flask" exposure of the spinal canal in an axial view. The view of the dural sac is enhanced if the spine is viewed from both sides of the patient during decompression. The view thus achieved is depicted by the arrows. The relatively narrow width of the ventral portion of the trough enhances stability by (1) minimizing bone removal and (2) allowing a snug fit for the subsequent bone graft (*stippled area*). (Source: Biomechanics of Spine Stabilization: Third Edition, © 2015 Thieme Medical Publishers, Inc.)

▸▸ **Answer 18**

Correct answer is D

It has been shown that most surgeons have a natural tendency to inadequately decompress the dural sac on the near side of the patient. This can be compensated for by using an "Erlenmeyer flask-like" approach with a narrow decompression ventrally and a wider decompression dorsally.

▸▸ **Answer 19**

Correct answer is A

One-third to one-half of the facet joint in the cervical spine can be resected without significant disruption to stability.[4]

Key Principles

- Ventral spine surgery may disrupt anterior and posterior longitudinal ligaments as well as the annulus fibrosis, affecting spinal stability.
- Instability secondary to bony decompression of the ventral spine may be minimized by resection of middle sagittal components or dorsal components and by limiting the volume of resection.
- Instability secondary to dorsal spinal decompression may be minimized by limiting the disruption of dorsal ligaments or by augmentation with spinal implants or laminoplasty.

References

[1] Chen TY, Crawford NR, Sontag VKH, Dickman CA. Biomechanical effects of progressive anterior cervical decompression. Spine 2001;26:6–13; discussion 14

[2] Steinmetz MP, Miller J, Warbel A, Krishnaney AA, Bingaman W, Benzel EC. Regional instability following cervicothoracic junction surgery. J Neurosurg Spine 2006;4:278–284

[3] Stoffman MR, Roberts MS, King JT. Cervical spondylotic myelopathy, depression, and anxiety: a cohort analysis of 89 patients. Neurosurgery 2005;57:307–313; discussion 307–313

[4] Raynor RB, Pugh J, Shapiro 1. Cervical facetectomy and its effect on spine strength. J Neurosurg 1985;63:278–282

12 Spine Fusion

Gabrielle Santangelo, Thomas A. Pieters, Daniel M. Sciubba

Learning Objectives

- Understand the advantages and disadvantages of bone grafts depending on the biomechanical region of their placement.
- Understand the concept and clinical implications of forces such as load bearing, load sharing, and translation.
- Understand the appropriate medical osteoporosis treatment options.
- Understand the limitations and applications of bone substitutes in fusions.

Questions

▸▸ Question 1

What is the correct order of placement of an interbody graft for a patient with a ventral compressive mass without evidence of tumor in the thoracic and lumbar spine?

- A. Decompression of neural elements, spinal stabilization, placement of ventral bone graft
- B. Spinal stabilization, placement of ventral bone graft, decompression of neural elements
- C. Placement of ventral bone graft, spinal stabilization, decompression of neural elements
- D. Decompression of neural elements, placement of ventral bone graft, spinal stabilization
- E. Placement of ventral bone graft, decompression of neural elements, spinal stabilization

▸▸ Question 2

Which of the following characteristics improves the integrity of a bone graft?

- A. Limiting surface area of contact of the graft
- B. Increasing cortical-to-cancellous bone ratio
- C. Freeze-dried bone
- D. Ethylene oxide sterilization of allograft graft
- E. Rapid rehydration with saline

▸▸ Question 3

What position is the most biomechanically advantageous placement of a ventral interbody bone graft?

- A. At the junction of the middle and posterior columns of Denis
- B. At the posterior column of Denis
- C. At the instantaneous axis of rotation (IAR) in the sagittal plane
- D. At the neutral axis when dorsal spinal element stability is adequate
- E. At the location of the middle column cortex

▸▸ Question 4

When considering the properties of the bone graft to the bone graft bed, which conditions should be met?

- A. Bone grafts should be denser and with greater integrity than the vertebral body
- B. Bone grafts should be selected to be the strongest link in the "stability linkage system"
- C. Bone grafts should be similar in density and integrity to the vertebral body
- D. Bone grafts should be less dense and with less integrity than the vertebral body
- E. Bone grafts should be selected to be the weakest link in the "stability linkage system"

▸▸ Question 5

Lumbosacral translational deformity can be understood using what principles?

- A. A shear force promotes bony healing
- B. Axial loading disrupts bony healing
- C. There is minimal inherent strength of the fibroligamentous complex between the vertebral bodies
- D. A deformity results in a parallelogram-like distortion of the ligamentous complex and the vertebral bodies
- E. If the disc interspace and fusion site are more sagittal oriented, then more shear forces are applied to promote fusion

▸▸ **Question 6**

Which of the following characteristics is true regarding dorsal spinal fusion?

- A. Dorsal spine fusions without instrumentation are not exposed to bone healing–enhancing compression and thus do not provide acute axial support for the spine
- B. Dorsal spine fusions tend toward a much faster fusion rate than ventral interbody fusions
- C. The integrity of a dorsal spine fusion does not degrade over time
- D. A fusion mass from a dorsal spine fusion typically does not experience any distraction during load bearing
- E. The success of a dorsal spine fusion is straightforward to assess on radiographic images

▸▸ **Question 7**

What can occur after dorsal spine fusion of the immature spine because of ventral spine growth?

- A. Osteoporosis
- B. Crankshaft phenomenon
- C. Osteophyte formation
- D. Translational deformation
- E. End-fusion degeneration

▸▸ **Question 8**

A postmenopausal woman who is more than 5 years past menopause and without menopausal symptoms who has a personal history of uncontrolled peptic ulcer disease and an extensive family history of breast cancer presents with significant bone pain associated with osteoporosis. What would be the most appropriate acute treatment for both her osteoporosis and the associated bone pain?

- A. Estrogen and progesterone
- B. Raloxifene
- C. Parathyroid hormone (teriparatide)
- D. Bisphosphonates (alendronate)
- E. Calcitonin salmon

▸▸ **Question 9**

What is true of bone substitutes?

- A. Only the use of autograft is associated with high fusion success rates
- B. Hydroxyapatite is associated with superior strength characteristics compared with autograft
- C. Bone substitutes can be added when the volume of autograft is not sufficient
- D. Allograft can present an increased risk for disease transmission
- E. There are high rates of long-term complications associated with harvesting autograft

▸▸ **Question 10**

Which of the following should be considered when using bone morphogenic protein as a bone graft substitute or graft extender?

- A. Bone morphogenetic protein-7 (BMP-7) has shown to be more effective than BMP-2
- B. The method of delivery of BMP to tissues is likely to not change in the future
- C. There is little research available on the benefit of BMP on fusion enhancement
- D. BMP has no effect of tissue inflammation
- E. BMP is associated with adverse events including radiculitis, heterotopic bone growth, and osteolysis

▸▸ **Question 11**

Which of the following is true in the postoperative phase regarding the use of nonsteroidal anti-inflammatory drugs (NSAIDs) after spinal fusion?

- A. Fixation devices eliminate the increased chances of pseudoarthrosis that are associated with the use of NSAIDs
- B. NSAIDs may interfere with revascularization during the entire healing period leading to pseudoarthrosis
- C. NSAIDs block prostaglandin E1 (PGE1) and PGE2 pathways, which are involved in both bone formation and absorption
- D. Using cyclooxygenase inhibitors may prevent the pseudoarthrosis associated with NSAIDs
- E. Radiation, steroids, chemotherapy, and tobacco usage affect a different phase of the healing process than NSAIDs

▸▸ Question 12

What is stress shielding?

- A. When a fixation device *allows* the fusion surface to "see" bone healing–enhancing forces
- B. Fixation devices eliminating the chance of pseudoarthrosis
- C. The enhancement of fusion by a fixation device
- D. When a fixation device prevents the fusion surface from "seeing" bone healing–enhancing forces
- E. Fixation devices increasing the chance of pseudoarthrosis

▸▸ Question 13

What osteoporosis medication has the lowest spine fracture risk reduction in patients without prior history of spinal fracture?

- A. Parathyroid hormone (teriparatide)
- B. Estrogen and progesterone
- C. Bisphosphonates (alendronate)
- D. Calcitonin salmon
- E. Raloxifene

▸▸ Question 14

What can reduce end-fusion degenerative changes?

- A. Neutral sagittal balance
- B. Positive sagittal balance
- C. Negative sagittal balance
- D. Successful bony spinal fusion
- E. Increase in intradiscal pressure by eccentric forces

▸▸ Question 15

A bone graft as the sole implant in the plane between two vertebral bodies ________.

- A. Supports the spine in sagittal loading
- B. Is enhanced by intact ligamentous integrity
- C. Provides forces that are always compressive
- D. Provides bidirectional force resistance in the immediate postoperative period
- E. Resists translational movement

▸▸ Question 16

A lateral/peripheral location of an interbody bone implant ________.

- A. Is improved by minimizing the surface area of contact
- B. Is associated with lower axial load bearing when compared with a centrally placed implant
- C. Resists sagittal stresses in the immediate postoperative period
- D. Is associated with greater subsidence resistance when compared with a centrally placed implant
- E. Is equal in axial load bearing and subsidence resistance when compared with a centrally placed implant

▸▸ Question 17

Which of the following is true regarding bone graft placement and the IAR?

- A. The further dorsal a bone graft is to the IAR, the greater the axial load–resisting ability it has
- B. The further ventral a bone graft is to the IAR, the greater resistance to flexion it provides
- C. Bone grafts placed directly at the IAR provide the greatest resistance to flexion and extension forces
- D. The further dorsal a bone graft is to the IAR, the shorter the moment arm becomes, providing lower resistance to flexion
- E. The further dorsal a bone graft is to the IAR, the greater resistance to flexion it provides

▸▸ Question 18

After a dorsal short segment pedicle screw fixation placed in distraction, when the patient is upright ________.

- A. Load sharing is increased and, thus, the implant is less likely to fail
- B. The implant is bearing only the weight of the torso
- C. The implant is bearing the sum of the load at time of surgery and the weight of the torso. Hence, it is more likely to fail

- D. The implant is bearing less than the weight of the torso due to the surgical offloading and is less likely to fail
- E. Load sharing is increased and the implant is more likely to fail

▸▸ Question 19

After a dorsal short segment pedicle screw fixation, which of the following is true when considering axial loads?

- A. Placement of the dorsal implant in compression allows sharing of the axial load between the dorsal implant and the ventral strut, reducing the strain on the dorsal implant
- B. Placement of the dorsal implant in compression prevents load sharing with the existing spinal axis
- C. Placement of the dorsal implant in distraction allows load sharing with a concomitant interbody strut
- D. Placement of the dorsal implant in distraction improves bone healing, an application of Wolff's law
- E. Placement of the dorsal implant in neutrally with regard to compression/distraction allows optimal load-sharing balance

▸▸ Question 20

Bone healing is ________.

- A. Improved by agents that reduce the inflammatory cascade
- B. Improved with direct current stimulation in both ventral weight-bearing and dorsal onlay scenarios
- C. Unaffected by NSAIDs after the inflammatory phase has completed
- D. Improved for both ventral and dorsal fusion with transcutaneous pulsed electromagnetic fields
- E. Diminished when compression is placed on an interbody graft

Answers

▸▸ Answer 1

Correct answer is A

The general principal in a ventral graft placement is to first perform decompression (see ▶ Fig. 12.1a,b) and spinal stabilization (see ▶ Fig. 12.1c), followed by the graft placement (see ▶ Fig. 12.1d,e,f). This allows for distraction of the pathologic segments with insertion of the bone graft in between, promoting load sharing between the dorsal instrumentation and the ventral bone graft. It also avoids possibly loosening the already placed bone graft with altered spinal biomechanics after decompression and instrumentation placement.[1]

▸▸ Answer 2

Correct answer is B

The integrity of a bone graft can be altered due to a number of factors. Autograft is superior to allograft; the greater cortical-to-cancellous bone ratio and greater surface contact of the graft with bone both improve the fusion potential, axial load-bearing ability, and resistance to movement. Processing of allograft material can change its integrity. While ethylene oxide sterilization does not affect strength, frozen bone that is thawed is preferred over freeze-dried bone due to its torsion and bending resistance, and slow rehydration improves the characteristics of this material.[2]

▸▸ Answer 3

Correct answer is C

The IAR in the sagittal plane is the optimal site of placement for a bone graft to increase the axial load resistance and the torso support. This is typically also at the junction or the anterior and middle columns of Denis in the location of the neutral axis (see ▶ Fig. 12.2, left). This is particularly true when the dorsal spinal element stability is deficient (most commonly); if it is sufficient, then a more ventral placement can be considered (see ▶ Fig. 12.2, right). The ventral cortex can bear axial loads more effectively than the middle column, and the anterior column can facilitate load sharing to prevent kyphotic deformity.

▸▸ Answer 4

Correct answer is C

The bone graft's density, integrity, and modulus of elasticity should be matched as closely with the bone graft bed (or vertebral body). In the "stability linkage system," bone grafts should neither be the strongest nor weakest link. One must recognize that stronger fusion masses may

Part IV

Spine Instrumentation Constructs: General Principles

IV

13 Implant Material Properties

Harel Deutsch

Implant failure is related to implant composition, morphology, and treatment. The surgeon's appreciation of implant material properties helps in deciding what implants are appropriate for different clinical demands.

Learning Objectives

- Understand the common materials used in spine implants and their different properties.
- Understand the surface characteristics of different implant materials.
- Understand the mechanisms of injury to different materials used in implants.
- Understand how the properties of nonmetallic implants such as ceramics, composites, or bone are different from metallic implants.

Questions

▸▸ Question 1

Resistance of implants to injury or deformation is related to which of the following factors?
- A. Implant composition
- B. Implant size
- C. Implant shape
- D. Material treatment of the implant
- E. All the above

▸▸ Question 2

What metal has the best imaging characteristics on computed tomography (CT) scan imaging?
- A. Titanium
- B. Stainless steel
- C. Cobalt-chrome
- D. Silver
- E. Iron

▸▸ Question 3

Which allograft preparation does not affect compression strength?
- A. Ethylene oxide sterilization
- B. Freeze dried
- C. Autoclave
- D. Radiation
- E. Iodine

▸▸ Question 4

Composites are defined as ________.
- A. Nonmetallic implants
- B. Plastic implants
- C. Biomaterials composed of a matrix material and a filler
- D. Titanium implants
- E. Cement

▸▸ Question 5

The main ceramic used in orthopedic surgery are all of the following except.
- A. Iron oxide
- B. Alumina (Al_2O_3)
- C. Zirconia (ZrO_2)
- D. Hydroxyapatite ($Ca_{10}(PO_4)_6(OH)_2$)
- E. Alumina matrix composite

▸▸ Question 6

Absorbable implants, usually composed of polylactide copolymers or a derivative thereof, have found limited utility in spine for which of the following reasons?
- A. Optimal biomechanics
- B. Toxicity related to breakdown products
- C. Favorably timed absorption
- D. Good visualization on X-ray
- E. Increasing utility in spine

▸▸ Question 7

Which element is commonly used in an unalloyed (pure) form?
- A. Aluminum
- B. Nickel
- C. Chromium
- D. Titanium
- E. Iron

▸▸ Question 8

The 0.2% tensile yield strengths of titanium depend largely on titanium's ________.

- A. Grade
- B. Temperature
- C. Density
- D. Age
- E. Color

▸▸ Question 9

Which of the following materials has the least stretch?

- A. Grade 1 titanium
- B. Grade 2 titanium
- C. Grade 3 titanium
- D. Grade 4 titanium
- E. 316 L stainless steel

▸▸ Question 10

Which material results in a relatively increased transfer of stress from the implant to bone and augments stress shielding when used with rigid systems?

- A. Grade 1 titanium
- B. Grade 2 titanium
- C. Grade 3 titanium
- D. Grade 4 titanium
- E. 316 L stainless steel

▸▸ Question 11

Stainless steel implants have fallen out of vogue because all of the following *except*:

- A. Greater risk of chronic infection
- B. Image properties on CT scans and MRIs
- C. Nickel allergies
- D. Cost
- E. Galvanic effect when combined with titanium

▸▸ Question 12

The converse of ductility is ________.

- A. Strength
- B. Weight
- C. Brittleness
- D. Deformability
- E. Hardness

▸▸ Question 13

Clinical implants usually fail due to ________.

- A. Load that exceeds the static strength of the implant
- B. Cyclic loading and implant fatigue
- C. Corrosion
- D. Local pH
- E. Implant surface structure

▸▸ Question 14

Which metal is most resistant to corrosion?

- A. 316 L stainless steel
- B. Co-Cr-Mo alloy
- C. Ti-6Al-4V alloy
- D. Titanium
- E. Ti-24Nb-4Zr-8Sn alloy

▸▸ Question 15

The purpose of shot peening surface treatment is to ________.

- A. Reduce corrosion
- B. Change the implant color
- C. Increased surface fusion
- D. Increased implant fatigue resistance
- E. Produce a titanium oxide film

▸▸ Question 16

Which of the following is true about notching?

- A. A 1% notch (a notch having a depth of 1% of the diameter of the implant) reduces the fatigue resistance of 316 L stainless steel by 10%
- B. Stainless steel is more prone to notching than titanium
- C. Braiding of many small wires increases the adverse effect of notching
- D. Notch sensitivity is defined as crack initiation that is secondary to an iatrogenically created stress concentration
- E. All the above

▸▸ Question 17

PEEK has found utility in spine surgery for which of the following reason?

- A. PEEK's Young's modulus of elasticity is 3,600 GPa, which is more similar to bone's 0.50 GPa than metals > 100,000 GPa
- B. PEEK is radio-opaque with less artifact on imaging studies
- C. PEEK has better bone integration due to surface properties
- D. PEEK is biologically inert and has low sterilization resistance
- E. PEEK has low tensile strength

▸▸ Question 18

Polymers such as ultra-high-molecular-weight polyethylene (UHMWPE) are most likely to be used in which spine surgery application?

- A. Lumbar fusions
- B. Adhesion barriers
- C. Implant surface treatment
- D. Cement augmentation
- E. Motion preservation

▸▸ Question 19

Which of the following is true about structural failure?

- A. Failure occurs due to cumulative effects of loading
- B. The average spine cycles 1 million times per year
- C. Metal failure usually begins without crack initiation
- D. Rod contouring does not affect rod strength
- E. Cracks are not affected by subsequent failure

▸▸ Question 20

Titanium has which of the following properties?

- A. Titanium is biologically active
- B. Titanium is less resistant to corrosion than stainless steel
- C. Shape memory alloys like nitinol (nickel-titanium) change shape under different environments
- D. Titanium is less notch-sensitive than steel
- E. Titanium causes more radiographic artifact than steel

▸▸ Question 21

What is the most common use of polymethyl methacrylate (PMMA) in spinal procedures?

- A. Kyphoplasty and vertebroplasty
- B. A surface coating to prevent metal corrosion
- C. Radiolucent implants
- D. Hemostasis
- E. Pedicle screws

Answers

▸▸ Answer 1

Correct answer is E

Different materials such as polyetheretherketone (PEEK), titanium, or stainless steel can have different strengths and resistance to deformation. The diameter of implants also affects their stiffness.

▸▸ Answer 2

Correct answer is A

Titanium appears to be imaged best with CT, whereas magnetic resonance imaging (MRI) is more suitable for porous titanium.

▸▸ Answer 3

Correct answer is A

Allograft processing, in general, adversely affects graft integrity. Ethylene oxide sterilization, however, does not affect compression strength. Bone that is frozen and then thawed is superior to freeze-dried bone for torsion and bending resistance. Of note, slow rehydration with saline improves the biomechanical characteristics of freeze-dried bone.

▸▸ Answer 4

Correct answer is C

Composite biomaterials are composed of a matrix material and a filler (reinforcement). This combination provides characteristics superior to those achieved with either component alone. Composite materials may have several phases. Some matrix materials may be combined with different types of fillers. Polymers containing particulate fillers are known as particulate composites.

▸▸ Answer 5

Correct answer is A

Ceramics are nonmetallic, inorganic solid compounds. Both alumina and zirconia are organized in dense, tightly packed repeating units known as crystals. The oxygen bonds in alumina and zirconia are extremely strong chemically speaking and among the most difficult to break. Thus, the crystalline structure helps to explain the hardness, strength, and chemical resistance of these ceramics. Clinically, hydroxyapatite ceramic has been shown to be effective as a bone graft extender in posterior spinal fusion surgery, but it is not effective as a standalone. Hydroxyapatite is brittle.[1]

▸▸ Answer 6

Correct answer is B

Absorbable implants, usually composed of polylactide copolymers or a derivative thereof, have found limited utility in spine surgical applications. Suboptimal biomechanical characteristics (e.g., strength), toxicity related to breakdown products, poor visualization on X-ray, and ill-timed absorption (e.g., before bone consolidation) have resulted in limited utility in spine. Polylactide copolymers have been used as adhesion barriers and have been used to prevent adhesions.

▸▸ Answer 7

Correct answer is D

A chemical element is a pure substance composed of atoms with the same number of protons. Metals are a group of elements that possess certain characteristic properties, including good thermal and electrical conductivity, malleability, and ductility. The mixing and melding of two or more elements yields an alloy that is useful in the manufacture of spinal implants. These elements include (with their standard abbreviations and atomic numbers in parentheses) the following: aluminum (Al, 13); titanium (Ti, 22); vanadium (V, 23); chromium (Cr, 24); manganese (Mn, 25); iron (Fe, 26); cobalt (Co, 27); nickel (Ni, 28); zirconium (Zr, 40); niobium (Nb, 41); and molybdenum (Mo, 42). Titanium is the only element that is commonly used in an unalloyed ("pure") form as an implant material. Alloys are engineered to combine the best properties of different elements, resulting in materials with superior characteristics. For example, combining iron with carbon produces steel, which is stronger and more durable than pure iron. Alloys often exhibit higher strength and hardness compared with pure elements. This is achieved by controlling the microstructure and crystal lattice of the alloy, making it more resistant to deformation and wear. Many alloys are designed to resist corrosion and oxidation better than individual elements. Stainless steel, for instance, contains chromium, which forms a protective oxide layer that prevents rusting and corrosion.

▸▸ Answer 8

Correct answer is A

The ultimate and 0.2% tensile yield strengths are the highest tolerable stress (to failure) and the stress that causes a 0.2% deformation, respectively. "Pure" (unalloyed) titanium is available in four grades. Each contains varying composition limits of multiple contaminants (including iron). Some of these contaminants are included by design; others are included because of difficulty of removal. Grade 1 is the purest and grade 4 the least pure. The strength of unalloyed titanium increases as the oxygen (a contaminant) content increases (0.18–0.40%). Although the density and modulus of elasticity of unalloyed titanium do not significantly change from grade to grade, the ultimate and 0.2% tensile yield strengths of titanium depend largely on its grade.

▸▸ Answer 9

Correct answer is A

The purest titanium (grade 1) is the softest pure titanium and is most ductile. The less pure titanium (grades 2–4) is similar in this regard to 316 L stainless steel. All have relatively high tensile strengths. Grade 4 has the highest strength and is used in aircraft components.

▸▸ Answer 10

Correct answer is E

316 L stainless steel is stiffer (i.e., has a higher modulus of elasticity) than all grades of unalloyed titanium. Therefore, it results in a relatively increased transfer of stress from the implant to bone.

This property augments stress shielding when 316 L stainless steel is used with rigid systems, such as fixed movement arm cantilever system. 316 L steel is a type of stainless steel, which is a group of alloys known for their excellent corrosion resistance. The "3" refers to the series: stainless steel is categorized into different series based on their chemical composition. The 300 series (e.g., 304, 316, 316L) contains a higher amount of chromium and nickel than other stainless steel series, making them more corrosion-resistant. The "16" refers to the percentage of chromium; 316 L stainless steel contains 16% chromium. Chromium is a key element that enhances the material's corrosion resistance by forming a protective oxide layer on its surface. The "L" stands for "low carbon": the "L" in 316 L indicates that this grade has a lower carbon content compared with standard 316 stainless steel. The reduced carbon content helps to improve its weldability.

▸▸ Answer 11

Correct answer is D

For many reasons, stainless steel implants have fallen out of vogue. These reasons include greater risk for chronic infection, image degradation, and nickel allergy. Ti-6Al-4V has now essentially replaced 316 L stainless steel for most spine implant applications. An accelerated form of corrosion that can occur in a mixed metal system, on account of the difference in electrochemical potential between the two metals, is galvanic corrosion.

▸▸ Answer 12

Correct answer is C

The term ductility describes, in a sense, the deformability of an object. A ductile object is one that can permanently deform before failure. The converse of ductility is brittleness. Brittle objects fail without permanent deformation. Metals may be elastically deformed until the yield point is reached. Plastic deformation ensues if further force is applied until ultimate failure occurs. Conversely, bone fractures without permanent deformation. The yield point of bone is equal to its ultimate failure point.

▸▸ Answer 13

Correct answer is B

Fatigue failure occurs because of the cumulative alterations of structure (damage) related to cyclical loading. The average spine cycles about 3 million times per year. Clinical implant failure rarely occurs after the application of a load that exceeds the static strength of the implant. Instead, implants usually fail after cyclical loading and implant fatigue.

▸▸ Answer 14

Correct answer is D

Corrosion is the degeneration of a metal by oxidation or a related process. Corrosion, with consequent metal weakening, is a potential complication of the exposure of an implant to a foreign environment. Corrosion resistance can be quantified by measuring the anodic polarization behavior of a specific metal against a control (e.g., a saturated calomel electrode in a physiologic [Hanks] solution). Titanium is much more resistant to corrosion than 316 L stainless steel. Cast Co-Cr Mo and Ti-6A1–4V are intermediate. All implants are chosen for their ability to resist corrosion in clinical applications. Protectivity against corrosion is related to titanium's characteristic development of surface film (oxide) (see ▸ Fig. 13.1). Iron contamination can significantly affect the corrosion process, especially in materials like stainless steel, where the presence of iron is critical to its properties. When stainless steel comes into contact with iron-containing materials, such as carbon steel or rusty surfaces, there is a potential for iron contamination. This can happen due to shared equipment, improper cleaning practices, or exposure to iron particles in the environment. The iron can act as a more active metal leading to localized corrosion and the iron can disrupt the stainless steel's oxide layer forming iron oxide on the stainless steel. Anodizing is an electrochemical process that enhances the corrosion resistance of certain metals, particularly aluminum and its alloys. A controlled oxide layer is formed on the surface of the metal. This oxide layer is known as "anodic oxide" or "anodic film." Anodizing increases the thickness of the natural oxide layer on the metal's surface. This thicker oxide layer acts as a barrier between the metal and the surrounding environment, hindering the penetration of corrosive substances and reducing the risk of corrosion. The anodic oxide layer is harder and more durable than the underlying metal, providing protection against mechanical damage and making the surface less susceptible to scratches. Fretting corrosion is a specific type of mechanical wear and corrosion that occurs at the

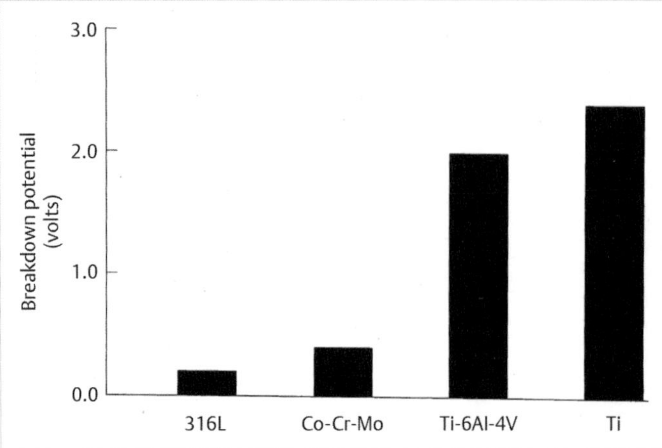

Fig. 13.1 Breakdown potential (volts) versus metal composition for implant metals in Hanks solution. The higher the breakdown potential, the greater the corrosion resistance. (Source: Data obtained from Disegi J. AO/ASIF Unalloyed Titanium Implant Material. 2nd ed. AO/ASIF Materials Technical Commission; 1991:3–25)

contact interface between two surfaces subjected to small, repetitive relative motions under load. It commonly occurs in tight-fitting components or in regions where two surfaces are in contact but experience slight movements, such as vibrations, oscillations, or micromovements. While stainless steel is known for its excellent corrosion resistance, it is also particularly prone to fretting corrosion because the micromovements can disrupt the stainless steel surface oxide layer. Crevice corrosion is a localized form of corrosion that occurs in narrow gaps, crevices, or confined spaces between two surfaces in contact with each other. The crevice provides for limited oxygen that results in accumulation of aggressive ions and an electrochemical cell corrosion effect due to the oxygen gradient.

▸▸ Answer 15

Correct answer is D

The surface characteristics of an implant material may affect its material properties. For example, the fatigue resistance of a metal may be enhanced by the process of shot peening.

Shot peening is a surface treatment in which small hard pellets are shot against the surface of a metal. This results in a compression deformation of the surface, which in turn results in an augmentation of the number of cycles required to cause failure.

▸▸ Answer 16

Correct answer is D

Notching is an injury to the surface of an implant that adversely affects structural integrity. Notch sensitivity is defined as crack initiation that is secondary to an iatrogenically created stress concentration. Titanium is known to be prone to the adverse effects of notching; in other words, it is very notch-sensitive. A 1% notch (a notch having a depth of 1% of the diameter of the implant) reduces the fatigue resistance of 316 L stainless steel wire by 63%, whereas bending, twisting, and knotting do not significantly affect fatigue resistance. This has obvious implications for the handling of wire during surgery. Twisting appears to be the optimal method of wire-to-wire approximation. The use of two full twists adds nothing to the security of the approximation. Commercial wire tighteners provide more consistent twists, with a concomitantly decreased chance of surface injury. The braiding or weaving of small strands of wire into a cable greatly reduces the danger posed by this phenomenon.

▸ Fig. 13.2 shows the relationship between the radius of curvature of a bend, the diameter of a wire, and the chance of notch-related failure. (**a**) A wire (or strand) that is bent will "fail" if the radius of curvature (R) of the bend is small enough. (**b**) If the diameter of the wire is increased, a lesser bend (greater radius of curvature) results in failure. (**c**) Therefore, a thin wire or strand can be bent at a sharper angle, with a smaller radius of curvature, than can a larger wire or strand. (**d**) Thus, a cable that is composed of many small strands can tolerate a bend with a very small radius of curvature (tight angle; upper) because it is composed of small-diameter strands (lower), whereas a solid wire cannot. R, R', R", radii of curvature.[2]

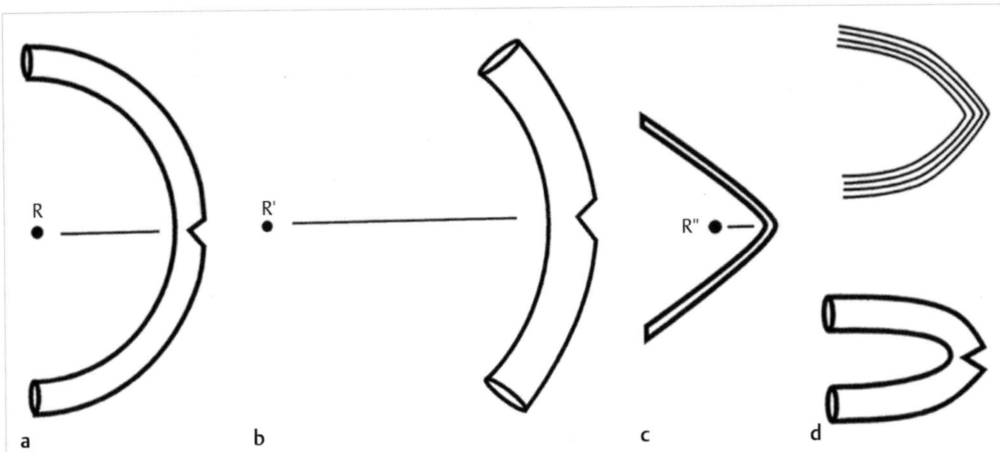

Fig. 13.2 The relationship between the radius of curvature of a bend, the diameter of a wire, and the chance of notch-related failure. **(a)** A wire (or strand) that is bent will "fail" if the radius of curvature (*R*) of the bend is small enough. **(b)** If the diameter of the wire is increased, a lesser bend (greater radius of curvature), results in failure. **(c)** Therefore, a thin wire or strand can be bent at a sharper angle, with a smaller radius of curvature) than can a larger wire or strand. **(d)** Thus, a cable that is composed of many small strands can tolerate a bend with a very small radius of curvature (tight angle; *upper*) because it is composed of small-diameter strands (*lower*), whereas a solid wire cannot. *R, R', R''* radius of curvature. (Source: Biomechanics of Spine Stabilization: Third Edition, © 2015 Thieme Medical Publishers, Inc.)

▸▸ Answer 17

Correct answer is A

PEEK has found utility in spine surgery due to its radiolucency, chemical stability, and superior sterilization resistance at high temperatures. PEEK can also be tailored into patient-specific implants for treating orbital and craniofacial defects in combination with additive manufacturing process. PEEK is bioinert, lacking osseointegration after implantation. Surface coating of PEEK implants can imbue the implants with biocompatible traits. Recent research has suggested that PEEK's biologically inert feature prevents bony ingrowth and results in delayed fusion. Although PEEK has an elastic modulus similar to natural bone, it exhibits deficient osseointegration after implantation.[3] Osseointegration is a biological process that refers to the direct structural and functional connection between living bone tissue and the surface of an artificial implant or medical device. Osteoblasts migrate to the implant's surface and start depositing a layer of bone matrix around the implant. This matrix eventually forms a direct contact between the bone and the implant surface. Over time, the newly formed bone matures and remodels to adapt to the mechanical stresses applied to it. This process continues for several months.

▸▸ Answer 18

Correct answer is E

UHMWPE is a semicrystalline polymer that has been used for over four decades as a bearing surface in total joint replacements. The mechanical properties and wear properties of UHMWPE are of interest with respect to the in vivo performance of UHMWPE joint replacement components. CoCr alloy metal-on-metal (MOM) hip bearings were used for joints to reduce long-term wear and short-term dislocation risk in hip arthroplasty, though long-term exposure to metal ions has been a concern with MOM for many decades. Orthopaedic literature reports of short-term revision due to metal hypersensitivity, osteolysis, and pseudotumor formation after implantation of MOM joints. In August 2010, DePuy Orthopaedics issued a voluntary worldwide recall for MOM joints due to a higher-than-expected revision rate. In May 2011, the FDA ordered orthopaedic manufacturers to perform postmarket surveillance studies for MOM joints. Highly cross-linked polyethylene materials were introduced and have since become the standard of care in hip arthroplasty. Highly cross-linked polyethylene reduces wear as well as the risk of osteolysis in total hip replacements. Research, however, has shown that cross-linking improves wear resistance but reduces the material's ductility and fracture resistance. Fractures of the cross-linked insert can result in the implant failure, and therefore, gamma inert sterilized polyethylene continues to be used in total knee and some disc replacements instead of highly cross-linked polyethylene.[4]

▸▸ Answer 19

Correct answer is A

Contouring can create tensile stresses and increase the risks of rod fracture. The greater the rod bending, the greater the rod strength is compromised. Fatigue failure occurs because of the cumulative effects of loading (the average spine cycles 3 million times per year). Metal failure begins with crack initiation. This may be associated with or encompass environmentally assisted cracking. The cracks progress if failure ensues.

▸▸ Answer 20

Correct answer is C

Titanium causes less radiographic artifact than steel. Titanium is inert but new technology with surface modification can alter biocompatibility. TiN coating can be used as a desirable blood-contacting material. Titanium surface modification is possible through plasma spray or physical vapor deposition. Osseointegration can be enhanced by changing roughness or coating Ti with a ceramic such as hydroxyapatite. More recently, the cellular effects of surface topography in the nanoscale range in titanium have been described.[5] Shape memory alloys (usually nickel–titanium alloys) change shape under differing environmental conditions. Changing temperature, for example, can alter shape.

▸▸ Answer 21

Correct answer is A

PMMA is also known as acrylic resin or acrylic glass. In vertebroplasty, PMMA is used as a cement-like material to stabilize fractured or collapsed vertebrae. Kyphoplasty is a similar procedure to vertebroplasty, but it involves an additional step. In kyphoplasty, a balloon-like device is inserted into the fractured vertebra and inflated to create a cavity before injecting PMMA. The MMA monomer is mixed with a polymerization initiator and the initiator breaks down, initiating the polymerization reaction. The free radicals react with the MMA monomer, causing it to join together, forming long chains of PMMA molecules. Once PMMA is injected, it quickly hardens or cures, forming a solid and stable mass within the vertebral body. The hardened PMMA provides immediate structural support to the fractured vertebra, stabilizing it and preventing further collapse.

Key Principles

- Implant failure is due to fatigue rather than static loading.
- Titanium is the most common implant material and stainless steel has fallen out of favor.
- Notching is a mechanism of spine instrumentation failure.
- UHMWPE is used in artificial disc technology because it reduces wear debris.

References

[1] Spivak JM, Hasharoni A. Use of hydroxyapatite in spine surgery. Eur Spine J 2001;10 Suppl 2(Suppl 2):S197–S204

[2] Dick JC, Bourgeault CA. Notch sensitivity of titanium alloy, commercially pure titanium, and stainless steel spinal implants. Spine 2001;26(15):1668–1672

[3] Liao C, Li Y, Tjong SC. Polyetheretherketone and its composites for bone replacement and regeneration. Polymers 2020;12(12):2858

[4] Kurtz SM, Toth JM, Siskey R, et al. The latest lessons learned from retrieval analyses of ultra-high molecular weight polyethylene, metal-on-metal, and alternative bearing total disc replacements. Semin Spine Surg 2012;24(1):57–70

[5] Chaput, CD. Surface treatments for spinal implants: a biological perspective. Spine 2018;43(7S):S6

14 Component–Component Interfaces

Rafid Kasir, Bobby Tay

Understanding the component interfaces in spine instrumentation is paramount to the development, successful application, and, when necessary, removal of these instruments.

Learning Objectives

- Understand examples and applications of anchors and longitudinal connectors in spine surgery.
- Understand the component–component locking mechanisms and differentiate between locking mechanisms.
- Understand advantages and limitations of constrained implants and semiconstrained implants.
- Understand how friction plays a role in component–component interfaces.
- Understand the two properties that influence the force of friction between components.

Questions

▸▸ Question 1

Which of the following is not considered an anchor in spinal implants?

- A. Hook
- B. Rod
- C. Lateral mass screw
- D. Wire
- E. Pedicle screw

▸▸ Question 2

Spinal implants rely on what force to resist failure at the component interfaces?

- A. Tension
- B. Gravity
- C. Friction
- D. Electromagnetic force
- E. Strong force

▸▸ Question 3

When designing a locking screw, adding what property would most increase the security of the screw–rod interface?

- A. Adding a smooth undersurface with minimal contact with the rod
- B. Lowering the maximal insertional torque that the locking screw can experience before failure
- C. Designing the screw to be placed end-on rather than tangential to the rod
- D. Adding a knurled surface to increase the surface area in contact between the rod and screw
- E. Increasing the modulus of elasticity of the screw

▸▸ Question 4

The force of friction is proportional to what?

- A. The second power of the coefficient of friction
- B. The first power of the mass of the object
- C. The first power of the normal force
- D. The third power of the distance between objects
- E. The charge between the two objects

▸▸ Question 5

A 45-year-old woman underwent a spine fusion for scoliosis in 1985. She has lived with continued back pain, and recent imaging has revealed that her Harrington rod has dislodged from the hook. Black residue is seen in the tissues surrounding the hook upon exploration. What factor is responsible for this finding?

- A. Implant corrosion due to the semiconstrained component–rod connector
- B. A reaction between an antibiotic she received for a pneumonia and the metal
- C. Implant loosening due to the overconstrained nature of the implant
- D. A platelet reaction to the callous formation
- E. Tissue naturally darkens with age

▸▸ Question 6

All of the following are examples of component–component locking mechanisms except:

- A. Three-point shear clamps
- B. Lock–screw connectors
- C. Circumferential grip connectors
- D. Pistol grips
- E. Constrained bolt–plate connector

▸▸ Question 7

A lock–screw connector may provide half of the pincer mechanism required for rod security. The other half of the pincer mechanism may be which of the following?

- A. Half of a circumferential grip connector
- B. Another lock–screw connector
- C. A constrained or semiconstrained screw–plate connector
- D. Constrained bolt–plate connector
- E. Constrained screw–plate

▸▸ Question 8

Which of the following are the two most widely used techniques to assess the integrity of spine component–component interfaces in the laboratory?

- A. Pulling and bending to failure tests
- B. Cyclical tension and axial loading
- C. Axial push strength and torsional strength
- D. Modulus of elasticity and time to fracture
- E. Stress and strain

▸▸ Question 9

A surgeon decides to use a constrained screw–plate construct with threads on the screw head and plate to affix two cervical vertebrae together during an anterior cervical discectomy and fusion. During the surgery, the surgeon finds that the hardware is prominent and there is a gap of a few millimeters between the plate and the bone. What strategy could have avoided this?

- A. Using larger-diameter screws
- B. Using shorter screws
- C. Using a semiconstrained screw–plate construct
- D. Placing the most proximal and distal screws first
- E. Minimizing osteophyte removal

▸▸ Question 10

Which of the following is the correct equation for calculating the coefficient of friction (μ) between two surfaces in spine surgery?

- A. $\mu = F_{normal}/F_{applied}$
- B. $\mu = F_{friction}/F_{normal}$
- C. $\mu = F_{applied}/F_{friction}$
- D. $\mu = F_{gravity} \times F_{applied}/F_{friction}$
- E. $\mu = F_{friction} \times F_{normal}$

▸▸ Question 11

Which of the following describes a component of constrained screw–plate constructs?

- A. Threaded screw heads and threaded plate
- B. Oblong shaped screw holes in the plate
- C. Plates that are machine-contoured to match the anatomy they are addressing
- D. Plates with a grooved undersurface
- E. Similar metals (e.g., using stainless steel screws with a stainless steel plate)

▸▸ Question 12

Which of the following describes a construct?

- A. A device used to stabilize the spine
- B. A combination of the implant and the spine segment encompassed
- C. A device used to connect two or more anchors
- D. A device that affixes two longitudinal members
- E. A device that affixes the bone to a longitudinal member

▸▸ Question 13

What is an advantage of constrained (rigid) screw–plate interfaces over semiconstrained interfaces?

- A. Additional points of fixation allow for a larger surface area for fixation
- B. They are stronger than their unconstrained counterparts
- C. They provide more versatility in instrumentation

- D. They are equal in cost to their unconstrained counterparts
- E. They allow the bone to be "sucked" onto the plate

▸▸ Question 14

A patient is undergoing a long posterior spine fusion and the surgeon decides to place semiconstrained hooks at the upper instrumented vertebrae. What is a property of the hook–rod interface in this scenario?

- A. The interface is strongest in flexion/extension
- B. The interface may be strengthened by selecting transverse process hooks over pedicle hooks
- C. The hook maybe placed percutaneously
- D. The interface allows for some motion
- E. The hook is permanently affixed to the rod and the rod must be cut appropriately

▸▸ Question 15

Which of the following is *not* a technique for creating a constrained interface between a screw and a plate?

- A. Expanding the head of the screw after placement
- B. A cam interface between the screw and plate
- C. A screw that threads into the plate
- D. Tightening the screw until the screw maximally pulls the bone to the plate
- E. Placing a cap into the screw and plate

▸▸ Question 16

Which of the following is a unit of force?

- A. Pound
- B. Joule
- C. Erg
- D. Meter
- E. Ohm

▸▸ Question 17

What may be a reason a surgeon chooses a cross-connector?

- A. To save costs
- B. To strengthen the construct in regard to rotational and axial stability
- C. To minimize the rate of adjacent segment disease
- D. To strengthen axial stability while sacrificing rotational stability
- E. Cross-connectors are necessary for fusions longer than three segments

▸▸ Question 18

A patient presents with ongoing back pain after a spinal fusion 30 years ago. Imaging reveals constrained bolt–plates were used for fixation and computed tomography (CT) scan shows no evidence of solid fusion with multiple loose metal nuts. Which of the following may have minimized the risk of this failure?

- A. Using bolts of varying heights
- B. Overtightening the nut past the manufacturer's recommendations
- C. Using angled washers for bolts placed in an oblique trajectory through the plate
- D. Overtapping the screw track
- E. Using a screw with a high outer to inner core diameter ratio

▸▸ Question 19

A patient is undergoing a revision L2–L5 posterior spinal fusion for a broken rod and pseudoarthrosis. The rod is found to be broken beneath the set screw and the smooth circumferential grip connector. What is a possible explanation for this?

- A. The surgeon who placed the instrumentation used a cobalt chrome rod rather than a titanium rod
- B. The surgeon failed to perform a laminectomy at the site of rod breakage
- C. This type of circumferential grip connector and set screw relies on slight deformation of the rod for security
- D. The original surgeon used a precontoured rod rather than manually bending the rod using a French bender
- E. The surgeon chose to use iliac crest autograft over allograft

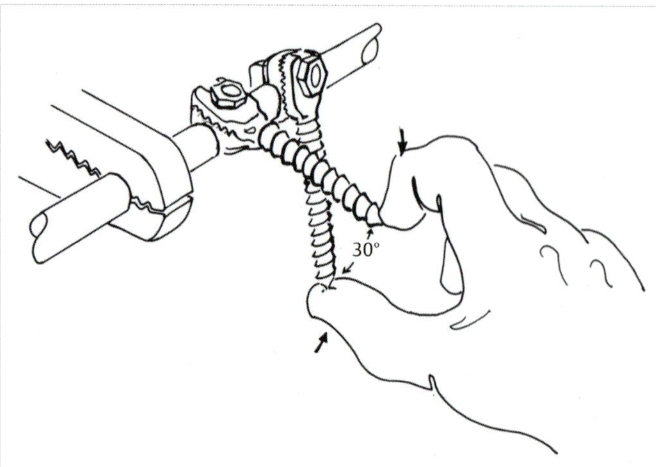

Fig. 14.1 Poor man's biomechanical testing. Apply two 50-mm screws to a rod (next to each other and divergent by 30 degrees) via the manufacturer's prescribed technique. Have an assistant hold the rod with locking pliers. Apply increasing degrees of force. Torsional strength can be graded according to the force required to cause the screw to rotate on the rod. In this manner, two or more systems can be compared. (Source: Biomechanics of Spine Stabilization: Third Edition, © 2015 Thieme Medical Publishers, Inc.)

▸▸ Question 20

▸ Fig. 14.1 depicts an individual applying a force to an anchor that has been locked on a rod. What is being tested?

- A. Axial strength
- B. Torsional strength
- C. Anchor pullout strength
- D. Rod strength
- E. Translational strength

Answers

▸▸ Answer 1

Correct answer is B

An understanding of the different types of anchors and longitudinal connectors is important before understanding the mechanisms by which they are connected. The anchors used in modern spinal instrumentation depend on clinical characteristics and desired biomechanical goals. Factors to consider are location of the desired fixation point on the vertebrae (i.e., pedicle, vertebral body, lamina), the nature of the bone (e.g., osteoporosis, postsurgical bone loss), and the desired stability. In posterior-based surgery, screws may be inserted in the pedicles, cervical lateral masses, or lamina. Hooks and wires may be fastened to the pedicles or around the lamina. Typically, screws are biomechanically superior to hooks and wires,[1,2,3] and screws inserted into the pedicle are most superior.[4] Contoured rods are then most commonly used and fastened to multiple anchors to limit motion between vertebrae.

▸▸ Answer 2

Correct answer is A

Friction is the force that opposes motion between two surfaces in contact. It is a fundamental force that plays a crucial role in our daily lives and the interface between spinal components are no exception. Friction is caused by the interlocking of microscopic irregularities on the surfaces of two objects in contact. When the two surfaces are pressed together, these irregularities create tiny bumps and ridges that resist motion, causing friction. Static friction is the focus of spinal fusion component interfaces.

A tension force is the force that acts on an object when it is being pulled or stretched. This may come into play when tensioning wires as anchors but is not the fundamental force at the wire–rod interface. The gravitational force is the force between two objects that have mass and is negligible between spinal components. The electromagnetic force is the force responsible for interactions between charged particles, not spinal implants.

▸▸ Answer 3

Correct answer is D

The principle force securing the rod and anchor in place in this example is the friction created by the set screw. Answer D is correct because it is the only answer that increases the force of friction. Answer A minimizes contact area, which decreases friction. Answer B minimizes the insertional force on the screw, which decreases the force of friction. Answer C describes end-on versus tangential screw placement, and tangential screw placement increases contact area between the screw and rod, which increases friction. Increasing the modulus of elasticity of the screw would have no effect on the stability of the screw and rod construct.

▸▸ Answer 4

Correct answer is C

The perpendicular application of force (normal force, N) to two surfaces causes friction to increase proportionally. The only other factor involved is the coefficient of friction, μ. The relationship of friction between two objects can be seen in ▸ Fig. 14.2. The perpendicular application of a force (N) to two surfaces (A and B) causes the friction (f) between the two surfaces to increase proportionally. The only other factor involved is the coefficient of friction (μ). This describes the frictional relationship between the two surfaces.

▸▸ Answer 5

Correct answer is A

Fretting corrosion is not an uncommon problem in semiconstrained spinal implants used in spine surgery. It occurs when small oscillatory movements between the implant components cause the release of metal debris due to friction, leading to corrosion. Semiconstrained component–rod connectors were historically typified by the Harrington distraction rod, the Harrington compression rod, and other relatively loose component–rod interfaces. The connections allow some toggling of the component on the rod where loosening and fretting corrosion may occur (see ▸ Fig. 14.3). The *dashed* and *solid lines* illustrate that the anchor can toggle on the rod.

▸▸ Answer 6

Correct answer is D

A longitudinal member may be connected to other implant components by one or more of the seven commonly used fundamental types of mechanisms: (1) three-point shear clamps; (2) lock–screw connectors; (3) circumferential grip connectors; (4) constrained bolt–plate connectors; (5) constrained screw–plate connectors; (6) semiconstrained screw–plate connectors; and (7) semiconstrained component–rod connectors (see ▸ Fig. 14.4).

▸▸ Answer 7

Correct answer is A

Lock–screw connectors work by using friction to lock the rod in place, preventing it from shifting or rotating. The set screw is inserted through a threaded hole in the pedicle screw and tightened against the spinal rod, creating a clamping force that holds the rod securely in place. Thus, the locking set screw provides half of the pincer mechanism required for security, and the other half of

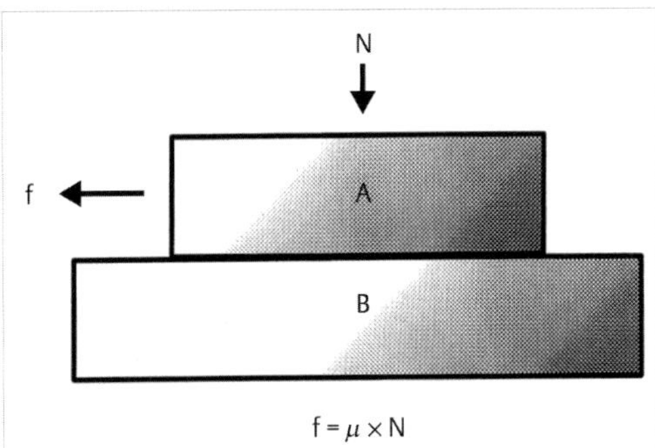

Fig. 14.2 The perpendicular application of a force (*N*) to two surfaces (*A* and *B*) causes the friction (*f*) between the two surfaces to increase proportionally. The only other factor involved is the coefficient of friction (μ). This describes the frictional relationship between the two surfaces. (Source: Biomechanics of Spine Stabilization: Third Edition, © 2015 Thieme Medical Publishers, Inc.)

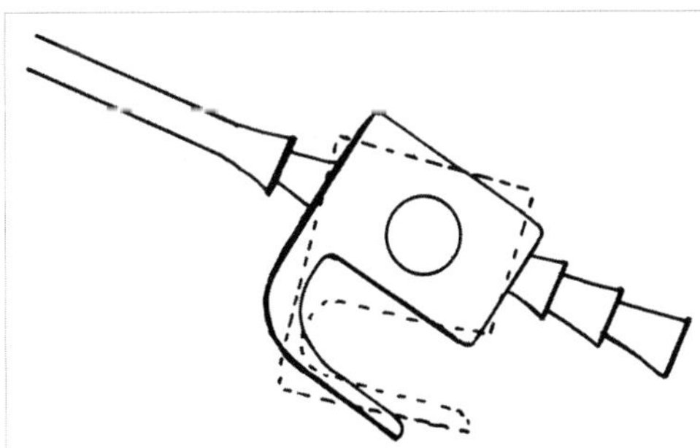

Fig. 14.3 An exaggerated depiction of a semiconstrained component–rod connector (Harrington distraction rod and hook) in extremes of the allowed toggle. The dashed and solid representation of the hook illustrates the fact that the hook can tilt on the ratcheted component of the rod. This then, functions to lock the hook's position on the rod and ideally secure fixation. (Source: Biomechanics of Spine Stabilization: Third Edition, © 2015 Thieme Medical Publishers, Inc.)

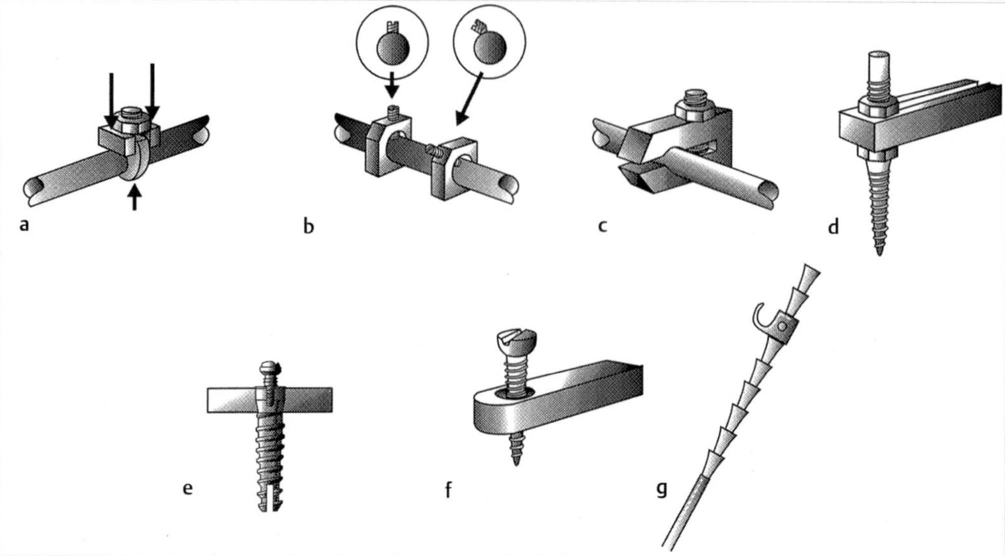

Fig. 14.4 The seven fundamental component–component locking mechanisms. **(a)** Three-point shear clamp. **(b)** Lock screw: end-on (*left*) and tangential (*right*). **(c)** Circumferential grip. **(d)** Constrained bolt–plate. **(e)** Constrained screw–plate. **(f)** Semiconstrained screw–plate. **(g)** Semiconstrained component–rod. (Source: Biomechanics of Spine Stabilization: Third Edition, © 2015 Thieme Medical Publishers, Inc.)

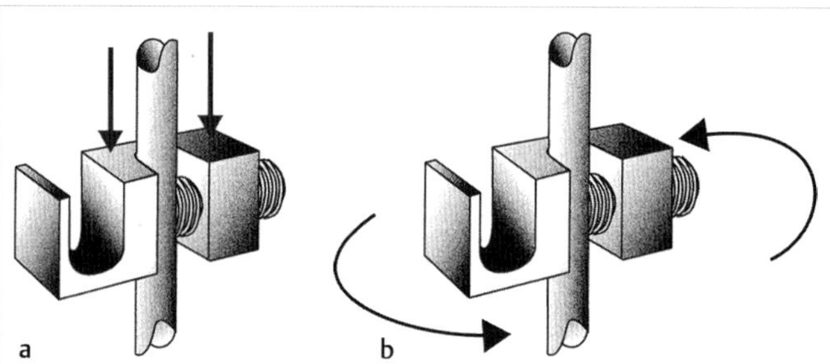

Fig. 14.5 **(a)** The axial push strength and **(b)** torsional strength methods of laboratory assessment. Arrows depict the forces applied by the testing device. (Source: Biomechanics of Spine Stabilization: Third Edition, © 2015 Thieme Medical Publishers, Inc.)

the pincer mechanism is either a three-point shear clamp or a circumferential grip connector. The lock–screw may be applied end-on or tangentially. There appears to be a mechanical advantage to tangential application. The lock–screw may be seated on a knurled surface, with a larger coefficient of friction, or on a smoother surface, relying mainly on a circumferential gripping force and slight component deformation.

▸▸ Answer 8

Correct answer is C

Axial push testing and torsional strength testing are two common laboratory tests used to assess the biomechanical properties of spinal implants. Axial push testing involves applying a compressive load to the implant along the axis of the screw or rod, while torsional strength testing involves applying a twisting force to the implant around its longitudinal axis (see ▸ Fig. 14.5). Shown in the figure is an axial push test (**a**) and a torsional strength test (**b**). Both tests can be performed in vitro using a specialized testing machine that measures the force and displacement of the implant under different loading conditions. Historic component–component connectors have axial push strengths ranging from 500 N for a Cotrel-Dubousset cross-link on a Cotrel-Dubousset rod to 3,400 N for a Texas Scottish Rite Hospital central post hook on a 1/4 inch shot penned rod with a Texas Scottish Rite Hospital top tightening T-bolt. For further reading, the American Society for the Testing of Materials (ASTM) provides industry standards for testing implants.[5]

▸▸ Answer 9

Correct answer is C

Constrained screw–plate constructs are biomechanically stronger than their semiconstrained counterparts.[6] These are commonly referred to as locking screws and plates versus nonlocking screws and plates, respectively. Of note is that this strategy (locking plate technique) does not allow the bone to be pulled tightly to the plate. In some regards, especially with minimally invasive fracture fixation, this is advantageous in that it allows the periosteum to be preserved. In cases where the desired result is that the plate be as close to the bone as possible, a semiconstrained screw–plate construct may be advantageous. Another alternative is to use a screw-capping construct, which both pulls the plate to the bone and constrains the screws to the plate (see ▸ Fig. 14.6).

▸▸ Answer 10

Correct answer is B

The coefficient of friction is defined as the ratio of the force of friction between two surfaces to the normal force pressing them together. In spine surgery, the force of friction between two implant components is an important consideration, as it can affect the stability and integrity of the implant. The coefficient of friction can be calculated by dividing the force of friction by the normal force, which is the force perpendicular to the surface of the two components in contact. The coefficient of friction increases as the interactions between the two objects increases. An analogy can be seen in tires and respective terrain; a mud tire has deep threads that interact with the mud, while a slick tire is most matched to a smooth road. In both cases the contact between the surfaces is increased. A smooth tire on a muddy road and a mud tire on a smooth road have diminished contact forces. Similarly, a circumferential grip connector is most matched to a smooth rod.

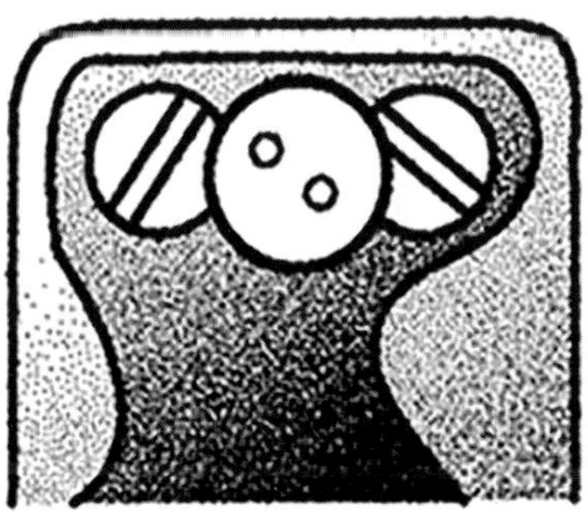

Fig. 14.6 Screw plate locking mechanisms. Screw-capping technique. (Source: Biomechanics of Spine Stabilization: Third Edition, © 2015 Thieme Medical Publishers, Inc.)

▸▸ Answer 11

Correct answer is A

Constrained screw–plate constructs have fixed angles between the screw and the plate. Locking the screw within the plate using a threaded screw head and threaded plate achieves this. Therefore, answer A is correct. Oblong shaped screw holes (B) allow for side-to-side motion of the plate as the screw head pushes against the plate. This is an example of a dynamic compression plate. Precontoured plates (C) are manufactured to better fit along different anatomic sites. Plates with a grooved undersurface (D) minimize the contact between the plate and the bone and are therefore thought to preserve vascularity—these are known as low contact plates.

▸▸ Answer 12

Correct answer is B

An implant is a device used to stabilize the spine via the connection of two or more spine components (segments). A construct is the combination of the implant and the spine segments encompassed by the implant (B). An assembly is the collection of components that together make up the implant. A longitudinal member (e.g., rod, plate) connects two or more anchors. An anchor (e.g., screw, wire, hook) affixes to the bone and to the longitudinal member. A cross-fixator affixes two (usually parallel) longitudinal members to each other.

▸▸ Answer 13

Correct answer is B

Locking plates are designed with specialized screw holes that allow the screws to engage the plate rigidly, forming a fixed-angle construct. This characteristic provides several advantages. The fixed-angle construct created by locking plates ensures that the screws do not rely on bone purchase for stability, thus reducing the risk of implant failure due to poor bone quality or inadequate screw purchase. They are biomechanically superior to semiconstrained implants (B). In orthopaedic trauma, for example, locking plates offer enhanced stability in these complex fracture patterns, allowing for early mobilization and potentially reducing the risk of nonunion or malunion.[7]

On the other hand, nonlocking plates, also known as semiconstrained screw–plate systems, rely on the friction between the plate and the bone to achieve stability. These plates are more commonly used in simple fractures with good bone quality, where the screw purchase is sufficient to hold the fracture fragments together. Points of fixation are not affected by constraint (A). Versatility of instrumentation (C) is unaffected by constraint. Constrained implants are typically more expensive than their semiconstrained counterparts (D).

▸▸ Answer 14

Correct answer is D

Hooks provide a more flexible fixation option when compared with pedicle screws, allowing for some degree of motion at the upper instrumented vertebrae. The motion can occur both at the hook–bone interface as well as the hook–rod interface, making choice D correct. This can be particularly beneficial in cases where adjacent segment degeneration is a concern in long fusion constructs, as it helps distribute the stresses along the fusion construct and potentially reduces the risk of adjacent level disease.[8]

Laminar hooks are designed to engage the bony lamina, pedicle hooks are designed to engage the pedicle, and transverse process hooks engage with the transverse process. The choice of hook type depends on various factors, including the surgeon's preference, the specific patient anatomy, and the goals of the surgery. The interface itself does not change with anatomic site selection for placing the hook, making choice B incorrect. Choice C is incorrect because soft tissues must be dissected to allow adequate hook placement.

▸▸ Answer 15

Correct answer is D

Constrained screw–plate designs and semiconstrained screw plate designs are two variations of spinal implant systems that offer distinct advantages and considerations in spine surgery. Constrained screw–plate designs involve the use of screws that are rigidly connected to the plate, restricting motion between the two components. This design provides a high level of stability and fixation, as the screws and plate act as a single unit, limiting any relative movement. The constrained configuration helps distribute the load more evenly along the construct, reducing stress concentration at the screw–bone interface. This design is particularly advantageous in cases where strong fixation and immediate stability are desired. Various techniques exist and are illustrated in ▸ Fig. 14.7, including an

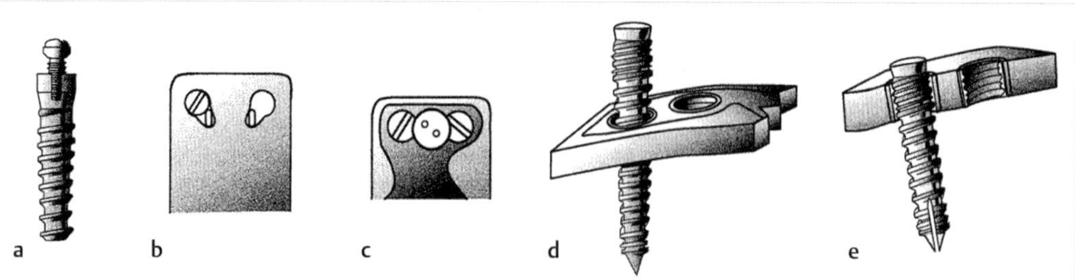

Fig. 14.7 Screw–plate locking mechanisms. **(a)** Expanding-head technique. **(b)** Cam technique. **(c)** Screw-capping technique. **(d)** Lockingplate strategy. **(e)** The latter uses a dual thread pitch design in which the machine thread pitch is half of the bone thread pitch. (Source: Biomechanics of Spine Stabilization: Third Edition, © 2015 Thieme Medical Publishers, Inc.)

expanding-head technique (**a**), cam technique (**b**), screw-capping technique (**c**), and a threaded locking plate strategy (**d**). Answer D is a property of semiconstrained screw–plate systems.

▸▸ Answer 16

Correct answer is A

A pound is commonly used as a unit of force, but it is important to note that in the International System of Units (SI), the unit of force is the newton (N). However, the pound as a unit of force is derived from its historical use in relation to gravity. Specifically, a pound is defined as the force required to accelerate a mass of 1 pound at a rate of 32.17405 feet per second squared (ft/s^2) in the presence of Earth's gravitational pull. This definition stems from Sir Isaac Newton's laws of motion, particularly the second law, which states that force is equal to mass multiplied by acceleration.

While the pound is not part of the SI system, it continues to be used in certain fields and regions, particularly in the United States, where customary units are still prevalent. In these contexts, the pound is often utilized in everyday measurements and practical applications involving force, such as weighing objects or describing weightlifting capacities. However, when it comes to scientific calculations and standardization, the newton is the preferred unit for measuring force, as it provides a consistent and globally recognized standard in the realm of physics and engineering. ▶ Table 14.1 illustrates various units of length, force, and energy.

Table 14.1 Units of measure pertinent to the mechanics of spinal stabilization constructs and conversion factors.

Measure of distance	
1 meter	39.37 inches
Measures of force (weight)	
1 newton	105 dynes
1 pound	16 ounces (avoirdupois)
1 pound	4.448 newtons
1 newton	0.225 pound
1 kilogram	9.8 newtons
1 kilogram	2.2 pounds
Measures of work (energy)	
1 inch-pound	quantity of energy required to raise a weight of 1 pound against gravity by a height of 1 inch
1 newton-meter	quantity of energy required to raise a weight of 1 newton against gravity by a height of 1 meter
1 erg	1 dyne-centimeter
1 inch-pound	0.083 foot-pound
1 joule	1 newton-meter
1 newton-meter	0.7375 foot-pound
1 newton-meter	8.85 inch-pounds
1 inch-pound	0.113 newton-meter

Source: Biomechanics of Spine Stabilization: Third Edition, © 2015 Thieme Medical Publishers, Inc.

▸▸ Answer 17

Correct answer is B

Cross-fixation is defined herein as the rigid fixation of bilaterally placed posterior fixation devices to each other in a rigid or semirigid manner to make the construct effectively a quadrilateral frame. There are various forms of cross-fixation. Historically, wires and acrylic cross-connectors were used to connect longitudinal connectors to prevent telescoping of the rods. Connecting modern longitudinal connectors that are anchored by toed in pedicle screws creates a triangular construct, which has substantial pullout resistance as well as resistance to sagittal plane translation and subluxation. Cross-fixation provides substantially greater stiffness and stability than that achieved without cross-fixation. This is especially advantageous with longer systems. Techniques of cross-fixation, however, consume valuable operative time, are associated with complications, and have diminishing advantage compared with modern-day fixed moment arm cantilever beam screw–rod fixation systems. ▶ Fig. 14.8 shows an example of a construct using cross-connectors.

▸▸ Answer 18

Correct answer is C

Answer C is correct. ▶ Fig. 14.9 illustrates constrained bolt–plate (e.g., Steffee plate) connectors. Note the rigid fixation of the screw to the plate by

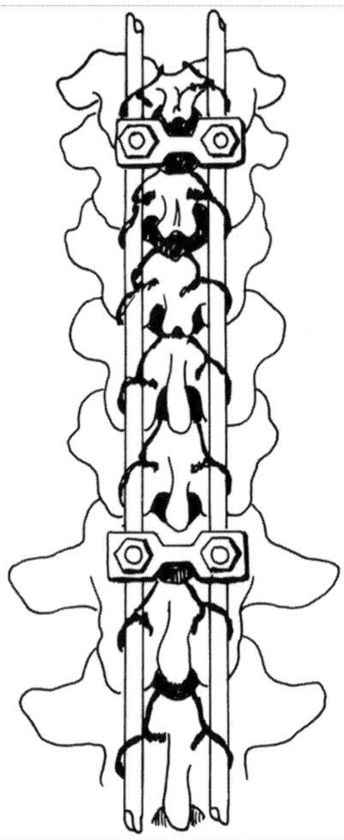

Fig. 14.8 Cross members are used to increase stability and to prevent one rod from telescoping past another in the Luque sublaminar wire technique. The use of two cross members near the junction of thirds provides a rectangular construct that can be fabricated in situ. Such strategies of cross fixation provided utility via the application of a quadrilateral frame construct in historical fixation systems, such as the Luque sublaminar wire technique, as depicted. This is not as much of an advantage today because of the rigid fixation achieved with bone via fixed moment arm cantilever beam screw–rod fixation techniques. (Source: Biomechanics of Spine Stabilization: Third Edition, © 2015 Thieme Medical Publishers, Inc.)

the bolt–plate mechanism. (**b, c**) The use of washers to compensate for screw height discrepancy and direction, respectively. If an angled washer is not used in a screw placed obliquely, this may result in inadvertent application of a moment arm to the vertebral body by the screw, resulting in (**d**) cutout (windshield wiper effect; *arrow*) or (**e**) an undesirable reorientation of the vertebral body. It may also result in inadequate tightening of the nut (**e**), which leaves a gap (*arrow*), thus fostering connector loosening. Unless the screw is perpendicular to the plate, the connection has not resulted in optimal tightness and security because of the inability to achieve an "in-line" configuration of the points of maximal contact between the plate and the hubs. Therefore, an optimally stable relationship between connector components is not achieved. *Straight arrows* depict points of contact of the nut and screw with the plate. Note the gaps and suboptimal contact realized when the screw is angled (**h**).

▸▸ Answer 19

Correct answer is C

Lock–screws may be seated on a knurled surface, relying mainly on friction between the two objects, or on a smoother surface, relying mainly on a circumferential gripping force and slight deformation of the rod. Answer C is therefore correct. Implant selection is important in successful spine surgery as well. Titanium and cobalt chrome are the two most common metals used in longitudinal rods, and while titanium has greater elasticity and decreases proximal junctional kyphosis rates, cobalt chromium has greater stiffness, therefore making choice A incorrect.[9] Laminectomy would actually theoretically remove area for bony fusion and promote pseudoarthrosis, making choice B incorrect. Contouring of rods plays a significant role in overall postoperative correction outcomes, as it can diminish their fatigue strength and increases the risk of rod fracture after implantation. Hand-held or French benders create significant stress risers and decrease the yield strength of the rod,[10] therefore making choice D incorrect.

▸▸ Answer 20

Correct answer is B

Answer B is correct. ▸ Fig. 14.1 illustrates a poor man's biomechanical test. Two screws are applied to a rod 30 degrees divergent to each other via the manufacturer's prescribed technique. The rod is held in place with locking pliers. Torsional strength can be graded according to the force required to cause the screw to rotate on the rod. In this manner, two or more systems can be compared. Axial strength can be tested by attempting to translate the screw along the length of the rod (answer A). Anchor pullout strength can be tested by attempting to remove the anchor from the bone (answer C). Rod strength can be tested by applying a force designed to bend or break the rod (answer D).

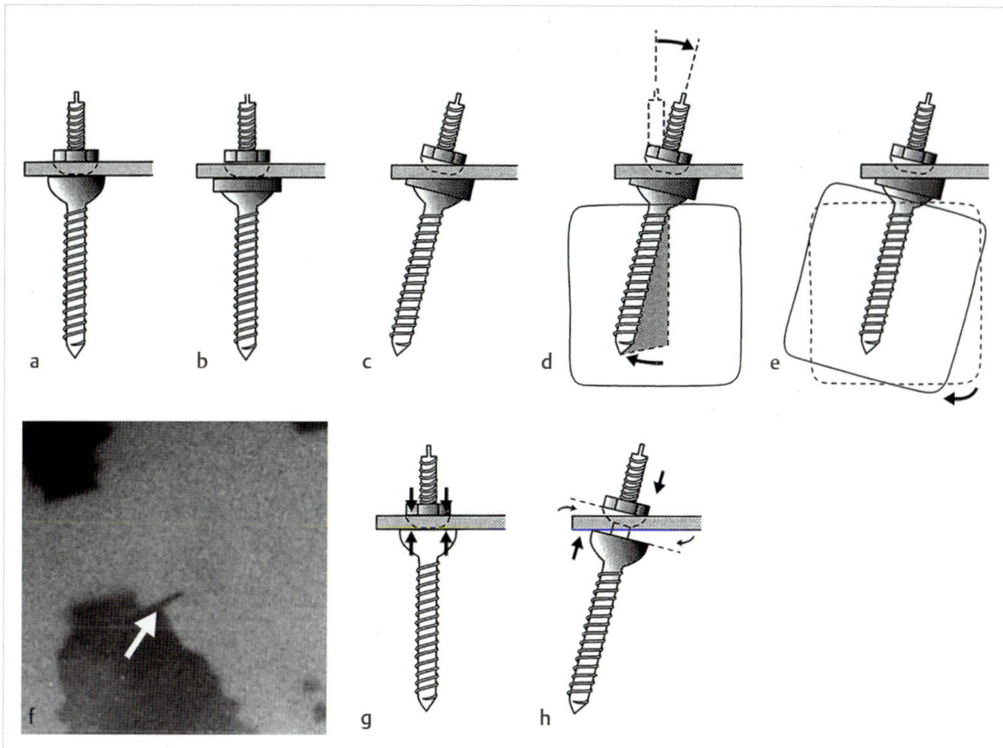

Fig. 14.9 **(a)** Constrained bolt–plate (e.g., Steffee plate) connectors. Note the rigid fixation of the screw to the plate by the bolt–plate mechanism. **(b, c)** The use of washers to compensate for screw height discrepancy and direction, respectively. An angled washer may not accurately compensate for the angle at the screw–plate junction. This may result in inadvertent application of a moment arm to the vertebral body by the screw, resulting in **(d)** cutout (windshield wiper effect; *arrow*) or **(e)** an undesirable reorientation of the vertebral body. **(f)** It may also result in inadequate tightening of the nut, which leaves a gap (*arrow*), thus fostering connector loosening. Contoured hub–plate interfaces provide some latitude in the latter regard. **(g)** However, unless the screw is perpendicular to the plate, the connection has not resulted in optimal tightness and security because of the inability to achieve an "in-line" configuration of the points of maximal contact between the plate and the hubs. Therefore, an optimally stable relationship between connector components is not achieved. Straight arrows depict points of contact of the nut and screw with the plate. **(h)** Note the gaps and suboptimal contact realized when the screw is angled. In **(g)** and **(h)**, the straight arrows portray the forces applied by the screw to the plate during tightening. The curve arrows in **(h)** portray the angular forces applied if the screw is not perpendicular to the plate and the abutting interfaces are not parallel. (Source: Biomechanics of Spine Stabilization: Third Edition, © 2015 Thieme Medical Publishers, Inc.)

Key Principles

- Longitudinal members connect two or more anchors to form an assembly of components that make up an implant.
- There are seven commonly used fundamental types of locking mechanisms: (1) three-point shear clamps; (2) lock–screw connectors; (3) circumferential grip connectors; (4) constrained bolt–plate connectors; (5) constrained screw–plate connectors; (6) semiconstrained screw–plate connectors; and (7) semiconstrained component–rod connectors.
- All locking mechanisms rely on friction between the components.
- Force of friction = coefficient of friction × normal (or perpendicular) force.
- Axial push strength and torsional strength are the most commonly used techniques to assess component–component interface integrity.

References

[1] Liljenqvist U, Hackenberg L, Link T, Halm H. Pullout strength of pedicle screws versus pedicle and laminar hooks in the thoracic spine. Acta Orthop Belg 2001;67(2):157–163

[2] Hitchon PW, Brenton MD, Black AG, et al. In vitro biomechanical comparison of pedicle screws, sublaminar hooks, and sublaminar cables. J Neurosurg. 2003;99(1):104–109

[3] Jones EL, Heller JG, Silcox DH, Hutton WC. Cervical pedicle screws versus lateral mass screws: anatomic feasibility and biomechanical comparison. Spine 1997;22(9):977–982

[4] Ito Z, Higashino K, Kato S, et al. Pedicle screws can be 4 times stronger than lateral mass screws for insertion in the midcervical spine: a biomechanical study on strength of fixation. J Spinal Disord Tech 2014;27(2):80–85

[5] American Society for the Testing of Materials (ASTM). Provisional Standard. Philadelphia, PA: ASTM; 1993

[6] Smith WR, Ziran BH, Anglen JO, Stahel PF. Locking plates: tips and tricks. J Bone Joint Surg Am 2007;89(10):2298–2307

[7] Meinberg EG, Agel J, Roberts CS, Karam MD, Kellam JF. Fracture and dislocation classification compendium—2018. J Orthop Trauma 2018;32(Suppl 1):S1–S170

[8] Metzger MF, Robinson ST, Svet MT, et al. Biomechanical analysis of the proximal adjacent segment after multilevel instrumentation of the thoracic spine: do hooks ease the transition? Global Spine J 2016;6(4):335–343

[9] Shega FD, Zhang HQ, Manini DR, et al. Comparison of effectiveness between cobalt chromium rods versus titanium rods for treatment of patients with spinal deformity: a systematic review and meta-analysis. Adv Orthop 2020;2020:8475910

[10] Demura S, Murakami H, Hayashi H, et al. Influence of rod contouring on rod strength and stiffness in spine surgery. Orthopedics 2015;38(6):e520-e523

15 Implant–Bone Interfaces

Christopher A. Sy, Terrence T. Kim, J. Patrick Johnson

The eventual success or failure of implants and associated hardware constructs can ultimately depend on physical interactions that occur along various points of contact between the implant and the bone. Implant material, shape, size, location, and overall relative geometry to the surrounding bone have an effect on an implant's strength and ability to resist external forces. Discussed here are the five fundamental types of implant–bone interfaces currently employed in spinal surgery—concepts that could help inform clinical decision making as well as surgical planning.

Learning Objectives

- Identify the five types of implant–bone interfaces including common examples of their use.
- Describe and discuss the attributes of screws.
- Understand the limitations of spinal implants and why screws have become predominant in modern practice.
- Understand what factors affect pullout resistance and how to optimize it.
- Understand the importance of geometry and force vectors.
- Appreciate the geometry and quality of bone as it pertains to the success of implant–bone interfaces.

Questions

▸▸ Question 1

A common location for abutting implant–bone interfaces is the interbody region (disc space) in between two vertebral bodies. What is true regarding the biomechanical properties of an implant used in the interbody region?

- A. Selecting an implant with a smaller surface area will decrease the likelihood that it will subside or "knife through" the vertebral body end plate
- B. Selecting an implant with a larger surface area will lead to a decreased ability to resist axial loading
- C. The edges of the end plate are the weakest portion of the end plate
- D. An implant's ability to resist axial loading is inversely related to cross-sectional area
- E. The center of the end plate is the weakest portion of the end plate

▸▸ Question 2

Newer generation disc arthroplasty devices are being designed with titanium–ceramic surfaces that contact the vertebral body end plates. The choice of material is based on knowledge regarding which of the five types of implant–bone interfaces?

- A. Penetrating
- B. Abutting
- C. Grabbing
- D. Osteointegration
- E. Conforming

▸▸ Question 3

Regarding the screw core (inner diameter), what can be said about its physical properties as it relates to the section modulus (Z)?

- A. As the core diameter increases, the pullout strength of the screw increases exponentially
- B. As the core diameter increases, the bending strength of the screw increases exponentially
- C. As the core diameter increases, the screw's ability to resist translational forces at the termination of screw tightening increases exponentially
- D. Screw core diameter is inversely related to the section modulus
- E. Screw core diameter has a minimal effect on the section modulus

▸▸ Question 4

The *arrow* in the ▸ Fig. 15.1 depicts a distance and physical property of screws known as what? What can be said about this property and how it affects the screw's capabilities?

- A. Screw threads; having decreased thread height leads to less bone compression during insertion, thus increasing pullout strength

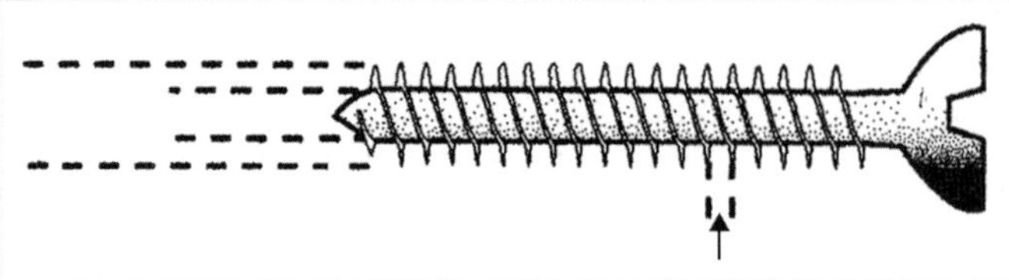

Fig. 15.1 The important anatomical aspects and characteristics of a screw: the head, the core, the thread, and the tip. (Source: Biomechanics of Spine Stabilization: Third Edition, © 2015 Thieme Medical Publishers, Inc.)

- B. Screw threads; pullout strength is determined only by thread height and not by thread shape or pitch
- C. Screw pitch; the pitch is directly proportional to the volume of bone between threads and thus to pullout resistance
- D. Screw pitch; the pitch is directly proportional to the insertional torque and thus to pullout resistance
- E. Screw pitch; the pitch is the only determinant of interthread bone volume but has no effect on screw lead or the distance the screw advances axially with each turn.

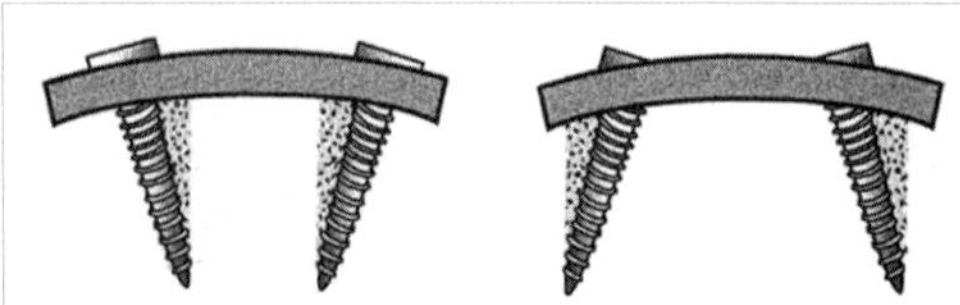

Fig. 15.2 (a) Toed-in and (b) toed-out screws in the axial plane resist pullout similarly if they provide a similar triangulation effect (depicted in the axial plane). However, they resist applied loads differently. (Source: Biomechanics of Spine Stabilization: Third Edition, © 2015 Thieme Medical Publishers, Inc.)

▸▸ Question 5

Current knowledge on tapping and screw insertion has demonstrated which of the following?

- A. Pretapped non–self-tapping and self-tapping screws, if used properly, provide similar pullout strengths
- B. Repeated removal and insertion of screws into cortical bone should be avoided as it has been shown to significantly weaken the screw's pullout strength
- C. Pretapping in cancellous bone strengthens the implant–bone interface
- D. Pretapping in cortical bone has been shown to increase the rate of microcracks around the screw threads
- E. Tapping is more important in cancellous bone and less important in cortical bone

▸▸ Question 6

▸ Fig. 15.2 depicts two different triangulation configurations of a screw and plate construct that are commonly employed. What is currently known about each configurations ability to bear/resist applied loads?

- A. Construct A likely has superior pullout resistance
- B. Construct B likely has superior pullout resistance
- C. Construct A has superior axial load resistance (perpendicular to the long axis of the screw)
- D. Construct B has superior axial load resistance (perpendicular to the long axis of the screw)
- E. Both constructs are equal in their ability resist axial loading (loads that are perpendicular to the long axis of the screws)

▸▸ Question 7

Conforming implant–bone materials such as PMMA can be useful because of which of the following properties?

- A. Since PMMA is able to match the contours of the bone, it has excellent osteointegration properties
- B. As long as PMMA is injected slowly (not pressurized), it can increase the bending strength of subsequent screw placement
- C. As long as PMMA is injected slowly (not pressurized), it will have more time to fill the interstices of bone before hardening
- D. When PMMA is injected with proper pressure, it can fill the interstices of the bone, effectively

increasing screw diameter and thus increasing pullout resistance
- E. Unlike other implanted materials (such as screws or hooks), conforming implants such as PMMA are able to conform precisely to the contours of the bone surface

▸▸ Question 8

Lag screws are useful for bringing two separate bony fragments closer together. In order for a screw to function as a lag screw, it should have which of the following properties?
- A. They should be fully unthreaded along the entire length of the screw
- B. They should have a far surface that is threaded and provides bony purchase, whereas the near surface is unthreaded and glides freely
- C. They should have a full-length flute, which collects bone debris as it is tightened
- D. They should have a small screw head so that it can glide through the near side fragment
- E. They should be made only with titanium since it has the best osteointegration properties

▸▸ Question 9

The triangulation demonstrated with the screw–bone implant shown in ▸ Fig. 15.3 should have maximum pullout resistance along which force vector?
- A. ↑
- B. ↓
- C. ←
- D. →
- E. ↔

▸▸ Question 10

Certain abutting interspace implants have been designed with added components that penetrate the adjacent bony end plates. What is the intended benefit of these abutting implants with penetrating components?
- A. Abutting implants that penetrate or subside are detrimental and are no longer used in modern practice

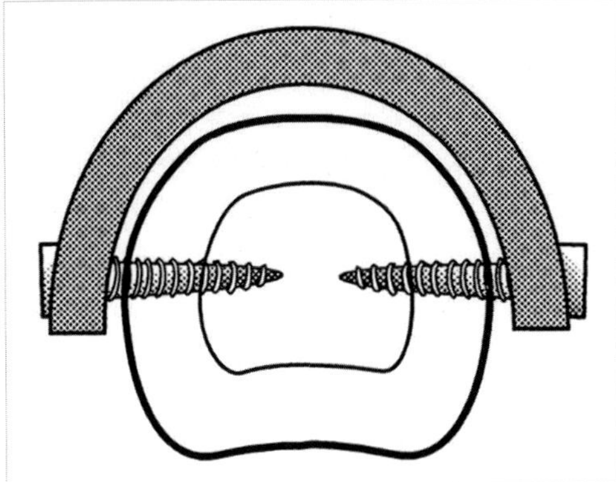

Fig. 15.3 The optimal orientation of a screw for pullout resistance via the triangulation effect is 90 degrees. (Source: Biomechanics of Spine Stabilization: Third Edition, © 2015 Thieme Medical Publishers, Inc.)

- B. Bony penetration allows for greater osteointegration properties regardless of the material used
- C. Abutting implants that penetrate adjacent bony end plates have been shown to have increased strength and are thus less likely to break or fail
- D. Abutting implants that penetrate adjacent bony end plates are more stable and never require additional pedicle screw instrumentation
- E. Abutting implants that penetrate adjacent bony end plates are less likely to migrate; this can minimize the chance of neural impingement and the chance of spinal deformation

▸▸ Question 11

Self-tapping screws only have a leading edge flute instead of a full-length flute. As a result, the initial drill hole (pilot hole) that is created should be slightly larger in diameter than the core diameter of the self-tapping screw that is subsequently placed. What is the reason for this?
- A. Self-tapping screws are inherently larger than tap screws
- B. The larger diameter allows for greater control of screw trajectory and minimizes the likelihood of a misplaced screw
- C. The larger diameter pilot hole increases bony purchase and thus pullout strength

- D. It facilitates accumulation of bony debris around the screw because the shorter flute cannot accommodate all the debris
- E. Self-tapping screws lack a tapered tap and will not fit in a smaller diameter hole

▸▸ Question 12

Which of the following components of a screw has no significant effect on pullout resistance?

- A. Major diameter
- B. Thread height
- C. Thread shape
- D. Thread pitch
- E. Head

▸▸ Question 13

Screw length does not routinely contribute to pullout resistance except under which of the following circumstances?

- A. Screw length contributes to pullout resistance when used in combination with injected PMMA
- B. Screw length contributes to pullout resistance only when combined with gripping implants such as laminar hooks
- C. Screw length contributes significantly to pullout resistance when they are part of a construct where they are rigidly triangulated
- D. Longer screws have increased pullout resistance only if the initial drill hole (pilot hole) is not pretapped
- E. Screw length contributes to pullout resistance only when titanium screws are used, which is why stainless steel screws are no longer used

▸▸ Question 14

Gripping implants such as hooks or sublaminar wires have substantial pullout resistance. Which of the following statements best explains this?

- A. Gripping implants are usually deployed within the disc space where they are less likely to migrate
- B. Gripping implants have greater contact surface and that contact is usually with cortical bone
- C. Gripping implants are designed to penetrate the bone and thus are more difficult to dislodge
- D. Gripping implants are easier to deploy by the surgeon and thus have less room for error
- E. Gripping implants are known more for their bending strength as opposed to their pullout resistance and are more often used in cantilever beam constructs

▸▸ Question 15

Which of the following strategies could be employed to best promote osteointegration?

- A. Application of a hydroxyapatite coating
- B. Use of smooth stainless steel surfaces instead of a matte or peened surface
- C. Injecting PMMA under pressure before screw insertion
- D. Using a nail instead of a screw, which causes more bone disruption
- E. Utilizing screws with the largest core diameter

▸▸ Question 16

Pretapping within cancellous bone before screw placement ________.

- A. Increases the rate of microfractures
- B. Has no significant effect
- C. Strengthens the implant–bone interface
- D. Is not needed if the bone is osteopoarotic
- E. Weakens the implant–bone interface

▸▸ Question 17

▸ Fig. 15.4 shows a short, curved plate construct (a) compared with a long curved plate construct (b). Which of the following statements correctly describes a significant drawback when utilizing one construct over the other?

- A. The screws used as part of construct “b” have increased pullout resistance
- B. Use of construct “b” will result in decreased pullout resistance as the screws are oriented more parallel and thus their triangulation effect is neutralized
- C. If both plates are made of titanium, then construct “a” is less likely to osteointegrate as the smaller plate has less titanium

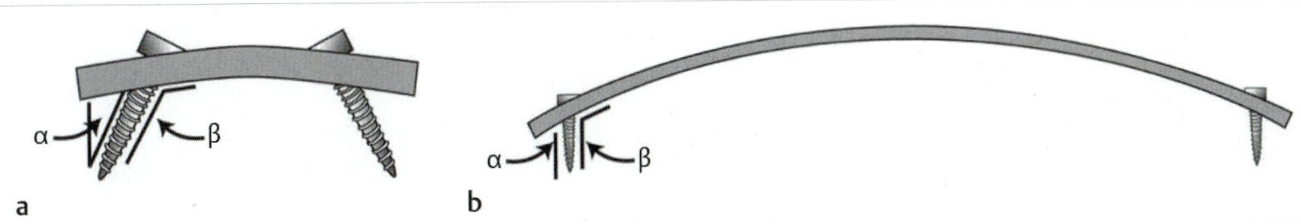

Fig. 15.4 (a) A short curved plate does not significantly alter the effective trajectory that the screw takes with the long axis of the spine. **(b)** If the plate is long, however, the angle (α) between the screw and the vertical axis differs from the corresponding angle (α) observed with a shorter plate even though the angle between the screw and the plate (β) does not change. This may adversely affect pullout resistance in a long implant. Note that the two screws in (B) are parallel to each other, whereas they are divergent in (A), which neutralizes the triangulation effect in longer implants. (Source: Biomechanics of Spine Stabilization: Third Edition, © 2015 Thieme Medical Publishers, Inc.)

- D. Greater angulation of the screws in construct "a" will make inserting screws into bone more challenging when compared with construct "b" where the screws have a straight trajectory
- E. Using construct "a" will have a significantly greater cost

▸▸ Question 18

What is important to note regarding the equation shown below, where y = insertional torque and x – pullout resistance?

$$y = \frac{x}{1142}\Big\} + 0.02$$

- A. Increasing insertional torque is the only way to increase pullout resistance
- B. Insertional torque is inversely related to pullout resistance
- C. Increasing pullout resistance is the only way to increase insertional torque
- D. It can lead to a false sense of security that an implant has high pullout resistance when it does not, especially with the use of conical-inner-diameter screws
- E. Outer diameter and thread design are less important when designing a screw with optimal pullout resistance

▸▸ Question 19

The compression screw–plate technique ________.

- A. Relies on sublaminar hooks or wires
- B. Utilizes screw triangulation with fixed moment arm screws
- C. Requires the use of PMMA that is pressure injected
- D. Is primarily designed to bear an axial load
- E. Causes translation of the vertebral body along the implant via a noncircular teardrop seat for a nonfixed moment arm screw

▸▸ Question 20

Which of the following strategies would best increase pullout resistance?

- A. Decreasing screw thread height
- B. Injecting PMMA slowly
- C. Bicortical purchase
- D. Inserting screws in parallel instead of triangulating them
- E. Using short screws with shorter thread pitch

Answers

▸▸ Answer 1

Correct answer is E

The center of the end plate is the weakest portion of the end plate and, conversely, the edges of the end plate are the strongest[1] (answer E is correct and answer C is incorrect). This is due to added strength from the cortical bone that makes up the edge/wall of the vertebral body. An important concept is that the ability to resist axial loading is *directly* related to cross-sectional area—thus, answer D is incorrect. Answers A and B are also incorrect statements that are related to the same concept. A smaller implant would actually *increase* the likelihood of subsidence. A larger implant would actually have *increased* ability to resist axial loading forces.

►► **Answer 2**

Correct answer is D

Titanium and ceramic materials have a capacity for bony ingrowth due to their high biocompatibility—a capability known as osteointegration.[2,3,4] Penetrating interfaces are a reference to certain implant shapes (nail/screw) that are designed to be driven into bone (answer A). Abutting surfaces refer to axial loading forces and the effect of implant cross-sectional area on axial load resistance (answer B). Gripping interfaces are those that physically wrap around a bony surface such as a hook or wire and thus is referring to the implant's configuration rather than material (answer C). Conforming is an implant's ability to accommodate the shape and contours of the bony surface, which usually refers to polymethylmethacrylate (PMMA) or some other injected acrylic that solidifies after a short time (answer E).

►► **Answer 3**

Correct answer is B

Bending strength is proportional to the section modulus (answer B). The section modulus (Z) is defined by the equation $Z = \pi D^3/32$, where D is the core diameter. Thus, core diameter has a substantial effect on section modulus[1] (answers D and E are incorrect). Pullout strength is determined more by the screw's outer diameter rather than the inner diameter (answer A is incorrect). Ability to resist translational forces at the termination of screw tightening is determined more by the screw head rather than the screw core (answer C is incorrect).[5]

►► **Answer 4**

Correct answer is C

The *arrow* depicts the *distance* between screw threads, which is known as screw pitch (answers A and B are incorrect). Increasing thread pitch is one strategy to increase the volume of bone between threads, which leads to increased pullout resistance (answer C is correct). Screw pitch is not directly related to insertional torque; the insertional torque can be increased by employing conical-inner-diameter screws (answer D is incorrect). Screw pitch is directly proportional to screw lead, so it determines both interthread bone volume and screw lead (answer E is incorrect). Furthermore, increasing screw pitch is only one strategy to increase interthread volume—other strategies are to increase thread height and to change thread shape.[6,7]

►► **Answer 5**

Correct answer is A

As long as proper technique is used, there is no difference in pullout strength between pretapped non–self-tapping screws and self-tapping screws[8] (answer A). Regarding cortical bone specifically, there is no significant effect on pullout strength with repeated removal and insertion using either screw type (answer B is incorrect). Pretapping cancellous bone weakens the implant–bone interface, but pretapping cortical bone decreases the incidence of microcracks.[9] Thus, pretapping is optimal in cortical bone but is less desirable and controversial in cancellous bone (answers C, D, and E are incorrect).

►► **Answer 6**

Correct answer is D

Both triangulation constructs have been shown to have equal pullout resistance, which is largely determined by the volume of bone (*shaded areas*) between the screw and plate[10,11] (answers A and B are incorrect). Configuration B most effectively resists axial loads that are perpendicular to the long axis of the screws due to optimal counteracting of component vectors (answer D is correct and answers C and E are incorrect).

►► **Answer 7**

Correct answer is D

PMMA can be useful when injected under pressure—only then is it able to fill the interstices of bone to potentially increase the effective diameter of a subsequently placed screw[12,13] (answer D is correct). PMMA does not have osteointegration properties and it does not precisely match the contours of bone—two very important limitations to understand regarding PMMA and other acrylic implants (answers A and E are incorrect). PMMA is unable to precisely match bone contours due to the presence of blood in the field, which can get in between the bone and the implant, as well as the effect of gravity, which can lead to PMMA flowing away from important interface points. PMMA has not been shown to increase screw bending strength (an inherent quality of the screw itself) nor does injecting slowly have any effect on hardening time (answers B and C are incorrect). Furthermore, the beneficial effects of PMMA have only been shown when injected under pressure (answer D).

▸▸ Answer 8

Correct answer is B

Lag screws have three conditions that must be met: (1) the near surface is unthreaded to allow the screw to glide freely through the bone fragment; (2) the far surface is threaded and provides bony purchase; and (3) when the screw is tightened, the head must make contact with the near surface fragment to halt longitudinal progression of the screw, effectively pulling the near fragment along the axis of the screw[14] (answer B is correct). Lag screws must be at least partially or fully threaded to provide some bony purchase (answer A is incorrect). A full-length flute is not required for a lag screw but is an important feature of a tap screw (answer C is incorrect). The screw head of a lag screw should be big enough to halt longitudinal progression of the screw instead of gliding through the near side bone fragment (answer D is incorrect). Technically, a lag screw can be made from any material as long as it exhibits the above-mentioned three conditions—titanium material or osteointegration capability is not a requirement for a lag screw (answer E is incorrect).

▸▸ Answer 9

Correct answer is A

The optimal orientation of a screw for pullout resistance based on the triangulation effect is 90 degree.[15] Thus, this construct would have maximum pullout resistance along a vector that is directed straight upward (answer A). Screws have the least pullout resistance along their long axis or 0 degrees (answers C, D, and E are incorrect). Answer B shows a force vector directed toward the bone that is the opposite of pullout.

▸▸ Answer 10

Correct answer is E

Abutting implants are most effective when they remain in the desired position and migration is minimized or eliminated (answer E). Not only does this minimize the chance of neural impingement and subsequent spinal deformation but also it optimizes the implant's load-bearing capabilities (as long as it is properly and optimally placed). Although it is true that implant subsidence is not desirable, certain implants that are still employed have been cleverly designed to have penetrating components, which limit migration while still limiting the likelihood of subsidence such as keels, spikes, or rigid wire stabilizers (answer A is incorrect). Osteointegration has more to do with implant material rather than bony penetration (answer B is incorrect). Bony penetration does not necessarily lend strength to an implant—that is more dependent on overall shape, size, and the materials used (answer C is incorrect). While it is true that abutting implants with penetrating components are designed to minimize migration and can thus be considered as more stable, it does not completely eliminate the need for additional instrumentation, which usually depends on a multitude of other patient factors (answer D is incorrect).

▸▸ Answer 11

Correct answer is D

Due to the shorter flute, self-tapping screws cannot accommodate all the bone debris that is created (answer D). Self-tapping screws and tap screws can be the same size (answer A is incorrect). Pilot hole diameter is not related to trajectory control and may actually lead to more deviation (answer B is incorrect). Larger pilot hole diameter does not directly lead to increased bony purchase and may actually decrease bony purchase if too much bone is drilled away (answer C is incorrect). Both self-tapping screws and tap screws have a tapered tip by design and the primary difference is the flute length (answer E is incorrect).

▸▸ Answer 12

Correct answer is E

Out of all these screw components, only the screw head has no significant effect on the screw's pullout resistance (answer E). The screw head plays a bigger role in resisting translational forces at the termination of screw tightening. The other screw components listed have a significant effect on pullout resistance and are all variables that are constantly optimized to maximize the pullout resistance of screws.[16,17,18,19]

▸▸ Answer 13

Correct answer is C

Screw length contributes significantly to pullout resistance primarily when they are part of a construct where they are rigidly triangulated, such as in ▶ Fig. 15.5 (answer C). The greater the shaded area under the curve, the greater the pullout resistance of the construct. When rigidly triangulated, longer screws result in a greater shaded area of bone, which translates to increased pullout resistance.[20] Injected PMMA can increase pullout resistance by increasing effective screw diameter and has less of a relation to screw length (answer A is incorrect). Although screw-hook constructs can have considerable pullout resistance thanks to the inherent properties of gripping implants, it has less to do with screw lengths used (answer B is incorrect). Pretapping before screw placement is usually associated with increased pullout strength if utilized appropriately (answer D is incorrect). Screw material has less of an effect on pullout strength but may have a greater effect on osteointegration—one of the reasons why titanium (high biocompatibility) is widely used as the material of choice in modern practice (answer E is incorrect).

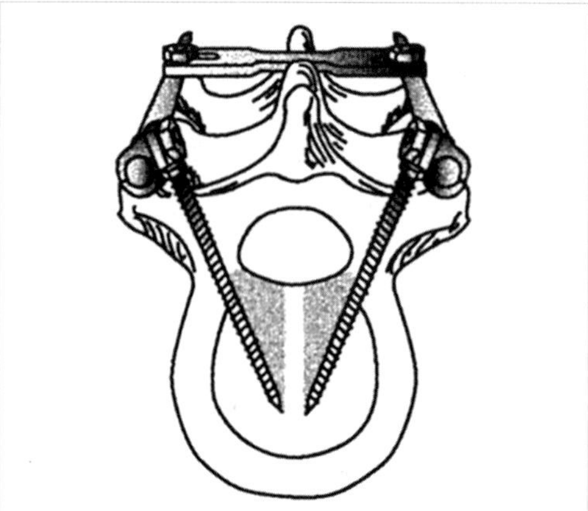

Fig. 15.5 Methods of minimizing screw pullout. Although screw length does not routinely contribute significantly to pullout resistance, it does contribute significantly when screws are rigidly triangulated. Note the increase in the shaded area. Increasing the screw angle (i.e., toe-in) also increases the size of the shaded area and thus pullout resistance. (Source: Data obtained from Bai B, Kummer FJ, Spivak J. Augmentation of anterior vertebral body screw fixation by an injectable, biodegradable calcium phosphate bone substitute. Spine 2001; 26: 2679–2683)

▸▸ Answer 14

Correct answer is B

Commonly used gripping implants such as hooks or wires do indeed have substantial pullout resistance and they derive this property mainly from the fact that they wrap around cortical bones structures such as the lamina or transverse processes, which have considerable cortical bone surfaces for contact[21] (answer B is correct and answer E is incorrect). They are not used in cantilever beam constructs. They are not utilized within the disc space where abutting implants are more commonly used (answer A is incorrect). Gripping implants do not penetrate bone by definition (answer C is incorrect). Ease of deployment is not a major factor in pullout resistance and there are situations where use of hooks or wires could be more challenging[22] (answer D is incorrect).

▸▸ Answer 15

Correct answer is A

Hydroxyapatite coating has been shown to improve osteointegration capability[23,24] (answer A). Matte or peened surfaces have greater osteointegration potential when compared with smooth surfaces (answer B is incorrect). PMMA does not enhance osteointegration and itself does not have osteointegration properties, although, if injected properly under pressure, PMMA can increase pullout resistance (answer C is incorrect). Nails have almost zero pullout resistance and are usually smooth and so they have low osteointegration potential (answer D is incorrect). Large core diameters contribute more to pullout resistance and are unrelated to osteointegration properties (answer E is incorrect).

▸▸ Answer 16

Correct answer is E

Pretapping within cancellous bone actually weakens the implant–bone interface[25,26] (answer E is correct and answers B and C are incorrect). Pretapping is more important in osteoporotic bone as it has been shown to decrease pullout resistance (answer D is incorrect). Pretapping actually decreases the rate of microfractures, although this applies to cortical bone and not to cancellous bone[27] (answer A is incorrect).

▸▸ Answer 17

Correct answer is B

Construct "b" has decreased pullout resistance because the screws are oriented in parallel and the triangulation effect is lost[28] (answer B is correct and answer A is incorrect). Plates, regardless of their length, are not usually intended for osteointegration (answer C is incorrect). Greater screw angulation does not necessarily increase difficulty of insertion; in fact, the longer plate may be more difficult to place due to its larger size (answer D is incorrect). Cost of materials should be considered but should not be the primary driver of clinical decision making; also construct "b" is more likely to have a greater cost since it is larger and requires more material to create (answer E is incorrect).

▸▸ Answer 18

Correct answer is D

Although this equation may be technically true, it can lead to a false sense of security, especially with the advent of conical-inner-diameter screws, which have substantial insertional torque but not necessarily high pullout resistance, which is dependent on other factors (answer D is correct). Pullout resistance is significantly affected by outer diameter and thread design[29,30,31] (answers A and E are incorrect). According to the equation, insertional torque is directly related to pullout resistance (answer B is incorrect). This only describes a mathematical relationship and does not describe a physical relationship that runs in both directions—increasing pullout resistance does not lead to increased insertional torque (answer C is incorrect).

▸▸ Answer 19

Correct answer is E

Compression screw techniques make use of nonfixed moment arm screws to translate an implant in relation to the vertebral body, as noted in ▸ Fig. 15.6 (answer E). (**a**) The compression screw technique uses a teardrop-shaped bed for the head of the screw. (**b**) As the screw is tightened and "snuggles" into the bottom of the bed, the head of the screw shifts the plate, allowing compression to be applied. *Arrows* represent the transition that occurs from a loose screw on the left to a tightened screw on the right. This is in contrast to the triangulation technique, which makes use of a fixed moment arm or rigid triangulation (answer B is incorrect). It does not depend on gripping implants such as hooks/wires nor does it rely on PMMA (answers A and C are incorrect). Unlike abutting implants, compression screw techniques are not primarily designed to bear axial loads but to apply compression forces between the bone and the implant (answer D is incorrect).

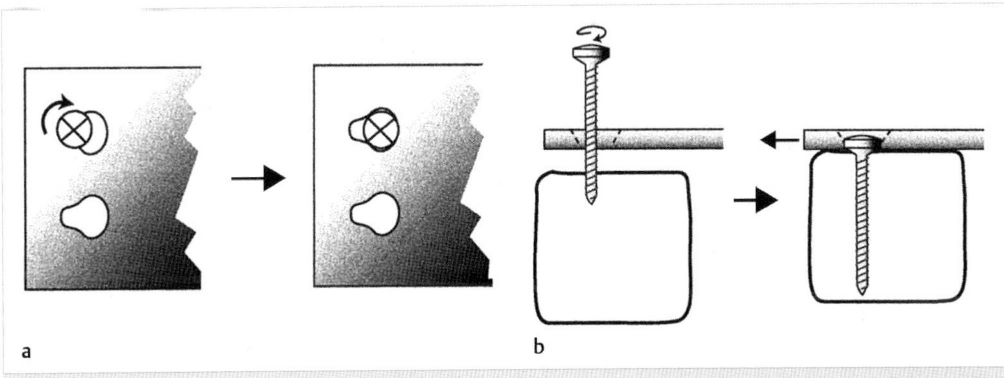

Fig. 15.6 (a) The compression screw technique uses a teardropshaped bed for the head of the screw. **(a, b)** As the screw is tightened and "snuggles" into the bottom of the bed, the head of the screw shifts the plate, allowing compression to be applied. Arrows represent the transition that occurs from a loose screw on the left to a tightened screw on the right. (Source: Biomechanics of Spine Stabilization: Third Edition, © 2015 Thieme Medical Publishers, Inc.)

▸▸ **Answer 20**

Correct answer is C

Of all these answers, only answer C is correct. Bicortical purchase is correlated with increased pullout resistance.[32] All the other answers would actually lead to decreased pullout resistance.

Key Principles

- All spinal implants have strengths and limitations, but screws have become dominant due to flexibility in their design and configurability.
- Pullout resistance is largely dependent on screw outer diameter, thread design, and triangulation.
- Cortical bone is stronger than cancellous bone but it is also more rigid (brittle).
- It is important to understand the force vectors that are present in any given situation—some are desired and should be encouraged, while others are detrimental and should be resisted.
- Ultimate success of implant–bone interfaces depends on a multitude of details and on proper utilization of the tools we have in our arsenal.

References

[1] Grant JP, Oxland TR, Dvorak MF. Mapping the structural properties of the lumbosacral vertebral endplates. Spine 2001;26:889–896

[2] Goodman SB, Davidson JA, Fornasier VL, Mishra AK. Histological response to cylinders of a low modulus titanium alloy (Ti-13Nb-13Zr) and a wear resistant zirconium alloy (Zr-2.5Nb) implanted in the rabbit tibia. J Appl Biomater 1993;4:331–339

[3] Mishra AK, Bucknell AL, Vaughn CM, et al. In vivo study of anodized commercially pure titanium and diffusion hardened Ti-13Nb-13Zr bone plates in a goat model. In: Proceedings of the Fifth World Biomaterials Congress; Toronto, Canada; June 1996:ii–797

[4] Seligson D, Mehta S, Mishra AK, et al. In vivo study of stainless steel and Ti-13Nb-13Zr bone plates in a sheep model. Clin Orthop Relat Res 1997;343:213–223

[5] Russell TA, Taylor JC, LaVelle DG, Beals NB, Brumfield DL, Durham AG. Mechanical characterization of femoral interlocking intramedullary nailing systems. J Orthop Trauma 1991;5:332–340

[6] DeCoster TA, Heetderks DB, Downey DJ, Ferries JS, Jones W. Optimizing bone screw pullout force. J Orthop Trauma 1990;4:169–174

[7] Sell P, Collins M, Dove J. Pedicle screws: axial pull-out strength in the lumbar spine. Spine 1988;13:1075–1076

[8] Foley WL, Frost DE, Tucker MR. The effect of repetitive screw hole use on the retentive strength of pretapped and self-tapped screws. J Oral Maxillofac Surg 1990;48:264–267

[9] Vangsness CT, Carter DR, Frankel VH. In vitro evaluation of the loosening characteristics of self-tapped and non-self-tapped cortical bone screws. Clin Orthop Relat Res 1981;157:279–286

[10] Barber JW, Boden SD, Ganey T, Hutton WC. Biomechanical study of lumbar pedicle screws: does convergence affect axial pullout strength? J Spinal Disord 1998;11:215–220

[11] Leong JCY, Lu WW, Zheng Y, Zhu Q, Zhong S. Comparison of the strengths of lumbosacral fixation achieved with techniques using one and two triangulated sacral screws. Spine 1998;23: 2289–2294

[12] Cohen DB, Cullinane D, Iizuka M, Walk N, Kostuik JP. Biomechanics of pedicle screw augmentation using polymethylmethacrylate. Paper presented at: 15th Annual Meeting of the North American Spine Society; New Orleans, LA; October 25–28, 2000:167.

[13] Wittenberg RH, Lee K-S, Shea M, White AA, Hayes WC. Effect of screw diameter, insertion technique, and bone cement augmentation of pedicular screw fixation strength. Clin Orthop Relat Res 1993;296:278–287

[14] Uhl RL. The biomechanics of screws. Orthop Rev 1989;18:1302–1307

[15] Benzel EC, Baldwin NG. Crossed-screw fixation of the unstable thoracic and lumbar spine. J Neurosurg 1995;82: 11–16

[16] Skinner R, Maybee J, Transfeldt E, Venter R, Chalmers W. Experimental pull-out testing and comparison of variables in transpedicular screw fixation. A biomechanical study. Spine 1990;15:195–201

[17] Krag MH, Beynnon BD, Pope MH, DeCoster TA. Depth of insertion of transpedicular vertebral screws into human vertebrae: effect upon screw-vertebra interface strength. J Spinal Disord 1988;1:287–294

[18] Maiman DJ, Pintar FA, Yoganandan N, et al. Pull-out strength of Caspar cervical screws. Neurosurgery 1992;31:1097–1101; discussion 110.1

[19] Smith SA, Abitbol JJ, Carlson GD, Anderson DR, Taggart KW, Garfin SR. The effects of depth of penetration, screw orientation, and bone density on sacral screw fixation. Spine 1993;18:1006–1010

[20] Ruland CM, McAfee PC, Warden KE, Cunningham BW. Triangulation of pedicular instrumentation. A biomechanical analysis. Spine 1991;16(Suppl):S270–S276

[21] Songer MN, Spencer DL, Meyer PR, Jayaraman G. The use of sublaminar cables to replace Luque wires. Spine 1991; 16(Suppl):S418–S421

[22] Cheung KMC, Luk KDK, Leong JCY. Radiographic assessment of pedicle hook placement. Spine 1997;22:2106–2111

[23] Sandén B, Olerud C, Johansson C, Larsson S. Improved bone-screw interface with hydroxyapatite coating: an in vivo study of loaded pedicle screws in sheep. Spine 2001;26:2673–2678

[24] Hasegawa T, Inufusa A, Imai Y, Mikawa Y, Lim TH, An HS. Hydroxyapatite-coating of pedicle screws improves resistance against pull-out force in the osteoporotic canine lumbar spine model: a pilot study. Spine J 2005;5:239–243

[25] Foley WL, Frost DE, Tucker MR. The effect of repetitive screw hole use on the retentive strength of pretapped and self-tapped screws. J Oral Maxillofac Surg 1990;48:264–267

[26] Misenhimer GR, Peek RD, Wiltse LL, Rothman SLG, Widell EH. Anatomic analysis of pedicle cortical and cancellous diameter as related to screw size. Spine 1989;14:367–372

[27] Vangsness CT, Carter DR, Frankel VH. In vitro evaluation of the loosening characteristics of self-tapped and non-self-tapped cortical bone screws. Clin Orthop Relat Res 1981;157:279–286

[28] Rodríguez-Olaverri JC, Hasharoni A, DeWal H, Nuzzo RM, Kummer FJ, Errico TJ. The effect of end screw orientation on the stability of anterior instrumentation in cyclic lateral bending. Spine J 2005;5:554–557

[29] Lieberman IH, Khazim R, Woodside T. Anterior vertebral body screw pullout testing. A comparison of Zeilke, Kaneda, Universal Spine System, and Universal Spine System with pullout-resistant nut. Spine 1998;23:908–910

[30] Brantley AGU, Mayfield JK, Koeneman JB, Clark KR. The effects of pedicle screw fit. An in vitro study. Spine 1994;19:1752–1758

[31] Wittenberg RH, Lee K-S, Shea M, White AA, Hayes WC. Effect of screw diameter, insertion technique, and bone cement augmentation of pedicular screw fixation strength. Clin Orthop Relat Res 1993;296:278–287

[32] Sell P, Collins M, Dove J. Pedicle screws: axial pull-out strength in the lumbar spine. Spine 1988;13:1075–1076

17 Quantitative Attributes of Spinal Implants

Bradley Schmidt, Garret Greeneway, Daniel Resnick

In order to surgically apply appropriate instrumentation constructs to the spine, it is critical to first have an understanding of the physics of the forces that these constructs have on the overall biomechanics of the spine.

Learning Objectives

- Understand the biomechanics behind how forces affect the spine depending on where they are applied in relation to the instantaneous axis of rotation (IAR).
- Understand the differences between a three-point bending (3PB) construct and a posterior tension band construct.
- Understand the maneuvers that can be performed to help prevent parallelogram-like effect of lateral translational deformation of posterior instrumentation.

Questions

▸▸ Question 1

When a simple compression instrumentation construct is used in the spine, the bending moment that results is _____ to the long access of the spine and is proportional to what?

- A. Parallel; proportional to the distance from the IAR
- B. Perpendicular; proportional to the distance from the facet joints
- C. Parallel; proportional to the distance from the facet joints
- D. Perpendicular; proportional to the distance from the IAR
- E. Perpendicular; proportional to the distance from the anterior longitudinal ligament (ALL)

▸▸ Question 2

Applying a distraction construct can result in no applied bending moment if the construct is placed where?

- A. In-line with the IAR
- B. In-line with the ALL
- C. In-line with the facet joints
- D. In-line with the spinous processes
- E. In-line with the lamino-facet line

▸▸ Question 3

You are seeing a patient with an operative burst fracture. There is retropulsion of bony fragments posteriorly seen on computed tomography (CT) scan. Which of the following spine constructs can decompress the ventral thecal sac through the use of indirect forces biomechanically created by the construct itself?

- A. Posterior tension band construct
- B. Simple distraction construct
- C. 3-point bending construct
- D. Load-sharing cantilever beam construct
- E. Interlaminar spacer construct

▸▸ Question 4

A 3PB construct can be used to correct a ventral deformity located near the end point of a construct by changing which parameter(s) in the bending moment mathematical equation ($M = [D_1 \times D_2 \times F_{3PB}]/D_{3PB}$)?

- A. F_{3PB}
- B. D_1 and D_2
- C. M
- D. D_{3PB}
- E. F_{3PB} and D_{3PB}

▸▸ Question 5

When considering implant placement and construct design, which of the following is true?

- A. The application of an implant so that it never applies (or bears) a load (force) is impossible
- B. Spinal implants can be placed in a way so that they never bear load
- C. Tension band constructs can be placed in a way so that they never bear load
- D. 3PB constructs can be placed in a way so that they never bear load
- E. Cantilever beam constructs can be placed in a way so that they never bear load

▸▸ Question 6

A patient presents with a severe burst fracture that exhibits progressive compression on upright X-ray imaging. A dorsal tension band construct alone ________.

- A. Is appropriate and is not dependent on the length of the construct
- B. Is appropriate but is dependent upon the length of the construct
- C. Is inappropriate because it cannot load share
- D. Is inappropriate because it depends on distance from the IAR
- E. Is inappropriate because burst fractures are stable

▸▸ Question 7

Two of the more common dorsal spine constructs used in surgery are the 3PB construct and the tension band. Regarding the bending moment, what is the key difference between these constructs?

- A. The bending moment applied by the 3PB construct changes in relation to the length of the construct, whereas tension band does not
- B. The bending moment applied by the tension band construct changes in relation to the length of the construct, whereas the 3PB construct does not
- C. The bending moment changes with the length of the construct in both the 3PB and the tension band constructs
- D. The bending moment does not change with the length of the construct in either the 3PB or the tension band constructs
- E. There is no bending moment created by the tension band construct

▸▸ Question 8

Tension band fixation (TBF) constructs can apply extension or flexion forces by what mechanism?

- A. TBF can only apply extension forces
- B. TBF can apply extension if tension band is dorsal to IAR and flexion if tension band is ventral to IAR
- C. TBF can apply extension if tension band is ventral to IAR and flexion if tension band is dorsal to IAR
- D. TBF can only apply flexion forces
- E. TBF applies neither flexion nor extension forces

▸▸ Question 9

TBF and 3PB constructs each generate moment arms as part of their overall construct design. What are the key principles surrounding the moment arms between these two constructs?

- A. Both TBF and 3PB construct moment arms are parallel to the construct/long axis of the spine
- B. Both TBF and 3PB construct moment arms are perpendicular to the construct/long axis of the spine
- C. Both TBF and 3PB construct moment arms are circumferential to the construct/long axis of the spine
- D. TBF construct moment arm is parallel and 3PB construct moment arm is perpendicular to the construct/long axis of the spine
- E. TBF construct moment arm is perpendicular and 3PB construct moment arm is parallel to the construct/long axis of the spine

▸▸ Question 10

Three months ago, you performed a pedicle screw fixation construct on a traumatic spine fracture. You obtain upright X-ray radiographs of the spine to see how the construct is healing after the passage of time. You notice that one of the most rostral screws has fractured right at the interface between the screw and rod. What type of construct was most likely created intraoperatively that resulted in this screw fracture?

- A. 3PB construct
- B. Fixed moment arm cantilever beam
- C. Nonfixed moment arm cantilever beam
- D. TBF
- E. Three-point tension construct

▸▸ Question 11

You are seeing a patient in clinic who was operated on at another institution. You notice on their upright spine X-rays that the rostral most screw has pulled out. Which of the following constructs was likely originally created that led to this construct failure?

- A. Long-segment 3PB construct for fracture dislocation
- B. Fixed moment arm cantilever beam for burst fracture
- C. Nonfixed moment arm cantilever beam for burst fracture
- D. Applied moment arm cantilever beam following pedicle subtraction osteotomy
- E. Three-point tension construct in setting of facet fracture

▸▸ Question 12

A patient presents to the emergency department after a motor vehicle accident with a T5–T6 fracture dislocation requiring surgical fixation. Six months postoperatively, you notice that a parallelogram-like translational deformation has occurred. Which maneuver could have been used intraoperatively to prevent this deformity from occurring?

- A. Toe-in of screws
- B. Toe-out of screws
- C. Toe-up of screws
- D. Toe-down of screws
- E. There is no maneuver that can be done to prevent this

▸▸ Question 13

There are a few maneuvers that can be performed intraoperatively during surgery to prevent parallelogram-like translational deformity formation. Which of the following is one of these techniques?

- A. Shortening the construct
- B. Toe-out of screws
- C. Rigid cross-fixation of the rod on each side to its counterpart
- D. Angling the screws directly parallel to the end plates
- E. There is no maneuver that can be done to prevent this

▸▸ Question 14

You perform a multilevel corpectomy on a patient for severe degenerative spondylotic myelopathy. You utilize a strut graft (bone or cage) and a plate with screws. Which of the following forces does this construct not tolerate well?

- A. Axial loading
- B. Extension
- C. Distraction
- D. Translation
- E. All of these forces are well tolerated via this construct design

▸▸ Question 15

A few days after you have performed a multilevel corpectomy utilizing a plate and screws for trauma, your patient suddenly develops neck pain and new neurologic symptoms including some weakness and numbness/tingling. You obtain a stat CT of the cervical spine. Which of the following do you expect to see on the scan if the problem was translational forces applied to the construct?

- A. Hematoma
- B. Kick-out of strut graft
- C. Screw malalignment
- D. Spinal cord infarction
- E. There will be nothing wrong seen on the scan

▸▸ Question 16

You need to perform a multilevel corpectomy for degenerative spondylotic myelopathy. You are worried about the translational forces that can risk graft kick-out. What technique can be used to help mitigate some of this risk?

- A. Adding an intermediate point of fixation
- B. Removing the plate
- C. Using only one screw per level
- D. Using fixed-angle screws
- E. Using a smaller plate

▸▸ Question 17

A nonfixed moment cantilever beam construct can gain some stability through what mechanism?

- A. Toe-out of screws
- B. Using shorter plates/rods
- C. Pulling the spinal elements into the plate
- D. Pushing the spinal elements away from the plate
- E. It is not possible to gain stability in a nonfixed moment cantilever beam construct

▸▸ **Question 18**

Why is understanding the location of the IAR critical when applying distracting forces with your spine construct?

- A. Distracting forces can result in either extension or flexion depending on where they are applied with respect to the IAR
- B. Distracting forces always result in extension with respect to the IAR
- C. Distracting forces always result in flexion with respect to the IAR
- D. Distracting forces can result in either axial loading or compression depending on where they are applied with respect to the IAR
- E. Distracting forces do not change their impact to the spine construct in regard to the IAR

▸▸ **Question 19**

You are performing a spinal fusion on an obese patient. You are worried about the effect that axial loading will have on the patient's construct once he is upright. What can you do with the construct to help with load bearing?

- A. Place the spinal implant in distraction
- B. Place the spinal implant in compression
- C. Place the spinal implant in extension
- D. Place the spinal implant in flexion
- E. Place the spinal implant in rotation

▸▸ **Question 20**

Why are cantilever beam fixation techniques useful for spine deformity surgery?

- A. Cantilever beam fixation should never be used in deformity surgery
- B. Cantilever beam fixation tolerates translational forces
- C. Cantilever beam fixation does not tolerate axial loading
- D. Cantilever beam fixation does not tolerate extension
- E. Cantilever beam fixation can be applied with either a flexion or extension moment arm

Answers

▸▸ **Answer 1**

Correct answer is D

Force vectors of a compression construct are applied at a finite distance from the IAR. The bending moment that is created from this applied force is proportional to distance of this applied force to the IAR. Additionally, the compressive force will be perpendicular to the long axis of the spine (see ▸ Fig. 17.1). The IAR is typically in the posterior third of the vertebral body and is not in association with the facet joints nor the ALL.

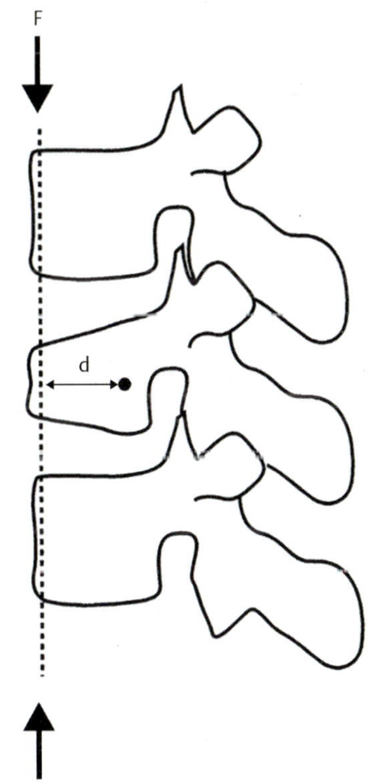

Fig. 17.1 A compressive force (*F*) applied at a finite distance (*d*) from the instantaneous axis of rotation (IAR; dot). (Source: Biomechanics of Spine Stabilization: Third Edition, © 2015 Thieme Medical Publishers, Inc.)

▸▸ Answer 2

Correct answer is A

An isolated distraction construct can be done from within the interbody region. When the interbody device is placed in-line with the IAR, the distraction force is being applied in the region of the neutral axis; therefore, no bending moment is created as there is no perpendicular distance from the IAR to the distracting force.

▸▸ Answer 3

Correct answer is C

3PB constructs typically involve instrumentation of multiple spinal levels. Biomechanically, this creates dorsally directed forces at the upper and lower levels and a ventrally directed force at the midpoint that is equal but opposite to the sum of the two dorsally directed forces. This therefore can be used to decompress the ventral aspect of the thecal sac by distracting the posterior longitudinal ligament. The resultant force pushes the bone and/or disc fragments ventrally and away from the thecal sac.

▸▸ Answer 4

Correct answer is B

In the bending moment equation, D_1 and D_2 are the distances from the fulcrum to the distal hardware/bone interfaces. D_{3PB} is the total distance of the construct (sum of D_1 and D_2). F_{3PB} is the ventrally directed force at the fulcrum of the construct (see ▸ Fig. 17.2). In a relatively even/centered construct, D_1 and D_2 will be roughly equivalent. This increases the bending moment. If one shortens D_1 and lengthens D_2, then the fulcrum of the construct moves toward the terminus nearest to D_1. This will then bring the ventrally directed force toward the terminus of the construct as well, which in turn will allow for a sagittal deformity correct at the terminus of the construct. Of note, in shortening D_1 and lengthening D_2, this will inherently lessen the bending moment mathematically, which should be taken into consideration during surgery.

▸▸ Answer 5

Correct answer is A

During the time of surgery, spinal implants can be placed in a neutral mode. This means that at the time of surgery, they apply no forces to the spinal column. However, as the patient is moved out of this surgical position, the implant will resist forces (to some degree) in all planes. Therefore, depending on the situation, the implant may act as a distraction device, tension band, cantilever beam, etc. Ultimately, the forces applied to an implant will vary depending on loading conditions.

▸▸ Answer 6

Correct answer is C

In the case described here, a tension band construct would not be ideal for the patient's surgical fixation. This is primarily because tension band

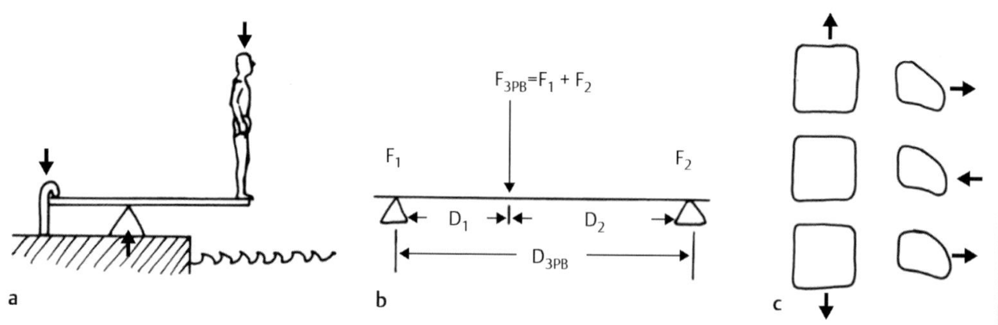

Fig. 17.2 (a) The force vectors at work when a person is standing on the end of a springboard. **(b)** These three-point bending forces are defined by Equation 1, $M = (D_1 \times D_2 \times F_3PB)/D_3PB$, in which D_1 and D_2 are the distances from the fulcrum to the terminal hook–bone interfaces, D_3PB is the sum of D_1 and D_2, and F_3PB is the ventrally directed force applied at the fulcrum. **(c)** Spinal three-point bending constructs (*horizontal arrows*) are usually applied in combination with another force vector complex—commonly, distraction (*vertical arrows*). (Source: Biomechanics of Spine Stabilization: Third Edition, © 2015 Thieme Medical Publishers, Inc.)

constructs cannot share axial load bearing. Therefore, in this patient with obvious load-bearing fracture instability (worsening of burst fracture on upright X-ray), the tension band would not properly support this instability. The surgeon should restore axial load-bearing ability through other means (dorsal tension band construct plus ventral corpectomy and interbody graft, use of a long-segment 3PB construct, use of a fixed moment cantilever beam construct, etc.). Not all burst fractures require surgery but evidence of instability on upright films would be an indication for fixation.[1]

▸▸ Answer 7

Correct answer is A

The bending moment applied by a 3PB construct is directly proportional to the length of the created construct, whereas the bending moment created by a tension band construct is independent of construct length and is only related to the distance of the tension band forces from the IAR.

▸▸ Answer 8

Correct answer is B

Dorsal spinal compression through TBF applies spinal compression forces at dorsal sites. This is the classic representation of a tension band. Since the compression is dorsal to the IAR, this results in extension forces being applied to the spinal column. However, ventral TBF constructs can also be created. For instance, a ventral cervical plate can act as a ventral TBF construct. This is due to the plate acting as a compression device, which is located ventral to the IAR. Therefore, it resists extension of the motion segment when the spine is extended. This can therefore exert flexion forces on the spinal column.

▸▸ Answer 9

Correct answer is E

The bending moment arms of TBF and 3PB constructs are not equivalent in regard to their direction. Specifically, the moment arm created by a TBF construct is perpendicular to the construct itself and the long axis of the spine, whereas the moment arm created by a 3PB construct is parallel to the construct itself and the long axis of the spine.

▸▸ Answer 10

Correct answer is B

A cantilever beam construct involves a beam that is affixed/supported at only one end. This can be represented by a screw that is affixed within the pedicle or a rigid plate construct. When first placed, these constructs bear no load. However, as the patient becomes upright, an axial load is inherently placed onto the system. This results in a significant stress placed onto the cantilever beam. The area of highest risk to feel this stress is at the screw–rod interface. As a result, if too much stress is ultimately applied, a screw fracture may occur at the interface between the rod and screw. Nonfixed moment arm cantilever beam constructs without adequate load-bearing support, 3PB constructs, and tension band constructs usually fail through screw pullout.

▸▸ Answer 11

Correct answer is C

Nonfixed moment cantilever beam constructs are represented by a beam that is affixed to a wall via a hinge. This construct therefore requires an accompanying ventral force vector that would oppose the hinge mechanism in an axial loading situation. If a pedicle screw or lateral mass screw is placed without sufficient ventral hold of the screw or if there is insufficient ventral support through other means (interbody cage or similar construct), then in the setting of an axial load, the nonfixed moment cantilever beam construct is insufficient to alone support this upright posture/axial load. This then can unfortunately result in screw pullout.

▸▸ Answer 12

Correct answer is A

Pedicle screw fixation constructs may fail to bear axial loads well due to a parallelogram-like translational deformation that can occur. Toe-in of the screws can prevent this type of construct failure. Biomechanical studies have been performed that demonstrate that the closer the pedicle-to-pedicle angle is to zero degrees, the less likely the construct will resist these internal forces.[2] Toe-out, toe-up, and toe-down of screws would not increase pullout strength of the screw constructs nor do they resist the parallelogram-like translational deformation.

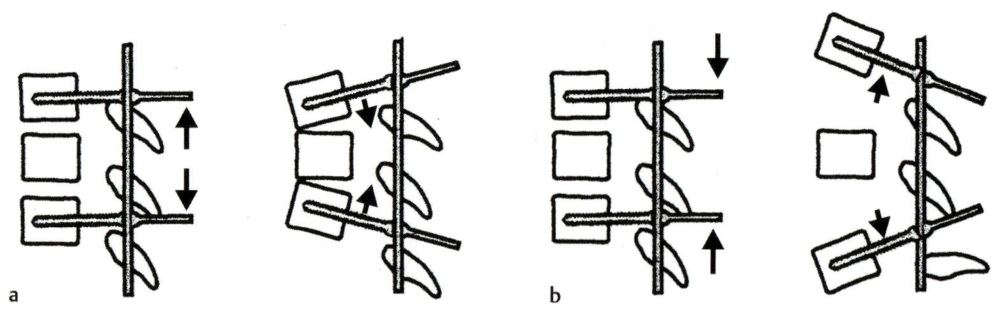

Fig. 17.6 (a) Applied moment arm cantilever beam construct in which a flexion moment is used. (b) Applied moment arm cantilever beam construct in which an extension moment is used. (Source: Biomechanics of Spine Stabilization: Third Edition, © 2015 Thieme Medical Publishers, Inc.)

▸▸ **Answer 20**

Correct answer is E

Cantilever beam fixation can be applied with either a flexion or extension moment arm. Depending on the deformity, inducing either flexion or extension can correct alignment and result in better patient outcomes. Cantilever beam fixation is typically rigid enough to accommodate these moment arms; however, one does have to be cautious not to exert too many stressors on the hardware or the bone, as this may result in implant/hardware failure (see ▸ Fig. 17.6).

Key Principles

- When utilizing spinal implants, the biomechanics of how the construct responds to external stressors (axial loading, translational forces, flexion/extension, etc.) is arguably as important as deciding who to operate on.
- Posterior TBF decreases its effectiveness with increased construct length, whereas 3PB construct increases its effectiveness with increased construct length.
- Cantilever beam constructs are useful for inducing flexion or extension and can therefore be useful in deformity correction.

References

[1] Lee JY, Vaccaro AR, Lim MR, et al. Thoracolumbar injury classification and severity score: a new paradigm for the treatment of thoracolumbar spine trauma. J Orthop Sci 2005;10(6):671–675

[2] Carson WL, Duffield RC, Arendt M, Ridgely BJ, Gaines RW. Internal forces and moments in transpedicular spine instrumentation. The effect of pedicle screw angle and transfixation—the 4R–4 bar linkage concept. Spine 1990;15:893–901

18 Construct Design

Megan Finneran, Paul M. Arnold

Understanding how to design a construct is an essential part of preoperative planning. There are several concepts to consider when creating a construct to maximize stabilization and fusion success.

Learning Objectives

- Understand how to formulate a blueprint for construct design.
- Understand the strengths, weaknesses, and indications for each type of implant component.
- Understand the balance of short- versus long-segment fixation.
- Understand the concept of load sharing.

Questions

▸▸ Question 1

Which of the following defines the term construct design?

- A. The combination of the implant and the portion of the spine to which it is attached
- B. An inserted device that is used to minimize or eliminate spinal segmental motion
- C. An implant that, via component–component attachments, can maintain its shape without assistance from the structure of the spine
- D. Making a blueprint
- E. The act of crafting an operative instrumentation plan for a case-specific instability problem

▸▸ Question 2

When should a lateral view be utilized as a component of the blueprint?

- A. For every fusion case
- B. Spondylolisthesis requiring posterolateral implant and pedicle screws
- C. Kyphotic deformity
- D. Fusion involving five levels or more
- E. Fusion crossing thoracolumbar junction

▸▸ Question 3

What construct type should be applied when addressing the convex side of a scoliotic deformity?

- A. Short fixed moment arm cantilever beam fixation
- B. Short nonfixed moment arm cantilever beam fixation
- C. Distraction fixation
- D. Tension-band fixation
- E. Neutral fixation

▸▸ Question 4

What are the three main components to consider when choosing a spinal implant?

- A. Anchor, longitudinal member, and cross member
- B. Cross member, screw type, and longitudinal member
- C. Longitudinal member, rod length, and cross member
- D. Anchor, longitudinal member, and sagittal balance
- E. Segment stability, anchor, and cross member

▸▸ Question 5

What is the most conventional orientation for a blueprint?

- A. Anterior–posterior, left side of drawing portrays right side of patient
- B. Anterior–posterior, left side of drawing portrays left side of patient
- C. Lateral, left side of drawing portrays anterior portion of patient
- D. Lateral, left side of drawing portrays posterior portion of patient
- E. Anterior–posterior and lateral views

▸▸ **Question 6**

What is the first label that should be added on the blueprint?

- A. Pedicle location
- B. Type of implant component
- C. Direction of axial load application
- D. Level of pathology
- E. Lower limit of construct

▸▸ **Question 7**

A patient has a T12–L1 translational deformity; the adjacent superior disc space is disrupted but the inferior is intact. What levels would be included in a 3A-2B plan?

- A. T10–L3
- B. T9–L3
- C. T10–L2
- D. T11–L2
- E. T11–L3

▸▸ **Question 8**

What is the general approach for construct design in an osteoporotic patient?

- A. Favor the use of hooks and sublaminar wires
- B. Increase construct length to an extra level above and below
- C. Use two rods on each side to maximize longitudinal member strength
- D. Use as few points of fixation as possible to minimize incision length
- E. Cross fixation between screws above and below the level of pathology

▸▸ **Question 9**

Which of the following would create a construct with approximately equal length above and below an unstable fracture at T8 with disruption of both adjacent disc spaces?

- A. T5–T10 pedicle screw fixation
- B. T5–T10 wire fixation
- C. T6–T10 hook fixation
- D. T6–T11 wire fixation
- E. T6–T11 pedicle screw fixation

▸▸ **Question 10**

For a T9–L3 pedicle screw fixation for a T12 fracture that extends into the T12 pedicle, where should cross members be placed?

- A. One cross member connecting the T11 screws
- B. One cross member connecting the L1 screws
- C. Three cross members at T9, L1, and L3
- D. Two cross members at T9 and L3
- E. Two cross members at T11 and L1

▸▸ **Question 11**

What type of load bearing is preferable when the sacrum is the terminal end of the construct?

- A. Simple distraction
- B. Three-point bending
- C. Tension-band fixation
- D. Fixed moment arm cantilever beam fixation
- E. Nonfixed moment arm cantilever beam fixation

▸▸ **Question 12**

What is a contraindication for a dorsal tension-band fixation construct?

- A. Fracture across a junctional segment
- B. Inability to place pedicle screws
- C. Ventral compressive lesion that cannot be accessed
- D. Scoliotic deformity
- E. Osteoporotic bone quality

▸▸ **Question 13**

Under what circumstances may screws be considered as the most appropriate anchor for a long construct in which an instrumentation–fusion mismatch is anticipated?

- A. A 45-year-old woman with metastatic lung cancer
- B. A 70-year-old woman with osteoporosis
- C. A 60-year-old man with ankylosing spondylitis
- D. A 19-year-old man with a Chance fracture after a motor vehicle accident
- E. A 30-year-old woman with a burst fracture causing retropulsion

▸▸ Question 14

In a T9–L3 construct with a cage implant at T12 and bilateral rods, which of the following fixation points is most likely to fail?
- A. T9
- B. T10
- C. T11
- D. L2
- E. L3

▸▸ Question 15

How can the orientation of hooks diminish a kyphotic deformity?
- A. Superior hook aimed superiorly, inferior hook aimed inferiorly
- B. Superior hooked aimed superiorly, inferior hook aimed superiorly
- C. Superior hook aimed inferiorly, inferior hook aimed inferiorly
- D. Superior hook aimed inferiorly, inferior hook aimed superiorly
- E. Superior hook–claw complex, inferior hook aimed inferiorly

▸▸ Question 16

What is a potential disadvantage of cross fixation that must be considered?
- A. Increased back pain
- B. Increased risk for infection
- C. Increased blood loss
- D. Increased risk of hook–bone interface failure
- E. Increased torsional deformation of rods

▸▸ Question 17

Which of the following is most vulnerable to pivoting bending moments?
- A. Short construct of hooks in compression mode
- B. Short construct of fixed-head pedicle screws
- C. Short construct of polyaxial pedicle screws
- D. Long construct of hooks in distraction mode
- E. Long construct of fixed-head pedicle screws

▸▸ Question 18

How does the use of a screw as the point of attachment allow for a shorter construct than hooks?
- A. Screws allow a greater range of choice for trajectory of the screw through the vertebral body
- B. The placement of a screw through the pedicle positions the screw in the lower half of the vertebral body
- C. Pedicle screws are more expensive, encouraging use of less instrumentation
- D. Screws require less exposure for placement than hooks
- E. Pedicle screws have greater rigidity of fixation than hooks

▸▸ Question 19

What kind of construct should be considered in a 40-year-old with an L2 fracture causing significant comminution of the vertebral body?
- A. Pedicle screw fixation one level above and one level below the fracture
- B. Interbody load-bearing strut
- C. Thoracic–lumbar–sacral orthosis
- D. L2 laminectomy to decompress the segment
- E. Hook fixation two levels above and two levels below

▸▸ Question 20

Which of the following is best managed by a long fixation construct?
- A. Traumatic L2 fracture with 4 mm of translational deformity
- B. T12 compression fracture with 1 mm of retropulsion
- C. L1 compression fracture with no retropulsion in the setting of osteoporosis
- D. L4–L5 spondylolisthesis causing radiculopathy
- E. Traumatic L3 fracture with significant comminution

Answers

▸▸ Answer 1

Correct answer is E

Answer choice E is the definition of construct design. A is the definition of construct, but not of construct design. B is the definition of an implant. C is the definition of an implant assembly. While D, making a blueprint, is a part of construct design, there is more to the concept that just outlining a blueprint.

▸▸ Answer 2

Correct answer is C

In general, a lateral view is not utilized for a blueprint. An anterior–posterior view is sufficient because it allows planning for both the left and right sides. The only time a lateral view should be encouraged is in cases of sagittal deformity or when both dorsal and ventral implants are needed. The lateral view allows demarcation of a plan in these cases that cannot be well-labeled on an anterior–posterior view. Of the answer choices, only a kyphotic deformity would benefit from inclusion of a lateral view on the blueprint due to its sagittal deformity. The other answer choices could be well-addressed with an anterior–posterior view only.

▸▸ Answer 3

Correct answer is D

The lateral bending of a scoliotic deformity requires addressing the concave and convex sides of the curve differently. Distraction fixation should be applied to the concave side (C), not the convex side. Compression fixation should be applied to the convex side in order to address the deformity. The mechanism of tension-band fixation is compression. Neutral fixation (E) will not correct the deformity. A short construct (choices A, B) should not be utilized to adequately address a scoliotic deformity.

▸▸ Answer 4

Correct answer is A

The main components are anchor (wire, hook, or screw), longitudinal member (rod or plate), and cross member (mechanism of cross fixation). B is incorrect because it specifies screw, instead of the broader possibility for anchor alternatives of wire or hook that should be part of the plan. C is incorrect because it omits the anchor and, while rod length will be a consideration intraoperatively, it is not an essential part of the preoperative planning. D is incorrect because it does not include cross member; while sagittal balance is an important consideration, this is not a main component for planning. E is incorrect because it omits longitudinal member; segment stability is part of the overall planning process when creating a construct design.

▸▸ Answer 5

Correct answer is B

An anterior–posterior drawing is the most conventional orientation, with the left side of the drawing portraying the left side of the patient because it aligns with the patient as viewed from behind. An operation performed in the prone position is the most common surgical approach, and thus the blueprint alignment reduces the chance of confusion. A is incorrect because it aligns with a patient in the supine position. C and D are incorrect because a lateral drawing does not show both the left and right sides of the spine, which may require differences in anchor choice and trajectory. E is incorrect; both views are only necessary when a sagittal plane deformity is to be addressed or both dorsal and ventral implants are be utilized.

▸▸ Answer 6

Correct answer is D

The level of pathology should be the first label represented on a blueprint because the plan will center around it. The location of the pedicle does not need to be identified on the blueprint (A). The type of implant component (B) and direction of load (C) should be included, but this information should be added after the pathology is identified. The upper and lower limits of the construct (E) should be represented, but they will depend on the level of the pathology.

▸▸ Answer 7

Correct answer is C

The first step in making a blueprint is identifying the level(s) of pathology. In this case, it is important to identify that the superior disc space, but not inferior, is disrupted. 3A-2B delineates a plan three levels above the pathology and two levels below it. This yields a plan from T10–L2 (option C). If, however, an unstable fracture occurs with disruption of the disc space above and below the vertebral body, the level of pathology includes the L1 vertebral body and inferior disc space, thus changing a 3A-2B plan to include T10–L3 instead of L2 (A). Answer choice B, in this case, would represent a 4A-3B plan, D would represent a 2A-2B, and E would represent a 2A-3B. A 3A–2B construct extends from T10 to L2. T10 is three segments above the T12–L1 disc interspace, and L2 is two segments below this interspace.

▸▸ **Answer 8**

Correct answer is A

Osteoporosis causes decreased bone quality and therefore decreased integrity of the implant–bone interface. Answer choice A is correct; hooks and sublaminar wires are favored because they resist pullout better than screws. This occurs because hooks and wires apply forces at a distance from the instantaneous axis of rotation. Multiple anchors should be used in an attempt to distribute and share the load between all components of the construct to decrease risk of failure (D is incorrect). While an increased construct length by an extra level above and below the level of pathology (B) may be advantageous, the strength of hooks and wires over screws is the most important concept. The increase of extra rods (C) and cross fixation (E) also may provide extra support but ultimately the choice of anchor is the most important to resist pullout.

▸▸ **Answer 9**

Correct answer is B

It is important to understand the difference between pedicle screws and wire/hook placement when planning a construct length. When using pedicle screws, an equal number of levels above and below the level of pathology will translate to an equal length of the construct above and below the pathology (choice A represents three above/two below and choice E represents two above/three below). However, when using wires or hooks, an additional level above the level of pathology must be added due to its caudal placement in order to create an equal construct (choice C represents two above/three below and choice D represents three above/three below). The attachment points for wires and hooks are at the caudal portion of the segment unlike for pedicle screws which are positioned at the upper half of the vertebral body.

▸▸ **Answer 10**

Correct answer is E

When using cross fixation, the most benefit is yielded by using two cross links approximately one-third from the top of the construct and one-third from the bottom. Two members are better than one (choices A and B are incorrect), and there is no added advantage from an additional cross member (choice C is incorrect). Choice D is incorrect because cross members should not be at the terminal ends of the segment.

▸▸ **Answer 11**

Correct answer is D

When the level of pathology is near the occiput or sacrum, there is less leverage applied by the terminus of the implant because a short lever arm is applied. That being said, a rigid implant–bone interface is preferable to maximize the strength of the implant. The most rigid interface is a fixed moment arm cantilever, which is less prone to failure from translation. Distraction (A) is best applied in pathology when height needs to be restored. Three-point bending (B) is best utilized over a long segment, which is not an option when pathology is close to the sacrum. Tension-band fixation (C) applies compressive forces to correct deformity. Nonfixed moment arm cantilever beam fixation (E) allows the angle of fixation to change and is less rigid than fixed.

▸▸ **Answer 12**

Correct answer is C

Tension-band fixation applies compressive forces to the spine. The dural sac must be adequately decompressed prior to the application of compressive forces that could worsen any existing neural impingement (C is correct). A fracture across a junctional segment (A), once any neural compromise is addressed, is not a contraindication. Inability to place pedicle screws is a challenge that can be overcome by using a different anchor

(B is incorrect). A scoliotic deformity could be well treated by tension-band fixation on the convex side (D is incorrect). Osteoporosis poses challenges to the surgeon with optimizing anchor strength, but tension-band fixation is not contraindicated (E).

▸▸ Answer 13

Correct answer is A

An instrumentation–fusion mismatch is a discrepancy between the number of levels of the spine instrumented and the number of levels actually fused. In general, it should be avoided when possible due to the risk of implant failure. When the mismatch does exist, some movement at the implant–bone interfaces of the instrumented but unfused levels is required to avoid failure. The rigidity of screws does not allow movement; when movement occurs, pullout of the screws occurs. Therefore, hooks and wires are more favorable in cases when mismatch cannot be avoided. The one exception to this concept is in patients with a limited life expectancy, in which screws can provide a short-term reliable fixation. Of the answer choices, A is the one with metastatic malignancy and inherently a short life expectancy.

▸▸ Answer 14

Correct answer is A

With a long construct, the rostral fixation points most commonly fail (A is correct). This is particularly true if the lever arm is shorter rostrally than caudally. The inferior (E) and middle (B, C, and D) points of contact are less likely to fail due to decreased tension on those points of fixation.

▸▸ Answer 15

Correct answer is D

The orientation of hooks can apply a distraction or compression force. A superior hook aimed inferiorly and an inferior hook aimed superiorly will work together to apply a compressive force, which will in turn diminish a kyphotic deformity (D is correct; see ▸ Fig. 18.1, image **c**). A superior hook aimed superiorly and an inferior hook applied inferiorly (choice A; image **b**) will apply a distraction force, which will increase the kyphotic deformity. Hooks aimed in the same direction will apply a neutral force (choices B, C). E is incorrect because aiming the inferior hook inferiorly will exaggerate a kyphotic deformity.

▸▸ Answer 16

Correct answer is B

Use of cross fixation can create dead space and thus increase the risk for infection (B is correct). Use of cross fixation does not increase back pain (A), and one study actually showed the use of cross links decreased back pain.[1] Cross fixation decreases, not increases, risk of hook–bone interface failure (D) and torsional deformation of rods (E) because all anchor points are rigidly interconnected. For the system to fail at the implant–bone

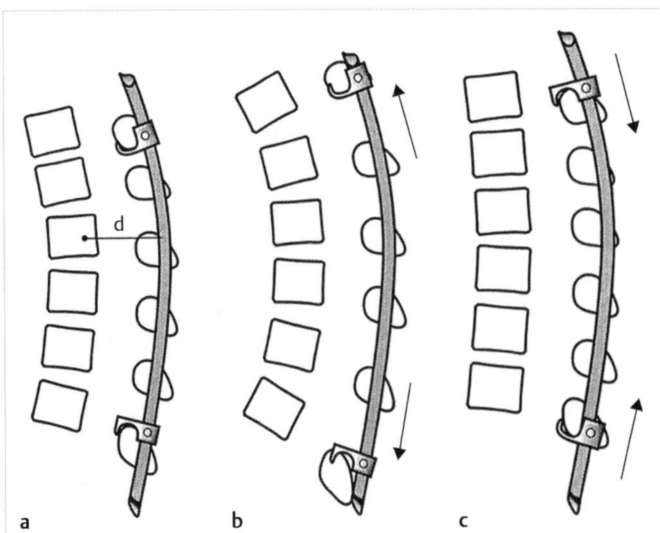

Fig. 18.1 (a) Applying a distraction with hooks along a kyphosis may exaggerate **(b)** the kyphosis. This is due to the application of a bending moment related (and proportional) to the length of the moment arm (*d*). **(c)** Conversely, applying a compression with hooks diminishes the kyphosis. (Source: Biomechanics of Spine Stabilization: Third Edition, © 2015 Thieme Medical Publishers, Inc.)

interface in the setting of cross fixation, multiple anchors would have to simultaneously fail. Cross fixation does not have any influence on blood loss (C).

▸▸ Answer 17

Correct answer is C

Longer constructs with more points of fixation are less vulnerable to pivoting bending moments. Fixed-head screws also eliminate pivoting bending moments as the fixed head does not allow movement of longitudinal segment. Therefore, the most vulnerable construct is a short one with polyaxial screws (C is correct). Choice A is incorrect because hooks in compression mode allow the spine and construct to share the axial load. Choice B is incorrect because fixed-head screws are able to resist pivoting. Choices D and E are incorrect because they are long constructs.

▸▸ Answer 18

Correct answer is E

It is true that pedicle screws have greater rigidity than hooks (E is correct), which in turn allows for a shorter construct. While it is true that the trajectory of a screw can vary (A), this does not influence the strength of screws over hooks. B is incorrect because the placement of a screw through the pedicle positions the screw in the upper part of the vertebral body, not the lower. While pedicle screws may be more expensive than hooks (C), this does not influence the decision making of the length of construct. Pedicle screws and hooks require an approximately equal width of exposure to place (D is incorrect), and this does not influence length of construct.

▸▸ Answer 19

Correct answer is B

When the vertebral body sustains a comminuted fracture, the dispersion of bone fragments diminishes the ability to heal due to soft tissues barriers that interfere. A corpectomy to remove the comminuted bone fragments with insertion of a load-bearing strut is the best option to promote healing (B is correct). Simple posterior fixation with pedicle screws (A) or hooks (E) could be used to create a robust posterior fusion, but the vertebral body may not be able to adequately bear an axial load. A laminectomy would not address the instability (D). The fracture is unlikely to heal without surgical intervention, so a brace (C) would not be adequate, particularly in a young patient.

▸▸ Answer 20

Correct answer is A

As a general principle, a shorter construct is favored whenever possible to avoid an instrumentation–fusion mismatch. One example that does require a long fixation is a posttraumatic fracture with more than 3 or 4 mm of translation deformity (A is correct and B is incorrect). A compression fracture without retropulsion in an osteoporotic patient would likely benefit most from a more conservative approach such as a kyphoplasty (C is incorrect). A one-level spondylolisthesis would likely benefit from a short construct (D is incorrect). A traumatic fracture with comminution would likely require an interbody strut (E is incorrect).

Key Principles

- Main principles of construct design include choice of implant construct, mode of application of the implant, and mechanism of load bearing.
- Construct design can be organized using a blueprint to identify the level of pathology, the levels of fusion, and the type of implants.
- Construct design should be catered to best address the patient's pathology.

Reference

[1] Mirzaei F, Iranmehr A, Shokouhi G, et al. The role of cross-link augmentation on fusion rate and patient satisfaction among patients with traumatic thoracolumbar spinal fracture: a randomized clinical trial. Neurocirugia (Astur: Engl Ed) 2022;33(3):105–110

19 Construct Failure and Prevention

Fabian Carballo Madrigal, Maxwell Boakye

Understanding why spinal implants fail is essential to successful spinal surgery practice. There are fundamental principles that can guide our approach to stabilizing the spinal column with an implant.

Learning Objectives

- Understand why and how implants fail.
- Understand the relationship between stress, bending moment, and section modulus.
- Understand how cantilever beam constructs (fixed moment arm vs nonfixed moment arm) differ in how and where forces are applied and how they behave when forces are applied.
- Understand how the stability of constructs can be improved.

Questions

▸▸ Question 1

It is important to understand the mechanisms that can cause the failure of spinal constructs. Which of the following is a likely cause of construct failure? Select the best answer.

- A. Addition of intermediate points of fixation
- B. Use of cobalt chrome implant
- C. Failure of the component–component interface
- D. Utilization of a rigid postoperative orthosis
- E. Use of polyetheretherketone (PEEK) implant

▸▸ Question 2

Understanding why and how implants fail is fundamental knowledge essential to successful spine surgery practice. Implants most likely fail at which of the following locations?

- A. At the point of maximum stress application
- B. At the location where a PEEK implant is inserted
- C. At the rostral screw location in rigid multisegmental constructs
- D. At intermediate points of fixation
- E. At the location of the highest section modulus

▸▸ Question 3

In the equation $\theta = M / Z$, what does Z represent?

- A. Section modulus
- B. Loading force
- C. Bending moment
- D. Torque
- E. Momentum

▸▸ Question 4

The section modulus is proportional to what?

- A. Third power of the outer diameter of a screw
- B. Second power of the outer diameter of a screw
- C. Third power of the inner diameter of a screw
- D. Second power of the diameter of the rod
- E. Fifth power of inner diameter of a screw

▸▸ Question 5

A 68-year-old woman has degenerative scoliosis with L2–L5 spondylolisthesis and stenosis that requires multilevel fusion. Her past history is significant for type 2 diabetes, hypertension, hypothyroidism, and Crohn's disease. The patient is on a hydrochlorothiazide diuretic and metoprolol for hypertension. Which of the following other chronic preoperative medications puts the patient at greatest risk for pseudoarthrosis and implant failure based on best peer-reviewed evidence?

- A. Metformin
- B. Humira
- C. Prednisone
- D. Gabapentin
- E. Synthroid

▸▸ Question 6

It is important to understand the differences between fixed moment arm and nonfixed moment arm cantilever beam constructs. Also, it is important to know the difference between the strength and stress characteristics of fixed inner diameter versus tapered inner diameter screws and their responses to bending moments.

With fixed moment arm constructs, screws are rigidly affixed to the plate or rod. With nonfixed moment arm cantilever beam constructs, screws may toggle in relation to the plate. Nonfixed moment arm cantilever beam screws are often exposed to forces very different from those applied to their fixed moment arm counterparts. It is important to understand where these implants differ in response to stress. This question also tests understanding of the graphical relationship between stress and the amount of bending moments at various distances from the tip of screws.

Which of the following is the best statement regarding fixed moment arm and nonfixed moment arm cantilever beam constructs?

- A. A fixed moment arm cantilever beam screw–plate construct with fixed inner diameter screw is more likely to fracture at the screw–plate junction
- B. Regarding the fixed moment arm cantilever beam with a fixed inner diameter screw, the bending moment rises exponentially with distance from the screw tip
- C. Regarding the fixed moment arm cantilever beam with a tapered inner diameter screw, the maximum stress is at the proximal screw
- D. Regarding the fixed moment arm cantilever beam with a tapered inner diameter screw, the bending moment rises exponentially with distance from the tip of the screw
- E. Regarding the nonfixed moment arm cantilever beam screws, the screws see the same force vectors (both in magnitude and direction) at various points along the screw

▸▸ Question 7

The "windshield-wiping" effect refers to what phenomenon? Select the best answer.

- A. Failure of constructs due to use of variable screws in traumatic spine fracture
- B. Bone degradation by toggling ventral nonfixed moment arm cantilever beam screws
- C. Screw loosening due to fixed-angle screws in osteoporotic spine
- D. Screw motion when a screw is placed through the bone graft
- E. Windshield-like motion of screws due to bicortical placed screws

▸▸ Question 8

Which of the following statements is correct regarding the strength characteristics of plates?

- A. Unlike the equation governing stress applied to screws, the strength a plate sees is governed by the equation $\theta = M/Z^2$
- B. The section modulus of a plate is a function of the cross-sectional area
- C. The strength of a plate is proportional to its bulkiness
- D. Plates break at intermediate points of fixation.
- E. Plates fractures at the point where the modulus is the greatest

▸▸ Question 9

It is important to understand the failure points of long segmental constructs and choose appropriate strategies to prevent failure at these points. Long fixed moment arm multisegmental constructs, e.g., T10–L5 pedicle instrumentation, tend to fail at what location?

- A. The most rostral screws
- B. The most caudal screws
- C. Screws in the middle of the construct
- D. Multiple locations
- E. None of the above

▸▸ Question 10

Which of the following is an excellent strategy to minimize multilevel implant failure in a 65-year-old woman with degenerative spondylolisthesis and scoliosis?

- A. Ensuring vitamin D_3 level is greater than 5 ng/mL
- B. Ensuring computed tomography (CT) scan (Hounsfield unit $\leq$ 75)
- C. Postconstruct pelvic tilt (PT) of 18, sagittal vertical axis (SVA) of 3.5 cm, and pelvic incidence–lumbar lordosis (PI-LL) mismatch of 9
- D. Using fruit- and nicotine-flavored vaping instead of cigarettes
- E. Use of hybrid constructs, including artificial discs with fusion

▸▸ Question 11

Regarding optimization of the implant–bone interface to minimize failure of multilevel cervicothoracic fusion constructs, which of the following strategies is best?
- A. Triangulation of screws
- B. Aim for postoperative T1 slope < 50
- C. Aiming for C2-SVA < 6 cm
- D. Adding intermediate fixation points to graft
- E. Ensuring DEXA T-score is less than −3.5

▸▸ Question 12

Axially dynamic implants ________.
- A. Rarely fracture.
- B. Bear axial loads, causing frequent fractures
- C. Are poor at resisting translation
- D. Are poor at resisting angulation
- E. Frequently fracture due to flexion forces

▸▸ Question 13

Which of the following statements regarding the benefits of additional points of fixation is correct?
- A. Additional points of fixation reduce load sharing
- B. Additional points of fixation reduce resistance to translation via a three-point bending mechanism
- C. Additional fixation points increase resistance to rotational forces
- D. Additional fixation points increase the implant's section modulus and reduce the implant's stress
- E. The integrity of fixation is independent of the number of high-quality fixation points

▸▸ Question 14

Regarding long bridging implants constructs used in multilevel corpectomies, select the best statement.
- A. They resist translational loads better than axial loads
- B. They are strengthened by adding intermediate fixation points through the native spine
- C. Anterior plating prevents graft loading in extension
- D. They are strengthened by adding an intermediate fixation point to the graft
- E. They are especially stable in the osteoporotic spine due to subsidence

▸▸ Question 15

Select the best statement regarding ventral multilevel fusions.
- A. Multilevel discectomies with fusion without an implant are associated with similar pseudoarthrosis failure rates than instrumented multilevel discectomies with fusion
- B. Using modern technology, careful crafting and optimization of the implant on the vertebral body is no longer necessary
- C. A three-level corpectomy with strut fusion/plating presents a biomechanically sound construct than four-level multilevel discectomies with fusion/plating
- D. The stability of a ventral multilevel corpectomy can be improved by adding a dorsal lateral mass fixation
- E. With modern instrumentation and biologics, fusion rates for multilevel discectomies are similar to single-level discectomies

▸▸ Question 16

The stability of a multilevel corpectomy can be enhanced by which of the following?
- A. Adding an intermediate point of fixation to the bone graft strut
- B. Adding an intermediate point of fixation to the native spine
- C. Allowing the bone graft to move with the implant using multiple screws through the graft
- D. Avoid any intermediate fixation to the graft or native spine
- E. Using variable-angle screws through the graft implant interface

▸▸ Question 17

Regarding the bone–bone interface, which of the following statements is correct?
- A. Subsidence and nonunion are encouraged by a poor fit between the bone graft and the vertebral body

- B. Small (in cross-sectional area) bone grafts subside less than larger grafts
- C. Grafts positioned in the center of the vertebral body will piston less than grafts positioned laterally
- D. Wider grafts that abut the cortical margins circumferentially are unstable
- E. Interbody bone–bone interface failure (e.g., nonunion of an anterior cervical corpectomy decompression and fusion) can be maximized by optimizing the lateral fit of the bone graft or cage within the lateral walls of the corpectomy trough

▸▸ Question 18

Which of the following regarding drilling and tapping is correct?

- A. Tapping cortical bone improves the integrity of the screw–bone interface
- B. Tapping cancellous bone improves the integrity of the screw–bone interface
- C. Drilling cancellous bone without tapping provides lower pullout resistance than that achieved with drilling and tapping
- D. Using an awl to prepare the hole compresses and weakens its integrity
- E. Placing bone chips in the hole or using pressurized polymethylmethacrylate can reduce the integrity of the screw bone interface

▸▸ Question 19

In the face of a preexisting cervical kyphotic deformity, select the correct statement.

- A. Laminoplasty and laminectomy without fusion are not useful clinical strategies to prevent deformity and failure
- B. The relative stiffness of laminoplasty is about the same as laminectomy without fusion
- C. Laminoplasty can be a good strategy if a patient is not osteoporotic
- D. Laminectomy is acceptable if facets are not violated
- E. Laminoplasty can usually prevent postoperative C5 palsy in kyphotic patients

▸▸ Question 20

Select the best statement regarding component–component interface failure.

- A. Occurs mainly due to patient noncompliance with bracing
- B. Occurs at least 12 months after implant placement
- C. Usually associated with PEEK implants
- D. Usually associated with the use of high-modulus implants
- E. Surgeon failure is one of the leading causes

Answers

▸▸ Answer 1

Correct answer is C

Constructs can fail because of implant failure (e.g., fracture of a plate), failure of the bone at the implant–bone interface, or failure at a component–component interface. Constructs can also fail due to improper surgical technique or judgment, e.g., asking too much of the implant or not optimizing bone density. Using a cobalt chrome implant, PEEK implant, or a rigid orthosis postoperatively should not cause an implant failure of a spinal construct if the decision to use is based on sound surgical judgment.

▸▸ Answer 2

Correct answer is A

Implant failure describes the fracture of an implant or failure of an implant component or degradation of the interface between the implant and the "native" bone. Implants usually fracture at the point of maximum stress application. Option A is correct. The intermediate point of fixation is not necessarily the point of maximum stress application; therefore, D is incorrect. Rigid multisegmental constructs tend to load the caudal screws more than the rostral screws; therefore, C is incorrect. In general, long fixed cantilever beam screw implants are associated with a relatively high failure rate. Implants fail at points of low modulus, not high. Implant fracture is a failure mechanism, to one degree or another, surgeon related. Either the surgeon improperly installed the implant or asked

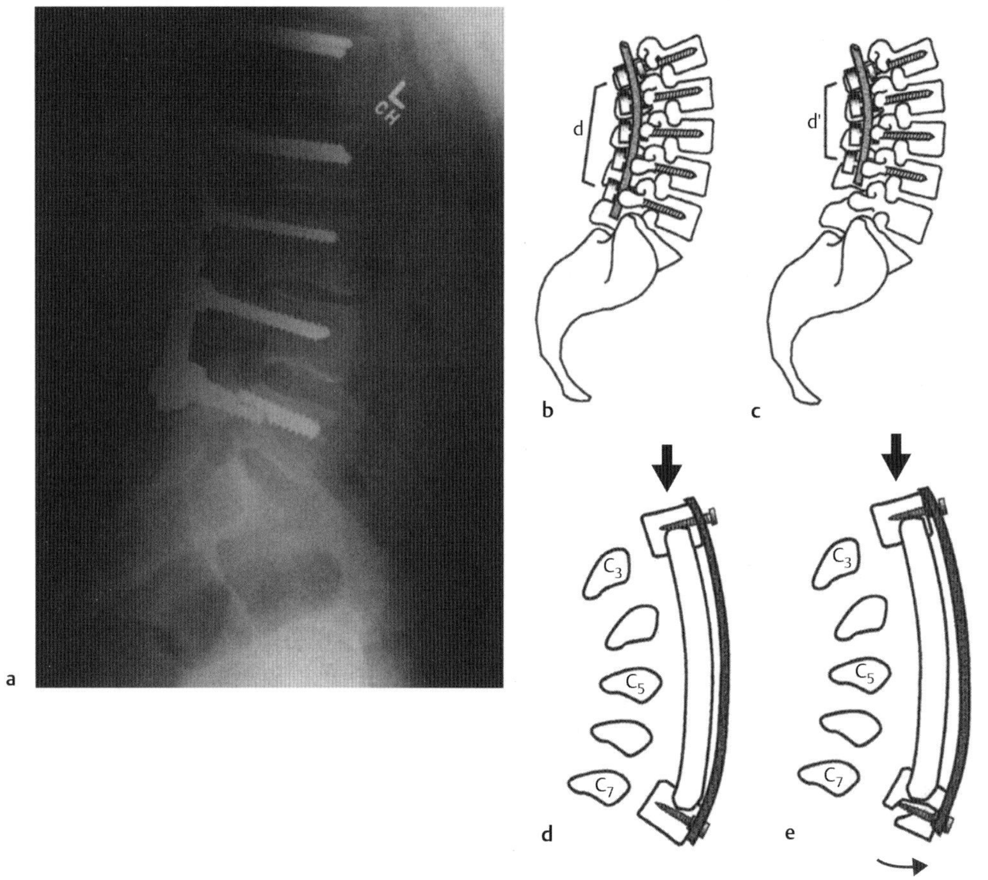

Fig. 19.7 (a) Long rigid (fixed moment arm cantilever beam) screw–rod multisegmental fixation tends to load the most caudal screws more than the rostral screws, as depicted in a clinical example. **(b, c)** In this situation, the use of a construct that extends one less segment caudally would have applied a lesser moment arm (*d* and *d'*) and a lesser bending moment. **(d, e)** This principle (i.e., the lower or most caudal portion of an implant is exposed the greatest stress) is shown in a cervical example. Note that the implant and strut kick-out (kick-through in this case) occurred at the caudal aspect of the construct. This is related to geometric and mechanical (physical) factors. (Source: Biomechanics of Spine Stabilization: Third Edition, © 2015 Thieme Medical Publishers, Inc.)

▸▸ Answer 10

Correct answer is C

The implant failure is often due to surgeon failure, poor optimization of bone density, inadequate bony preparation, spine gardening, poor geometry of constructs, poor postoperative sagittal balance, lumbopelvic parameters postmedical optimization—vitamin D_3 levels < 20 ng/mL, CT Hounsfield unit < 97.5, DEXA scan T-score < −2.5 are associated with risks of implant failure after spinal instrumentation. There is no evidence that vaping decreases the risk of nicotine-associated pseudoarthrosis compared with regular cigarettes. Artificial discs are only approved for limited indications and have minimal impact on the overall stability of spine constructs. Using hybrid constructs in multiple-level lumbar fusion for degenerative scoliosis is experimental and not standard of care. Postoperative pelvic parameters of PT 18, SVA 3.5 cm, and PI-LL mismatch of 9 are good outcomes for a 65-year-old. Adjacent-level deformity

(deformity that occurs at a level adjacent to a prior fusion) and segmental degeneration occur with much less frequency when normal alignment is present following a fusion; thus, C is the correct answer.[2]

▸▸ Answer 11

Correct answer is A

Screw geometry can be modified to enhance pullout resistance. A classic example of this concept is the triangulation of screws (option A is correct). Correcting deformity is an excellent example of normalizing or optimizing the geometry of native spine or implants to improve the stability of constructs. The recommendations are to keep C2-SVA less than 4 cm and T1 slope less than 30 degrees; therefore, B and C are incorrect. Stability is enhanced by adding intermediate fixation points to the native spine, not graft; therefore, D is incorrect. As in the lumbar spine, optimizing bone density improves bone integrity. It is recommended to avoid implants when the DEXA T-score is < 2.5.[2]

▸▸ Answer 12

Correct answer is A

Any strategy that offloads the implant minimizes the chance of implant failure. Axially dynamic implants, by the nature of their application, bear minimal axial load and allow load sharing by allowing natural subsidence (making option A correct and option B incorrect). They resist translation, rotation, and angulation but not axial loading (option C, D, and E are incorrect).

▸▸ Answer 13

Correct answer is C

The integrity of fixation is proportional to the number of "high-quality" fixation points in "native bone," which increases load sharing (options A and E are incorrect statements). The ability to resist spinal deformation in more than one plane and by more than one mechanism is illustrated in ▸ Fig. 19.8 using the example of a rigid ventral construct acting as a fixed moment arm cantilever

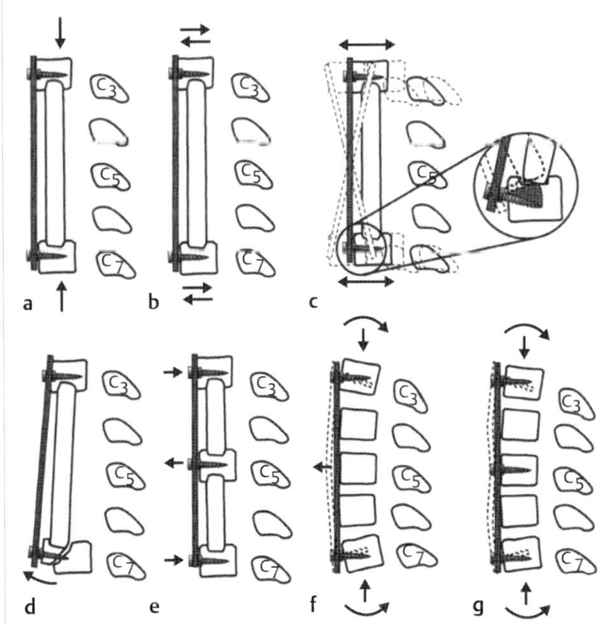

Fig. 19.8 A rigid fixed moment arm cantilever beam implant with two screws at each end. **(a)** This is a bridging implant, a construct that resists axial loads (*vertical arrows*) well. However, loads are usually applied from a variety of orientations—in addition to simple axial loading. **(b)** Shear loads (horizontal arrows) can cause translation. (*Shaded area*, **c**) This may cause the screw–bone interface to degrade and **(d)** ultimately to fail, usually as a result of axial loading. (*Arrows*, **e**) The addition of a third (intermediate) point of fixation causes the implant to more effectively resist these loads (e.g., translation) via a three-point bending mechanism. The threepoint bending effect resists shear-producing loads in all planes. Axial loads can also be resisted more effectively by using an intermediate fixation point. **(f)** The flexibility of an implant bearing an axial load is significantly diminished by **(g)** using an additional intermediate point of fixation. (Data obtained from16) The intermediate fixation point minimizes flexibility (as depicted by the dashed implant in F and G). (Source: Biomechanics of Spine Stabilization: Third Edition, © 2015 Thieme Medical Publishers, Inc.)

beam (**a**). In this circumstance, in which two screws are employed at either endpoint of the implant, axial loads are borne well, if not equally, as is shown with a single-level anterior cervical decompression fusion with plating (**a**). However, implants and implant–bone interfaces rarely fail following simple one-dimensional loading. They usually fail following repetitive loading (fatigue) via multiple orientations. This has been shown to occur regarding implants that are applied without intermediate fixation points to the "native spine." The loads are usually applied from a variety of angles and orientations. These include transverse, rotational, and shear loads. As already stated, the implant depicted in part **a** bears axial loads well. However, it does not effectively resist translational and rotational loads (**b**). This is so because the long moment arm associated with the long implant applies significant stress to the spine when such loads are applied. This may cause degradation of the screw–bone interface (**c**) and ultimately a failure because of axial loading (**d**). The longer the implant, the more prone the implant becomes to these effects. The addition of intermediate fixation points allows the implant to resist these translational loads via a third fixation point and three-point bending mechanical strategies (**e**); thus, option B is incorrect.

The additional fixation points permit axial loads to be borne more effectively and increase the resistance to translation, rotational, and shear forces; thus, option B is incorrect, and C is the correct statement and right answer. This is the case in the lumbar spine with the employment of pedicle screws. Axial loads can be borne more effectively with additional intermediate fixation points into the "native spine," as well. Consider the fact that most implants are flexible (**f**). The extent of deformation (bowing) of a flexible implant is significantly limited using an intermediate fixation point (**g**). These intermediate points of fixation must be to the "native spine." The section modulus is an intrinsic property of the screws or implant and is related to the inner diameter's third power and not influenced by the number of fixation points; therefore, option D is a false statement.

▸▸ Answer 14

Correct answer is B

Long bridging constructs after corpectomy, in which two screws are used at each terminus of the implant, bear axial loads well. However, implants and implant–bone interfaces rarely fail following simple one-dimensional loading. Long bridging implant constructs used in multilevel corpectomies usually fail following repetitive loading (fatigue) via multiple orientations (option A and C are incorrect statements). Adding an intermediate point of fixations to the native spine but not to graft is necessary to improve translational and rotational stability (option B is correct). The bone graft does not provide a biomechanically sound foundation for a screw. Adding a fixation point to the bone graft degrades the integrity of the construct. Furthermore, the bone graft is weakened by a screw, with the screw taking up a significant cross-sectional area of the graft. Finally, the bone graft, in such a construct, is forced to move with the implant. This can cause excessive motion at the strut–vertebral mortise, degrading the bone–implant interface.

Stand-alone strut graft is loaded in flexion and unloaded in extension. Adding an anterior plate reverses this and increases graft compression in extension (option C is incorrect). This can be prevented by additional fixation points. Osteoporosis will worsen the stability of any long bridging construct; therefore, E is wrong.[3]

▸▸ Answer 15

Correct answer is D

Multiple-level discectomies with fusion without an implant have high failure rates due to pseudarthrosis (option A is incorrect). Careful bone preparation is mandatory, lest suboptimal contact be achieved between the implant and the vertebra (see ▸ Fig. 19.9a). Careful sculpting of the contact surface ("gardening") should maximize the surface area of contact (▸ Fig. 19.9b). Interbody bone–bone interface failure can be minimized by considering factors that predispose to subsidence. "Fit is important." A careful consideration of mortise geometry and precise "carpentry" should minimize gap formation. Small sectional area grafts piston more than large cross-sectional area grafts (option B is incorrect).

Multiple-level discectomies with plating (with screws placed at each level) present a biomechanically very sound construct, whereas multiple-level consecutive corpectomies with strut fusion, with or without bridging implant plating, do not (option C is incorrect).

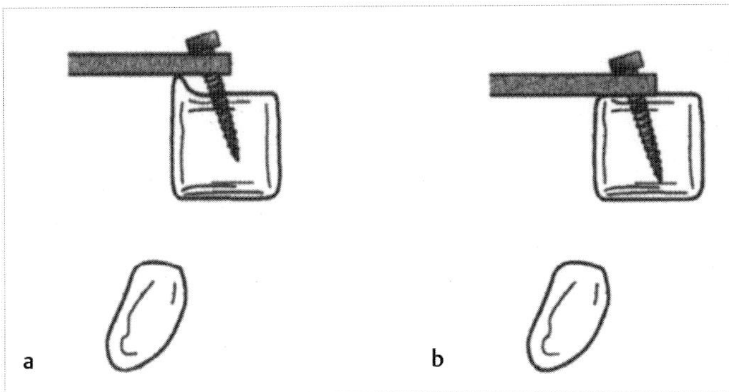

Fig. 19.9 (a) Careful bone preparation is mandatory, lest suboptimal contact be achieved between the implant and the vertebra. (b) Careful sculpting of the contact surface ("gardening") should maximize the surface area of contact. (Source: Biomechanics of Spine Stabilization: Third Edition, © 2015 Thieme Medical Publishers, Inc.)

The ability of the implant to resist failure is in part related to its ability to distribute loads (load sharing), so that no single portion of the implant or spine bears excessive portion of the load (load bearing). It is optimal if applied loads are distributed over multiple points of contact with the spine. One such way is to provide additional implant–bone interfaces (option D is correct).

Multilevel cervical discectomies result in more number of fusion surfaces to heal and increased loads at the caudal end of the construct, therefore increasing the risk of implant failure or pseudoarthrosis at the caudal level (option E is incorrect).

▸▸ Answer 16

Correct answer is B

In the case of a long ventral corpectomy with decompression operation, attaining an intermediate point of fixation to the parent spine may be achieved in the cervical spine by "leaving" an intermediate vertebral body. ▶ Fig. 19.10 shows that (**a**) long cervical decompression (e.g., C4–C6 inclusively) can be accomplished with a C4 and C6 corpectomy accompanied by a C3–C5 and a C5–C7 interbody fusion. (**b**) This provides a solid vertebral body site (C5) for intermediate screw fixation in "native bone" while providing (*dashed arrows*, **c**) adequate visualization for dural sac decompression. This may (and probably does) offset the disadvantages associated with the increased number of fusion interfaces that must heal. Another method of achieving the same biomechanical advantage (i.e., intermediate fixation points) is employing a ventral and a dorsal operation (ventral corpectomies plus dorsal lateral mass fixation). However, the lateral mass fixation points are not as solid as an intermediate vertebral body. A second operation is also required, with its associated morbidity and potential mortality. Nevertheless, corpectomies at three or more levels with strut graft fusion may be effectively augmented by adding a dorsal implant.

Intermediate bone graft attachment sites are effective only if placed in (**a**) a vertebral body ("native spine") rather than in (**b**) the bone graft (see ▶ Fig. 19.11). The bone graft does not provide a biomechanically sound foundation for the screw. Furthermore, the bone graft is weakened by the screw, with the screw taking up a significant cross-sectional area of the graft. (**c**) Finally, the strut graft, in such a construct, is forced to move with the implant. This can cause excessive motion at the strut–vertebral mortise, further degrading the integrity of the construct. Adding a fixation point to the bone graft impairs the integrity of the construct. Stability is not enhanced by adding an intermediate fixation point to a bony strut. Stability is lessened. Furthermore, the bone graft is weakened by a screw, with the screw taking up a significant cross-sectional area of the graft. Finally, the bone graft, in such a construct, is forced to move with the implant. This can cause excessive motion at the strut–vertebral mortise, degrading the bone–implant interface. Therefore, A, C, and D are incorrect. Adding screws to the graft weakens the construct regardless of whether they are fixed or variable screws. Therefore, E is wrong. In the case of a long ventral corpectomy with decompression operation, attaining an intermediate point of fixation to the parent spine may be achieved in the cervical spine by "leaving" an intermediate vertebral body; therefore, B is correct.

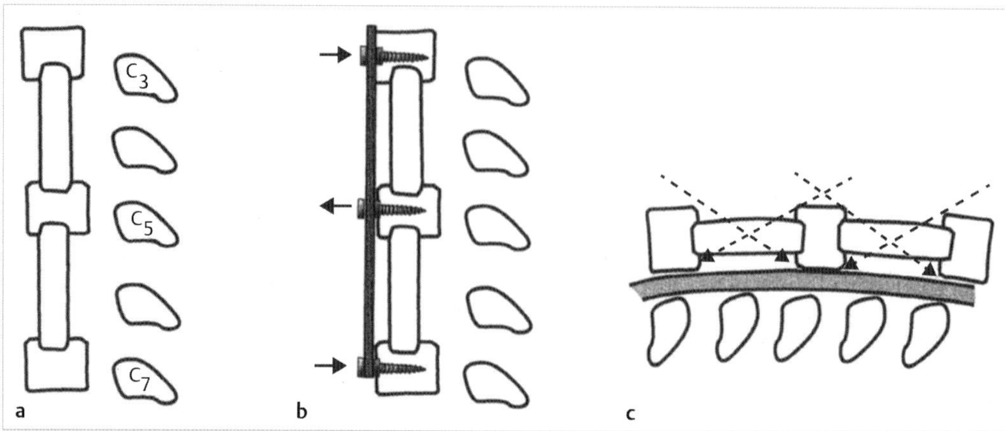

Fig. 19.10 **(a)** A long cervical decompression (e.g., C4–C6 inclusively) can be accomplished with a C4 and C6 corpectomy accompanied by a C3–C5 and a C5–C7 interbody fusion. **(b)** This provides a solid vertebral body site (C5) for intermediate screw fixation in "native bone" while providing (*dashed arrows*, **c**) adequate visualization for dural sac decompression. (Source: Biomechanics of Spine Stabilization: Third Edition, © 2015 Thieme Medical Publishers, Inc.)

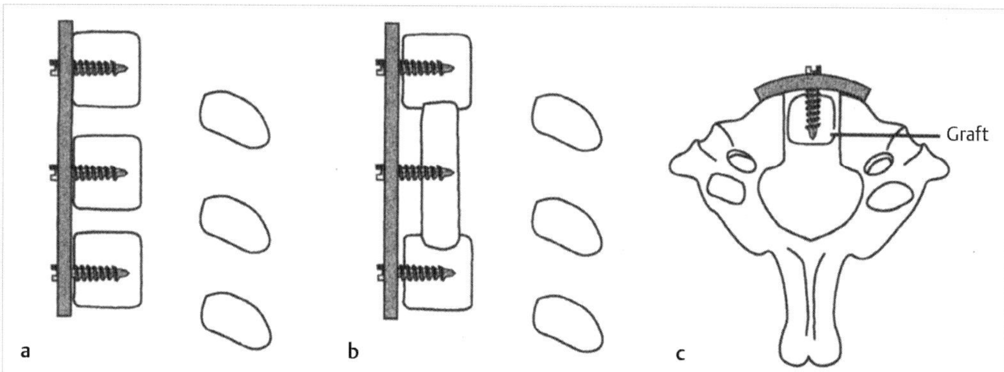

Fig. 19.11 Intermediate bone graft attachment sites are effective only if placed in **(a)** a vertebral body ("native spine") rather than in **(b)** the bone graft. The bone graft does not provide a biomechanically sound foundation for the screw. Furthermore, the bone graft is weakened by the screw, with the screw taking up a significant cross-sectional area of the graft. **(c)** Finally, the strut graft, in such a construct, is forced to move with the implant. This can cause excessive motion at the strut–vertebral mortise, further degrading the integrity of the construct. (Source: Biomechanics of Spine Stabilization: Third Edition, © 2015 Thieme Medical Publishers, Inc.)

▸▸ Answer 17

Correct answer is A

The interface between the interbody bone graft or strut and the vertebral body is prone to failure. Subsidence and nonunion are encouraged by a poor fit between the bone graft and the vertebral body (option A is true). Grafts positioned in the center of the vertebral body will piston more than grafts positioned laterally (option C is false). Wider grafts that abut the cortical margins circumferentially are stable (option D is false). Optimizing the lateral fit of the bone graft or cage within the lateral walls of the corpectomy trough is a strategy to minimize bone–bone interface failure (option E is false). Small (in cross-sectional area) grafts subside more than larger grafts (option B is false).

▸▸ **Answer 18**

Correct answer is A

Tapping cortical bone (pedicles of a vertebral body) improves the integrity of the screw–bone interface (option A is true), although tapping cancellous bone weakens it (option B is incorrect). Tapping cancellous bone weakens the purchase of a screw and diminishes its pullout resistance. Simply drilling cancellous bone without tapping provides greater, not lower, pullout resistance than that achieved with tapping (option C is incorrect). Appropriately done, drilling does not increase the size of the screw hole and therefore does not diminish its pullout resistance.

Using an awl to prepare the hole compresses the areolar cancellous bone, thus improving, not weakening, its integrity, as opposed to drilling and removing the bone debris and/or tapping (option D is incorrect). Placing bone chips in the hole or using pressurized polymethylmethacrylate can also augment integrity (option E is wrong). Note that nonpressurized polymethylmethacrylate lessens the integrity of the screw–bone interface.

▸▸ **Answer 19**

Correct answer is A

The effect of laminoplasty on spinal integrity has not been adequately investigated. Although spinal stiffness may be increased (compared with stiffness after laminectomy), deformity progression may not be impeded, particularly if kyphosis was present preoperatively. The relative spinal stiffness associated with laminoplasty (e.g., vs that after laminectomy without fusion) is not known and, as such, should not be assumed to be greater than that associated with laminectomy (option B is incorrect). Deformity progression is expected because of the bending moment created by existing kyphosis. Hence, neither laminectomy nor laminoplasty is an optimal strategy in the face of an existing kyphosis, regardless of its extent (option A is correct and options C and D are incorrect). The incidence of C5 palsy is not necessarily prevented by choosing laminoplasty, irrespective of the presence or absence of kyphosis (option E is incorrect).

▸▸ **Answer 20**

Correct answer is E

Component–component interface failure can occur as a result of (1) improper surgical techniques (e.g., improper implant installation), (2) acute failure of a properly installed implant, or (3) failure via fatigue of a properly installed implant in which a fusion was not acquired. All, to one degree or another, are surgeon-related failures rather than patient noncompliance with bracing; therefore, A is wrong. The surgeon either improperly installed the implant or asked too much of the implant–bone interface. It is the surgeon's responsibility to understand what to expect from the implant—and not to ask too much of the implant. The use of a PEEK implant or high-modulus implant is safe if chosen and guided by appropriate surgical judgment; therefore C and D are wrong. Failure can occur acutely even with proper installation; therefore, B is wrong.

Key Principles

- Implants always fail at the point of maximum stress application.
- Stress = bending moment/section modulus.
- Cantilever beam constructs (fixed moment arm vs nonfixed moment arm) differ significantly in how and where forces are applied.
- Constructs with multiple points of fixation are generally able to provide greater load sharing and resist translational forces and rotational deformation.

References

[1] McConnell M, Shieh A. Polypharmacy in osteoporosis treatment. Clin Geriatr Med 2022;38(4):715–726

[2] Dimar J, Bisson EF, Dhall S, et al. Congress of Neurological Surgeons systematic review and evidence-based guidelines for perioperative spine: preoperative osteoporosis assessment. Neurosurgery 2021;89(Suppl 1):S19–S25

[3] DiAngelo DJ, Foley KT, Vossel KA, et al. Anterior cervical plating reverses load transfer through multilevel strut-grafts. Spine (Phila Pa 1976) 2000;25:783–795

Part V

Spine Instrumentation Constructs: Region Specific Considerations

V

20 Craniocervical and Upper Cervical Constructs

John Williams, Andrew M. Hersh, Nicholas Theodore

The anatomical and clinical complexities of the upper cervical spine and craniocervical junction pose significant challenges for the managing surgeon, including (1) the high risk of treatment failure, (2) the significant multiplanar forces affecting this region, and (3) the difficulties associated with achieving solid fusion in the upper cervical spine–occiput region (i.e., the craniocervical junction).

Learning Objectives

- Understand the anatomical/geometric and multiplanar motion characteristics of the craniocervical junction that pose unique challenges to achieving successful fusion.
- Learn how historical craniocervical fixation techniques have shaped our understanding of the above-mentioned concepts and improved current fixation and fusion techniques.
- Recognize the advantages and limitations of various techniques to achieve craniocervical stabilization.
- Appreciate how the biomechanics of the craniocervical spine inform methods that improve the safety of instrumentation and fusion techniques.

Questions

▸▸ Question 1

How much combined flexion/extension movement is allowed by the occiput–C1 joint and C1–C2 joint, respectively?

- A. 20 degrees, 20 degrees
- B. 10 degrees, 5 degrees
- C. 5 degrees, 40 degrees
- D. 25 degrees, 20 degrees
- E. 5 degrees, 10 degrees

▸▸ Question 2

Which of the following C1–C2 fixation strategies best resists the multiplanar motion allowed by the craniocervical junction to promote fusion?

- A. Dorsal C1–C2 wire fixation alone
- B. Dorsal C1–C2 wire fixation with dorsal bone graft spacer
- C. C1–C2 transarticular screws augmented by C1–C2 wire fixation
- D. C1–C2 transarticular screws augmented by dorsal bone graft spacer
- E. C1–C2 transarticular screws with both dorsal bone graft spacer and C1–C2 wire fixation

▸▸ Question 3

According to Wolff's law and its corollaries, which of the following effects improves bone healing?

- A. Torque generates positive charge, which recruits osteoclasts
- B. Compression creates a negative charge that stimulates osteoblast activity
- C. Torque creates a negative charge that stimulates osteoblast activity
- D. Increased cancellous bone use promotes new blood vessel growth
- E. Compression increases osteoblast–osteoblast contact synchronizing activity

▸▸ Question 4

What are the major challenges to ventral fixation in the upper cervical region?

- A. Risk of infection with transoral approaches; suboptimal trajectory with transoral and extrapharyngeal approaches; juxtaposition of vascular and neural structures; sufficient bone for screw placement
- B. Risk of infection with transoral approaches; increased risk of high-flow cerebrospinal fluid (CSF) leak; sufficient bone for screw placement
- C. Risk of infection with transoral approaches; suboptimal trajectory with transoral and extrapharyngeal approaches; juxtaposition of vascular and neural structures; increased traction on the recurrent pharyngeal nerve
- D. Risk of infection with transoral approaches; juxtaposition of vascular and neural structures; sufficient bone for screw placement; increased traction on the recurrent pharyngeal nerve

- E. Risk of infection with transoral approaches; juxtaposition of vascular and neural structures; increased risk of high-flow CSF leak; increased traction on the recurrent pharyngeal nerve

▸▸ Question 5

What are three situations in which odontoid screw fixation should be avoided?

- A. Patients over age 75 years; uncontrolled diabetes mellitus; significantly comminuted fractures
- B. Odontoid height < 10 mm; diagonal or angulated fractures; concomitant nondisplaced C1 anterior ring fractures
- C. Old fractures with fibrous nonunion; diagonal or angulated fractures; significantly comminuted fractures
- D. Patients over age 75 years; old fractures with fibrous nonunion; diagonal or angulated fractures
- E. Odontoid height < 10 mm; old fractures with fibrous nonunion; significantly comminuted fractures

▸▸ Question 6

What is a unique advantage of ventral strut grafting strategies?

- A. The ability to visualize the vertebral arteries
- B. The ability to decompress and fuse/apply an implant through a single approach
- C. Superior ability to resist rotation compared with posterior approaches
- D. Superior ability to resist flexion/extension compared with posterior approaches
- E. Superior ability to resist translation compared with posterior approaches

▸▸ Question 7

What is a common method of mitigating "cheese cutting" or loosening of wires and cables in dorsal constructs?

- A. Spinous process wiring
- B. Increasing the gap between rod and bone
- C. Creating a greater angle of exposure of wire to bone
- D. "Burying" the wire or cable in cut bone troughs
- E. Using parallel double wires or cables

▸▸ Question 8

Which type of occipital bone fixation provides significant bone–interface integrity?

- A. Lateral
- B. Foramen magnum
- C. Midline
- D. Inverted
- E. Bicortical

▸▸ Question 9

How can the working area for a dorsal C1 lateral mass screw be expanded?

- A. Drilling the caudal insertion of the dorsal arch of C1
- B. Unroofing the medial transverse foramen
- C. Drilling the cranial insertion of the dorsal arch of C1
- D. C1 laminectomy
- E. Drilling the caudal and cranial insertion of the dorsal arch of C1

▸▸ Question 10

What are two ways in which the lag effect can be achieved in occipitocervical fusion constructs?

- A. Oversizing screws and craniocaudal angulation
- B. Craniocaudal angulation and tapping screw trajectories
- C. Bicortical screw purchase and oversizing screws
- D. Overdrilling proximal bone with fully threaded screw and using partially threaded screws
- E. Overdrilling distal bone with fully threaded screw and bicortical screw purchase

▸▸ Question 11

What length of a C2 pedicle screw and a C2 pars screw, respectively, will fall short of contacting the vertebral artery?

- A. 15–16 mm; 9–10 mm
- B. 12–14 mm; 18–20 mm

- C. 18–20 mm; 12–14 mm
- D. 9–10 mm; 15–16 mm
- E. 14–15 mm; 18–20 mm

▸▸ Question 12

Safe insertion of a C1–C2 transarticular screw can be augmented by aligning (1) the insertion site, (2) the dorsal–rostral aspect of the C2 facet, and (3) the upper one-third of the ventral C1 arch. If these points are not aligned, which two points should be used?

- A. The insertion site and the ventral vertebral artery foramen
- B. The dorsal–rostral aspect of the C2 facet and the medial portion of the groove for the vertebral artery of C1
- C. The lateral aspect of the C2 lateral mass and the cranial one-third of the odontoid process
- D. The lateral aspect of the C2 lateral mass and the upper one-third of the ventral C1 arch
- E. The insertion site and the dorsal–rostral aspect of the C2 facet

▸▸ Question 13

Midline occipital screw fixation provides solid fixation but is not ideal in resisting which challenge to occipital cervical fusion?

- A. Long flexion moment arm
- B. Pullout force resistance in flexion
- C. Rotation
- D. Cortical drift
- E. Sagittal loading stress

▸▸ Question 14

How are the bones of the occiput and the upper cervical laminae and spinous processes comparable?

- A. Cortical-to-cancellous ratio: the occiput is predominantly compact and cortical; the cervical posterior elements are softer
- B. Cortical-to-cancellous ratio: the occiput is predominantly cancellous and soft; the cervical posterior elements are compact and cortical
- C. Trabecular density: the occiput is characterized by small-cell, high-density trabeculae; the posterior cervical elements are large-cell, low-density
- D. Trabecular density: the occiput is characterized by large-cell, low-density trabeculae; the posterior cervical elements are small-cell, high-density
- E. The relatively large, low-angle curve surface of the occiput allows for a more favorable baseline bone–implant interface potential

▸▸ Question 15

What is a limitation of ventral upper cervical plating techniques for "free-standing" stabilization?

- A. Limited craniocaudal surface area for fixation, leading to the "windshield wiper" effect
- B. C1–C2 ventral plates dictate the screw entry point, which may provide suboptimal fixation
- C. The soft bone of the clivus is more susceptible to "cheese cutting" by the ventral plates
- D. A lack of true cortical bone along the ventral face of the body of C2
- E. Repeated microtrauma leading to stress failure from esophageal contact during swallowing

▸▸ Question 16

What is an advantage provided by crossed translaminar C2 screw fixation techniques?

- A. Minimal triangulation effect
- B. An interface to allow for short screw insertion to augment C2 pars fixation
- C. No safety advantage when compared with C2 pars and pedicle fixation strategies
- D. No risk to the vertebral arteries
- E. Easy integration into longitudinal constructs

▸▸ Question 17

In which of the following scenarios should C2 lateral mass fixation be used?

- A. Adjoining C1 lateral mass screws in C1–C2 constructs
- B. When standard C2 fixation points are not readily available
- C. When short-segment constructs are favored
- D. Anchoring the cranial portion of a cervical–upper thoracic long construct
- E. Treating patients with congenital spinal canal narrowing

▸▸ Question 18

Which feature is provided by occipital button fixation?

- A. Better flexion/extension resistance with bicortical contact
- B. Mass effect for traumatic occipital durotomy tamponade
- C. Significant lateral skull surface area of contact
- D. Marginal lateral modulus of elasticity
- E. Inverted triangulation effect

▸▸ Question 19

What is a feature of extension of occipitocervical fixation constructs to C7?

- A. Facilitates safe, early construct termination above the thoracic spine
- B. Increases patient satisfaction with preserved motion
- C. Resists pullout strain on the caudal screws
- D. Reduces postoperative kyphotic deformity by preserving ligamentous posterior tension bands
- E. Places significant stress on the cervicothoracic junction

▸▸ Question 20

Why are wire and cable techniques particularly susceptible to loosening via "cheese cutting?"

- A. Relatively small surface area of contact between the bone and the wire or cable
- B. Inferior material strength of wires and cables compared with rods and screws
- C. Technical error during placement
- D. Stretching or creep from metal cables
- E. Continuous bone remodeling

Answers

▸▸ Answer 1

Correct answer is D

Solid arthrodesis can be difficult to achieve in the craniocervical region due to the multiple motion orientations that must be restricted by the implant and the geometry and characteristics of the ligamentous soft tissue and bone. The other answers suggest lesser degrees of flexion/extension and are incorrect. Flexion, extension, and rotation about the long axis of the spine are extensive in the upper cervical spine (see ▸ Table 20.1). Rotation may interfere with the fusion process enough to render it unsuccessful. For example, dorsal C1–C2 wire fixation strategies provide adequate resistance in flexion and extension relatively effectively, but poor resistance in translation and rotation, which can cause fusion failure.

Table 20.1 Movements allowed in the craniocervical region

Joint	Motion	Range of motion (degrees)
Occiput–C1	Combined flexion and extension	25
	Lateral bending (unilateral)	5
	Axial rotation (unilateral)	5
C1–C2	Combined flexion and extension	20
	Lateral bending (unilateral)	5
	Axial rotation (unilateral)	40

(Biomechanics of Spine Stabilization: Third Edition), © 2015 Thieme Medical Publishers, Inc.

▸▸ Answer 2

Correct answer is E

As noted previously, flexion, extension, and rotation are extensive in the upper cervical spine. Transarticular screws are very effective in resisting C1–C2 rotation and translation, and are superior to dorsal fixation alone, eliminating answer choices A and B. Resistance to flexion is enhanced by the addition of wire fixation, while resistance to extension is enhanced by a dorsal bone graft spacer. The other answer choices (C and D) include wire fixation or dorsal bone graft spacers alone and are less effective than their combination.

▸▸ Answer 3

Correct answer is B

Wolff's law maintains that bone heals best under compression, which produces a negative surface charge, which stimulates osteoblastic activity, thereby improving the healing process. The other choices reference incorrect mechanisms. The lag screw effect, such as that employed with odontoid screw fixation, can be used to achieve compression. The order of steps in the operation are of the utmost importance, as deviations can result in fusion failure. For example, if C1–C2 transarticular screws are placed prior to a dorsal C1–C2 wire tightening, the dorsal bone graft may initially be placed in compression, but the laminae will revert to their prewired position as the wires relax or "cut" into bone.

▸▸ Answer 4

Correct answer is A

Ventral craniocervical and upper cervical constructs include odontoid screw fixation, ventral short fusion strategies, plate fixation, and transarticular screw fixation. Anterior surgeries require oral or high extrapharyngeal surgical approaches, which can be difficult. Despite the obvious advantage to achieving decompression and stabilization through the same approach, biomechanical and anatomical restrictions often limit the utility of such a strategy (see ▸ Fig. 20.1). These approaches do not inherently have a higher risk of CSF leak; however, CSF leaks in this anatomical region are more difficult to repair. Moreover, the risk of meningitis is increased, owing to direct contact with the oropharyngeal space.

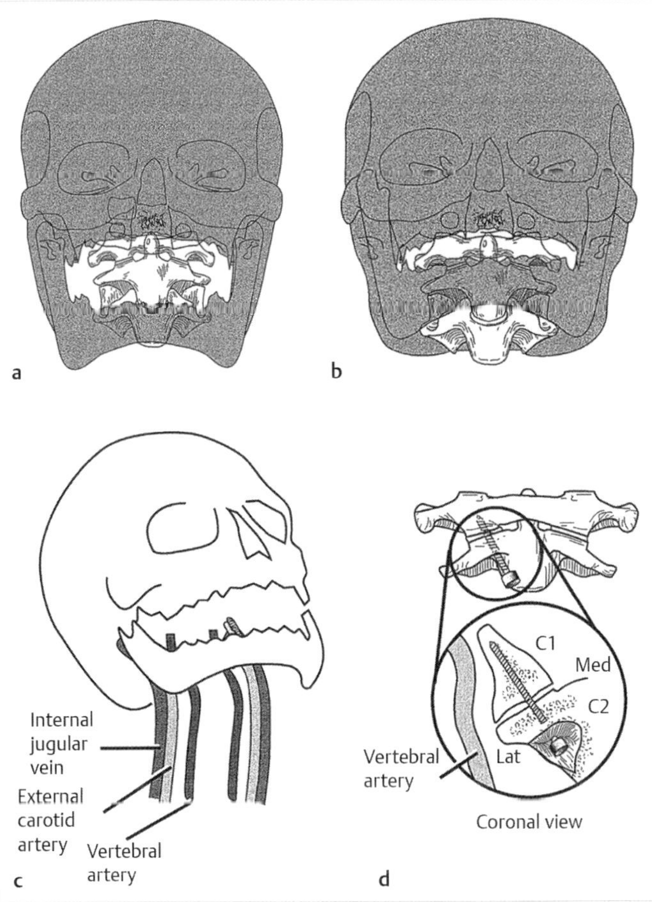

Fig. 20.1 Ventral fixation in the upper cervical region poses significant challenges to the surgeon. These include **(a)** the risk for infection with transoral approaches, **(a, b)** the suboptimal trajectory with transoral and extrapharyngeal approaches, **(c)** the juxtaposition of vascular and neural structures, and **(d)** the adequacy of bone in which to place screws. (Source: Biomechanics of Spine Stabilization: Third Edition, © 2015 Thieme Medical Publishers, Inc.)

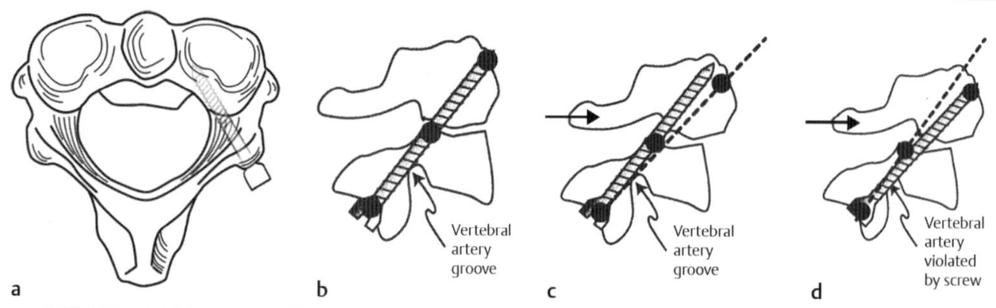

Fig. 20.4 The C2 pedicle provides a relatively safe site for C2 screw fixation. An appreciation of its anatomy is critical. **(a)** An axial view of the C2 pedicle illustrates the anatomy. **(b)** The safety of C1–C2 transarticular screw fixation can be augmented by aligning three points in the sagittal plane (*dots*): (1) the insertion site, (2) the dorsal–rostral aspect of the C2 facet, and (3) the upper one-third of the ventral C1 arch. **(c)** However, if these points are not linear (in line), the first two points (screw trajectory) instead of the first and third points (*dashed line*) should be used. **(d)** This avoids infringement of the vertebral artery foramen by the screw (screw trajectory), which will not occur if the first two points have been used (*dashed line*). The surgeon should also keep in mind that the vertebral artery foramen is usually more laterally than medially situated. Therefore, a relatively medial trajectory is generally safer. (Source: Biomechanics of Spine Stabilization: Third Edition, © 2015 Thieme Medical Publishers, Inc.)

▸▸ Answer 14

Correct answer is A

The bone of the occiput differs in consistency from that of the upper cervical laminae and spinous processes, especially regarding the cortical-to-cancellous ratio. Bone graft recipient beds are often significantly separated (e.g., occiput–C1 and C1–C2), presenting substantial challenges to fusion. Moreover, the compact nature of the bone of the occiput makes early union less likely, thereby decreasing likelihood of arthrodesis. An appreciation of the size and caliber of implant anchor sites of affixation is critical, particularly in the pediatric population.

The early structural integrity of upper and occipital fusions may be imparted by the bone graft. The cortical portion of the bone graft contributes a substantial portion of the initial integrity. A spinal implant may provide the early stability that the cortical bone of a dorsal bone graft might initially provide, thus making the cortical portion of the bone graft less necessary.

▸▸ Answer 15

Correct answer is B

C1–C2 ventral cervical plates dictate the screw entry point, which may provide suboptimal fixation. Therefore, a solid knowledge of the anatomical relationships between the fixator and the intrinsic spine anatomy on a case-by case basis is essential, and several ventral upper cervical plating techniques have been devised. These techniques are complicated by two predominant factors: (1) the relatively weak screw fixation points and (2) the risk for infection stemming from transoral contamination. The subarticular atlantoaxial locking plate provides an optimal biomechanical advantage, but the above features limit its use. Additionally, transoral upper cervical plate fixation is less stable compared with combined anterior and posterior reconstruction procedures and is therefore limited as a "free-standing" stabilization strategy.

▸▸ Answer 16

Correct answer is D

Crossed translaminar C2 screw fixation techniques provide relatively safe sites of fixation in comparison to pedicle and pars interarticularis approaches (answer choice C is incorrect). They provide a substantial triangulation effect (answer choice A is incorrect) and allow the use of long screws (28–32 mm) (answer choice B is incorrect). Additionally, they are inserted under direct vision and palpation, often eliminating the need for image assistance or guidance. Insertion of C2 translaminar screws poses no risk to vertebral arteries compared with the other techniques. However, the hardware can appear asymmetrical on anteroposterior and lateral radiographic images. The surgeon must use the bony anatomical structures as they lie for optimal fixation, which sometimes result in an asymmetrical image.

▸▸ Answer 17

Correct answer is B

C2 lateral mass fixation points are not ideal for use with occipitocervical fixation, particularly in osteoporotic bone. Long applied moment arms and substantial loads place significant stress on these screw–bone interfaces. Therefore, a strategy that includes a long implant and pedicle fixation may provide superior construct integrity. If shorter constructs are indicated, the elimination of C1–C2 rotation via C1–C2 transarticular screws or C1 lateral mass and C2 pedicle screws that are rigidly attached to the occiput with a rod or plate may provide optimal fixation.

Occasionally, standard C2 fixation points may not be readily available. The lateral mass of C2 can provide a safe, albeit less robust, C2 fixation alternative. The standard starting point for the C2 facet screw is similar to that of subaxial facet screws just medial to the middle of the facet joint. However, the trajectory differs. A lateral and caudal trajectory is optimal to avoid injury to the vertebral artery from a lateral and rostral approach. Bony purchase is usually more than adequate. The C2–C3 facet joint may be "violated" by the downward- and outward-facing screw; therefore, drilling into the C3 facet may be required if C3 facet joint purchase is desired.

▸▸ Answer 18

Correct answer is C

Occipital button fixation provides significant lateral skull surface area of contact. Pullout and other forms of failure are much less likely compared with other skull fixation techniques. Direct dural visualization minimizes the chance of excessive dural compression.

▸▸ Answer 19

Correct answer is E

C1–C2 transarticular screw fixation or the use of C1 lateral mass and C2 pedicle screws facilitates the termination of an occipitocervical construct at C2. Concomitant pathology, such as a tumor or degenerative change, may mandate caudal extension of the construct.

These constructs can generally be extended caudally to C5 or C6; however, extending these constructs to C7 places significant stress on the cervicothoracic junction (see ▶ Fig. 20.5). Extension of the constructs to T2 or T3 may facilitate fixation integrity in these situations, thereby including the cervicothoracic junction and allowing fixation to C7–T1, T2, and T3. However, motion is significantly restricted by including these additional vertebral levels.

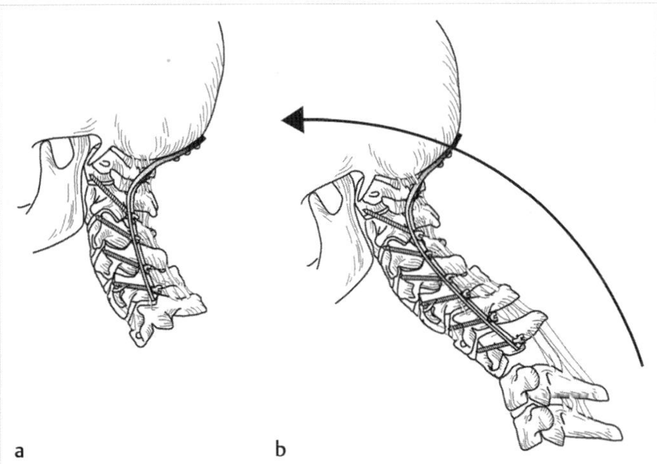

Fig. 20.5 (a) Occipitocervical constructs can be extended caudally to C5 or C6 without significant concern. **(b)** However, extension to C7 places significant stress on the cervical thoracic junction, potentially resulting in junctional instability. (Source: Biomechanics of Spine Stabilization: Third Edition, © 2015 Thieme Medical Publishers, Inc.)

▸▸ **Answer 20**

Correct answer is A

As noted previously, wire and cable fixation to the occipital bone, laminae, and spinous processes is a clinically proven method of bone anchoring. Wires and cables tend to loosen via “cheese cutting” through bone. This effect is due predominantly to the relatively small surface area of contact between the bone and the wire or cable, which can be increased by using parallel double wires or cables. In general, cables are stronger and more resistant to notching and fatigue failure than wires. Stainless steel is stronger than titanium. Polyethylene cables have as much tensile strength as stainless steel cables but are much more susceptible to stretching or creep.

Key Principles

- Wolff's law maintains that bone grows and remodels under mechanical stress. Consequently, compression should be sought when possible. A lag screw effect or the application of compressive loads can achieve such compression.
- Ventral constructs allow the surgeon to decompress, fuse, and/or apply an implant through one approach, but anatomical and biomechanical constraints increase the complication rate compared with dorsal constructs, which offer greater stabilization potential.
- Careful consideration of the patient's spinal biomechanics is critical to decision making for upper cervical constructs. Poor biomechanics, as can be seen in the elderly, increases the risk of complications in craniocervical surgery.
- Caudal extension of occipitocervical constructs to C7 can place significant stress on the mobile cervicothoracic junction. Extension to T2 or T3 reduces range of motion but can improve fixation integrity.

Reference

[1] Rampersaud YR, Simon DA, Foley KT. Accuracy requirements for image-guided spinal pedicle screw placement. Spine (Phila Pa 1976). 2001;26(4):352–359

21 Ventral Subaxial Spine Constructs

Sanjay Dhawan, Mayur Sharma

Learning Objectives

- Understand spinal instrumentation constructs from a biomechanical viewpoint.
- Understand the biomechanical forces responsible for implant failure.
- Understand ventral compression and ventral distraction spinal fixation.
- Understand the significance of multisegmental spinal fixation.

Questions

▸▸ Question 1

Which of the following statements is correct regarding the historically used Dwyer and Zielke devices to reduce spinal deformities?

- A. Used to apply distraction forces at the concave side of the scoliotic curve of the spine
- B. Used to apply compression forces at the convex side of the scoliotic curve of the spine
- C. Used to apply distraction forces at the convex side of the scoliotic curve of the spine
- D. Used to apply compression forces at the concave side of the scoliotic curve of the spine
- E. Used on both the convex and concave sides of the spine

▸▸ Question 2

The application of distraction forces to the spine does not always result in the same net force direction and output. Which of the following is true regarding distraction forces application?

- A. Determined by location of instantaneous axis of rotation (IAR) in relation to points of instrumentation-related force application
- B. Is independent of location of IAR
- C. If distraction force is ventral to IAR, forces applied are in same orientation to dorsal tension-band fixation
- D. If distraction force is in line with IAR, forces applied are in opposite orientation to dorsal tension-band fixation
- E. If distraction force is dorsal to IAR, forces applied are in same orientation to dorsal tension-band fixation

▸▸ Question 3

Tension-band forces necessitate the use of an applied moment arm to achieve their desired result. The length of the moment arm is the perpendicular distance from the point of application of the forces (by the construct) to ______.

- A. Midpoint of the instrumented vertebral body at same level
- B. IAR
- C. Junction of anterior two-thirds and posterior one-third of the width of instrumented vertebral body at same level
- D. Junction of anterior one-third and posterior two-thirds of the width of instrumented vertebral body at same level
- E. Posterior edge of the instrumented vertebral body

▸▸ Question 4

A dorsal screw–plate construct is effective in resisting axial loads and spinal extension, but it is not as effective in resisting flexion. Which of the following statements is correct regarding screw–plate constructs?

- A. Screw–plate constructs are cantilever beam constructs that always use screws in fixed moment arm
- B. Semiconstrained screw–plate devices do not require adequate dorsal spinal stability
- C. Plate bending or fracture or screw cutout may occur following flexion with screw–plate constructs
- D. Dorsal spinal stability does not determine the extent of complications with screw–plate constructs
- E. Cantilever beam constructs are a type of dorsal distraction implants that always use screws in a nonfixed moment arm mode

▸▸ **Question 12**

Which of the following is the prerequisite for ventral cantilever beam constructs to be considered ventral compression fixation devices?

- A. Applied in distraction, and resist compression and/or extension of the spine
- B. Applied in distraction, and resist compression and/or flexion of the spine
- C. Applied in compression, and resist distraction and/or flexion of the spine
- D. Applied in compression, and resist distraction and/or extension of the spine
- E. Applied in compression, and resist translation and/or rotation of the spine

▸▸ **Question 13**

Which of the following is the most plausible explanation for ventral compression fixation devices to fail in flexion, much as their distraction counterparts failing in extension?

- A. Inherent ability of ventral compression fixation devices to compensate for absent or lost dorsal tension-band force applications
- B. Inherent inability of ventral compression fixation devices to compensate for absent or lost dorsal tension-band force applications
- C. Inherent ability of ventral compression fixation devices to compensate for absent or lost ventral tension-band force applications
- D. Inherent inability of ventral compression fixation devices to compensate for absent or lost ventral tension-band force applications
- E. Inherent inability of ventral compression fixation devices to compensate for absent or lost dorsal tension-band force applications

▸▸ **Question 14**

Compression force application by the construct allows load sharing with the spine and/or interbody strut. This can be enhanced first by distraction of the spine, followed by placement of the interbody strut, and then the application of compression of the implant onto the strut. What additional advantages are provided by the compression of the implant onto the previously placed interbody strut?

- A. Increased security of strut–mortise interface and load sharing between the implant and the strut
- B. Decreased augmentation of bone healing–enhancing forces
- C. Higher chances of pole vaulting
- D. Decreased load sharing between the implant and the strut
- E. No additional effect on security of strut–mortise interface

▸▸ **Question 15**

Implant security may be enhanced in some cases by the addition of a cantilever beam construct to a ventral interbody fusion. How does the use of an intermediate point of spine fixation enhance implant security?

- A. Decreases resistance to translation deformation
- B. Decreases axial loading bearing via cantilever beam fixation
- C. Increases axial loading bearing via cantilever beam fixation and resistance to translation deformation by applying three-point bending forces
- D. Increases resistance to rotational deformation and decreases axial loading
- E. Increases rotational load bearing via cantilever beam fixation

▸▸ **Question 16**

Terminal bending moments may become apparent in situations in which excessively long tension-band fixation forces are applied to the ventral spine. Which of the following interventions can virtually eliminate this phenomenon?

- A. Using thicker screws
- B. Extending the length of the fusion
- C. Performing multisegmental fixation
- D. Using long plating systems with terminal screw fixations with no intermediate points of fixation
- E. Terminal bending movements cannot be eliminated irrespective of additional measures

▸▸ Question 17

Which of the following statements is true regarding implantation of rods and mechanics of the construct in thoracolumbar region?

- A. Interbody struts or cages increase the tension on the rods
- B. Smaller rods offer no additional facilitation in the ease of insertion compared with their larger counterparts
- C. Interbody struts or cages do not provide offloading of rods
- D. Smaller rods incorporated in dual-rod system significantly affect the mechanics of the construct
- E. Diameter of the rods incorporated in dual-rod system does not significantly affect the mechanics of the construct

▸▸ Question 18

Which of the following statements is incorrect about dual-rod system implants in thoracolumbar spine?

- A. Dual-rod systems provide stiffer constructs than their single rod counterparts particularly in torsion and flexion–extension loading
- B. Addition of cross-connectors to the dual-rod system helps in improved mechanics of the system
- C. Dual-rod systems provide unequivocally improved mechanics over that achieved with single-rod systems
- D. Dual-rod systems provide significantly better lateral bending stiffness than single-rod systems
- E. Addition of interbody strut increases stiffness in flexion with single-rod systems. This effect is also evident with dual-rod systems

▸▸ Question 19

Parallelogram deformation as shown in ▸ Fig. 21.3 can occur with ventral screw–rod system. Which of the following interventions can help prevent such deformations?

- A. Rigid cross-fixation of the rods
- B. Extension of the fusion both rostrally and caudally
- C. Using single-rod system eliminates this deformity

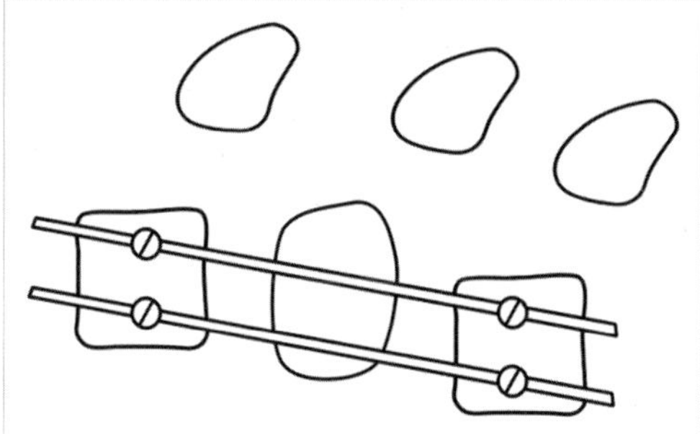

Fig. 21.3 Parallelogram deformation can occur with ventral screw–rod systems. (Source: Biomechanics of Spine Stabilization: Third Edition, © 2015 Thieme Medical Publishers, Inc.)

- D. Smaller rods decreased the chances of parallelogram deformity
- E. Using shorter screws decreases the chances of parallelogram deformity

▸▸ Question 20

Implant-derived bending moments result from implant-derived force applications to the spine by means of a moment arm. The bending moment is proportional to what?

- A. Diameter of the rods
- B. Length of the screws
- C. Length of the moment arm
- D. Number of instrumented vertebral levels
- E. Diameter of the screws

▸▸ Question 21

Some ventral devices can be placed in either a distraction or a compression mode. The distraction and subsequent compression of the spine on an interbody bone graft is facilitated by the smooth rod technique. Which of the following interventions can prevent overcompression?

- A. Using an interbody that compresses the end plate more in the inferior direction
- B. Using a flat-faced cage
- C. Using dual-rod system
- D. Using screws with larger diameter
- E. Using interbody cage with serrated edges apposed with the inferior end plate

Answers

▸▸ Answer 1

Correct answer is B

The Dwyer device, or a modification of it made by replacing the cable with a rod (Zielke apparatus), was used in the past to achieve deformity correction by the application of compression forces (tension-band fixation) on the convex side of a scoliotic curve via multisegmental points of fixation, as shown in ▶ Fig. 21.4. Recently, ventral multiple-level screw–rod fixation strategies have become increasingly popular.

▸▸ Answer 2

Correct answer is A

The characterization of the force application is determined by the location of the IAR in relation to the points of instrumentation-related force application. If the point of application of a distraction force by an implant is ventral to the IAR, forces opposite in orientation, but similar in nature, to dorsal tension-band fixation are applied. These are usually applied via cantilever beam constructs. If the point of application of the force by the construct is in line with the IAR, the distraction and tension band–like forces (bending moments) are not applied to the spine, as shown in ▶ Fig. 21.5. Such constructs are simple distraction (buttress) constructs.

▸▸ Answer 3

Correct answer is B

The length of this moment arm is the perpendicular distance from the point of application of the forces (by the construct) to the IAR. If this type of force is applied in the opposite direction (i.e., in a distraction mode), either distraction with extension or a three-point bending type of fixation is achieved. The distraction with extension is a kind of tension-band distraction fixation or distraction fixation applied at a perpendicular distance from the IAR.

▸▸ Answer 4

Correct answer is C

Cantilever beam constructs are a type of ventral distraction implants that use screws in either a fixed

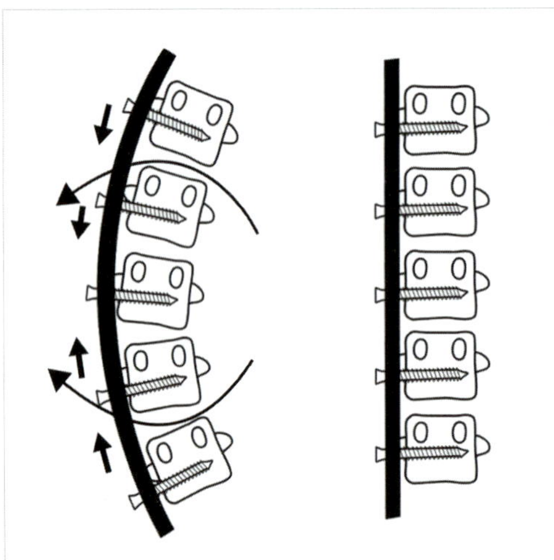

Fig. 21.4 The Dwyer and Zielke devices were historically used to apply compression fixation (tension-band fixation) at multiple levels of the spine (*left*). They were applied on the convex side of a scoliotic curve to reduce the deformity (*right*). Straight arrows depict implant force applications; curved arrows depict resulting bending moments. (Source: Biomechanics of Spine Stabilization: Third Edition, © 2015 Thieme Medical Publishers, Inc.)

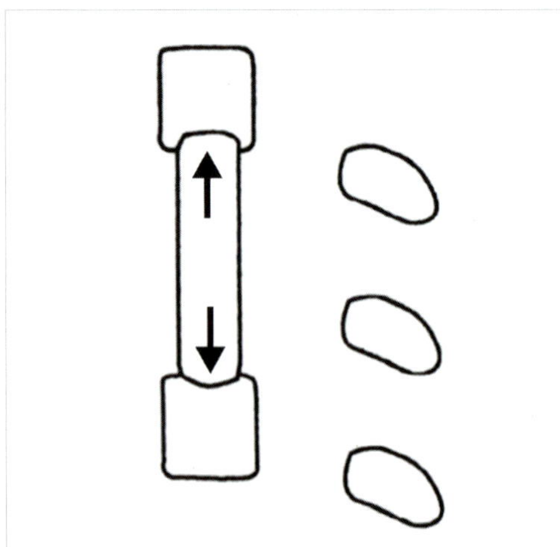

Fig. 21.5 The application of a distraction force to the mid-vertebral body region (in the region of the neutral axis) results in buttressing of the spine, without the application of a moment arm. (Source: Biomechanics of Spine Stabilization: Third Edition, © 2015 Thieme Medical Publishers, Inc.)

moment arm or a nonfixed moment arm mode. Distraction, as applied by a semiconstrained (semirigid or dynamic) screw–plate device, requires that adequate dorsal spinal stability be present. In this situation, plate bending or fracture or screw cutout may occur following flexion. Dorsal spinal stability, to a certain extent, determines the extent of complications associated with ventral screw–plate constructs. If dorsal spinal stability is present or created, these complications are less likely. A screw–plate construct, regardless of the mode of application, is effective in resisting axial loads and spinal extension, but it is not as effective in resisting flexion.

▸▸ Answer 5

Correct answer is B

Nonfixed moment arm cantilever beam implants transfer a greater percentage of axially applied load through the spine compared with their fixed moment arm counterparts. This is related to their diminished stiffness as well as to implant design characteristics. This must be considered in the selection of a rigid (fixed moment arm cantilever beam) versus a more dynamic (nonfixed moment arm cantilever beam) implant.

▸▸ Answer 6

Correct answer is D

Ventral plates cause unloading of an interbody strut in flexion and loading in extension. This is related to the fact that IAR moves toward the implant, thus causing more loading in extension (see the ▸ Fig. 21.6) and unloading in flexion (see ▸ Fig. 21.7); these forces may be reduced by using dynamic implants or buttress plates.

▸▸ Answer 7

Correct answer is A

The impaction of a graft in a vertebral body can occur in osteoporotic bone. The creation of a mortise, however, may have significant advantages for such a construct. It may help prevent one of the most common complications of this type of fixation, the "pole vaulting" of adjacent vertebral bodies past each other (**a**). This may result in screw loosening (if a cantilever beam implant, such as a cantilever beam plate, is used in conjunction with the interbody strut) and ultimately failure. This can be prevented by using a different construct altogether (e.g., a multilevel fixation construct) by creating a deeper mortise for an interbody construct or by using an additional accompanying construct (e.g., a dorsal fixation procedure). Fixation to three or more vertebrae automatically results in the application of three-point bending forces to the spine. The application of a ventral

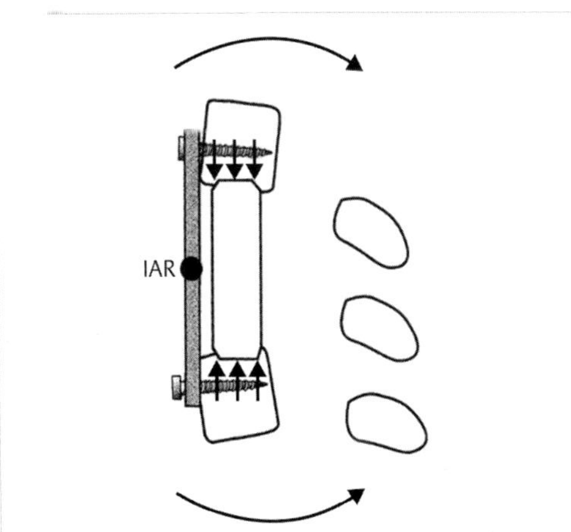

Fig. 21.6 The bone graft is loaded in compression (*arrows*). (Source: Biomechanics of Spine Stabilization: Third Edition, © 2015 Thieme Medical Publishers, Inc.)

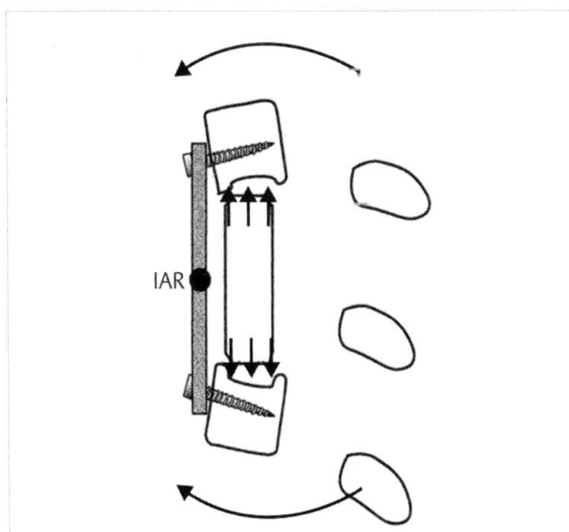

Fig. 21.7 If it is flexed, the bone graft is unloaded (*arrows*). This is related to the fact that the instantaneous axis of rotation (IAR; *dot*) is located in or about the implant in such constructs. Therefore, angular motion rotates about the IAR. (Source: Biomechanics of Spine Stabilization: Third Edition, © 2015 Thieme Medical Publishers, Inc.)

screw–plate construct in a three-point bending mode can be used to alter spine configuration. However, it may result in screw pullout, screw cutout, or plate fracture. Contouring the plate (**b**) or the shape of the bone ("gardening", **c**) may minimize the occurrence of these complications.

▸▸ Answer 8

Correct answer is B

Plates usually fracture at the point of maximum stress application (option B), which is a function of the bending moment and the strength of the implant. Site of screw attachment or the midpoint of the plate may not be the site of maximum stress application. Therefore, options C, D, and E are incorrect.

The inadvertent application of a three-point bending force to the spine may result in excessive force application that could result in (1) improper seating of the plate, (2) retropulsion of an intervening vertebral body, or (3) screw pullout or cutout, as shown in ▶ Fig. 21.8.

▸▸ Answer 9

Correct answer is C

Long bridging plates (long, multisegmental plates with screw anchors at both ends and with no intermediate fixation points) are associated with significant complications, most notably failure at the screw–bone interface. This appears to be, at least in part, related to their rigid nature (so option A is incorrect), their inability to allow subsidence (option B is incorrect), and their inability to effectively resist translation and rotation (option C is correct; option E is incorrect).

▸▸ Answer 10

Correct answer is A

The decompression itself can cause neurologic complications, which may be related to a "shifting" of neural structures resulting from the decompression. C5 radiculitis is such a complication. The C5 nerve root is particularly prone to this complication because of its nearly perpendicular projection from the spinal cord, which results in exposure of the C5 nerve root to more tension than adjacent nerve roots (option A is correct; options B, C, and D are incorrect). This, combined with a shifting of the neural elements following decompression, may contribute to the neurologic syndrome. In the literature, posterior movement of the thecal sac after cervical spine decompression has been postulated as one of the causes of C5 radiculitis and C5 nerve palsy (option E is incorrect).[1,2]

▸▸ Answer 11

Correct answer is B

Soft tissue complications, such as dysphagia and recurrent laryngeal nerve injuries, are known to occur after anterior cervical decompression and fusion procedures. Low-profile plates can diminish the incidence of dysphagia.[3] Female gender and multiple-level procedures seem to be associated with an increased incidence.[4] Anterior cervical

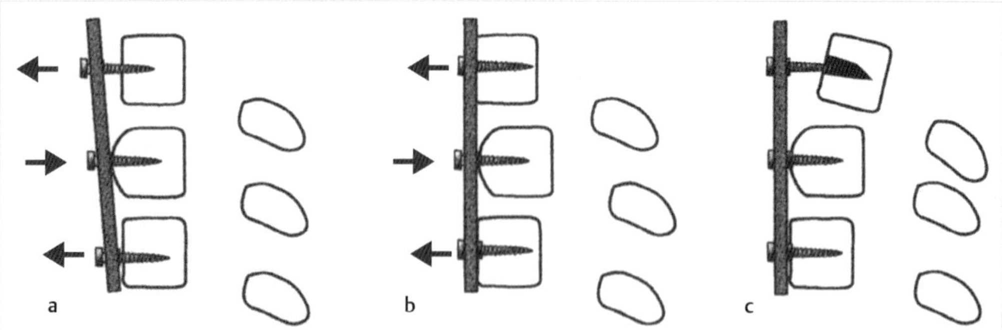

Fig. 21.8 (a, b) The inadvertent application of a three-point bending force (*arrows*) to the spine may result in excessive force application unbeknownst to the surgeon. **(a)** Improper seating of the plate or **(b)** retropulsion of an intervening vertebral body can occur. **(c)** Screw pullout or cutout. (Source: Biomechanics of Spine Stabilization: Third Edition, © 2015 Thieme Medical Publishers, Inc.)

decompression and fusion surgery at upper surgical levels at C3–C5 have been shown to be associated with greater risk of dysphagia.[5] Airway compromise should be carefully watched for in patients with prolonged procedures (lasting more than 5 hours), involving more than three vertebral segments and associated with more than 300 mL of blood loss.[6]

▸▸ Answer 12

Correct answer is D

Ventral cantilever beam constructs (fixed or nonfixed moment arm cantilever beams) are considered ventral compression fixation (tension-band fixation) devices if they (1) are applied in a compression mode, (2) resist distraction of the spine, and/or (3) resist extension of the spine (option D is correct, and options A, B, and C are incorrect). This concept is similar, but opposite in orientation, to those forces and mechanisms associated with noninterbody ventral distraction fixation.

▸▸ Answer 13

Correct answer is E

Ventral compression fixation devices may fail in flexion, much as their distraction counterparts may fail in extension. This has to do primarily with their inherent inability to compensate for absent or lost dorsal tension-band (compression) force applications (option E is correct, and options A, B, C, and D are incorrect).

▸▸ Answer 14

Correct answer is A

Compression force application by the construct allows load sharing with the spine and/or interbody strut. This can be enhanced first by distraction of the spine, then placement of the interbody strut, and finally the application of compression of the implant onto the strut. Not all techniques allow this because of the physical limitations of most implants and the anatomical limitations of the spine (which are region-specific). Compression of the implant onto the previously placed interbody strut provides (1) increased security of the interbody strut–mortise interface, (2) load sharing between the implant and the strut, and (3) the augmentation of bone healing–enhancing forces (i.e., compression) (option A is correct; options B, C, D, and E are incorrect).

▸▸ Answer 15

Correct answer is C

Implant security may be enhanced in some cases by the addition of a cantilever beam construct to a ventral interbody fusion via an intermediate point of fixation to a retained intervening vertebral body. This is depicted in the form of a fixed moment arm cantilever beam construct that also applies three-point bending forces (see ▸ Fig. 21.9). The use of an intermediate point of spine fixation provides for axial load bearing via cantilever beam fixation and for resistance to translation deformation via a three-point bending force application.

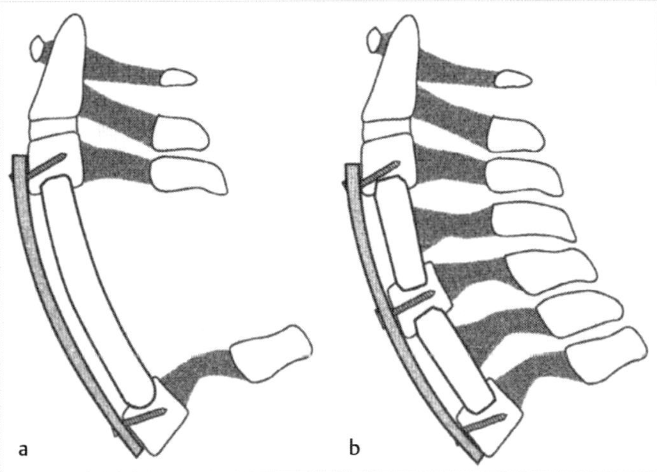

Fig. 21.9 Implant security may be enhanced in some cases by the addition of a cantilever beam construct to a ventral interbody fusion. **(a)** This is depicted in the form of a fixed moment arm cantilever beam construct. **(b)** The use of an intermediate point of spine fixation provides for axial load bearing via cantilever beam fixation and for resistance to translation deformation via three-point bending force application. (Source: Biomechanics of Spine Stabilization: Third Edition, © 2015 Thieme Medical Publishers, Inc.)

▸▸ Question 4

What is the prototype of dorsal three-point bending fixation?
- A. Knodt rod
- B. Cerclage wiring technique
- C. Harrington rod
- D. Dorsal cantilever beam fixation
- E. Dorsal cervical plate–screw fixation

▸▸ Question 5

How does the direction of force applied to the spine by tension-band fixation construct compare with that of the force applied by three-point bending constructs?
- A. Differs by 45 degrees
- B. Differs by 90 degrees
- C. Differs by 180 degrees
- D. Differs by 360 degrees
- E. Equal direction, different magnitude

▸▸ Question 6

In a dorsal compression or tension-band fixation construct to stabilize a flexion deformity, as in image a of ▸ Fig. 22.2, what anatomical structure must be intact for appropriate fixation?
- A. Anterior longitudinal ligament
- B. Lamina
- C. Facet joints
- D. Intervertebral disc
- E. Posterior longitudinal ligament

▸▸ Question 7

Dorsal tension band by cerclage wiring most effectively resists which movement or force?
- A. Anterior translation
- B. Posterior translation
- C. Lateral translation
- D. Extension
- E. Flexion

▸▸ Question 8

In the use of a Harrington rod construct, the addition of sleeves can directly increase ________.
- A. Compression
- B. Distraction
- C. Shear
- D. Fusion
- E. Stress shielding

▸▸ Question 9

The application of isolated dorsal spinal distraction forces is most likely to exaggerate ________.
- A. Neuroforaminal stenosis
- B. Kyphotic deformity
- C. Dynamic instability
- D. Coronal deformity
- E. Disc herniation

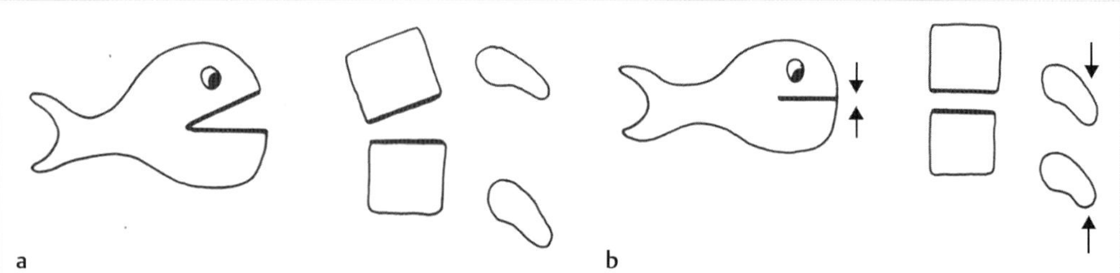

Fig. 22.2 (a) The analogy between a fish's open mouth and a flexion deformity. **(b)** The fish's mouth can be closed (or the deformity reduced) by a tension-band fixation mechanism. (Source: Biomechanics of Spine Stabilization: Third Edition, © 2015 Thieme Medical Publishers, Inc.)

▸▸ **Question 10**

What affects the length of the moment arm in a dorsal tension-band fixation construct?
- A. The distance between the points of attachment
- B. The total length of the construct
- C. The number of points of attachment
- D. The distance from the IAR to the point of attachment of the construct
- E. Nothing, because there is no moment arm

▸▸ **Question 11**

Dorsal tension-band techniques have an added mechanical advantage due to the anatomy of the subaxial cervical spine relative to other spine regions; to what is this advantage due?
- A. The normal cervical lordosis
- B. The orientation of the cervical facets
- C. The bifid cervical spinous processes
- D. The shorter cervical pedicles
- E. The shorter height of the vertebral bodies

▸▸ **Question 12**

Altering a three-point bending technique in which way would diminish the load applied to terminal implant–bone interfaces?
- A. Shorten the construct
- B. Lengthen the construct
- C. Use of a sleeve
- D. Use of crosslinks
- E. Use of terminal hooks

▸▸ **Question 13**

How would altering a multisegmental fixed cantilever beam fixation construct have prevented the screw fracture, as seen in ▸ Fig. 22.3?
- A. Shorten the construct
- B. Lengthen the construct
- C. Use of a sleeve
- D. Use of crosslinks
- E. Use of terminal hooks

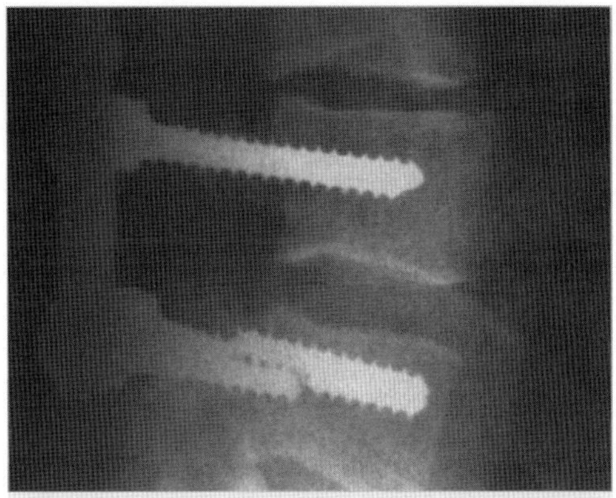

Fig. 22.3 The lower screw of a long screw rod construct may fail by fracture. This screw is loaded more than all other screws. A shorter construct (one less lumbar segment) rather than a longer construct might have prevented this. This would have allowed the fusion of one less "vital" motion segment and the application of a shorter moment arm to the most caudal screw. (Source: Biomechanics of Spine Stabilization: Third Edition, © 2015 Thieme Medical Publishers, Inc.)

▸▸ **Question 14**

Which of the following is *not* a technique to decrease or prevent lateral translation deformation (parallelogram-like) in a fixed moment arm cantilever beam pedicle fixation construct?
- A. Toe-in configuration of pedicle screws
- B. Rigid cross-fixation of the two longitudinal members (cross-link)
- C. The addition of fixation with an intervening segment
- D. Increasing the length of the fixation to include more segments
- E. Increasing screw length

▸▸ **Question 15**

▸ Fig. 22.4 is representative of which type of fixation?
- A. Fixed moment arm cantilever beam construct
- B. Nonfixed moment arm cantilever beam construct
- C. Applied moment arm cantilever beam construct
- D. Dorsal compression fixation
- E. Three-point bending cantilever beam construct

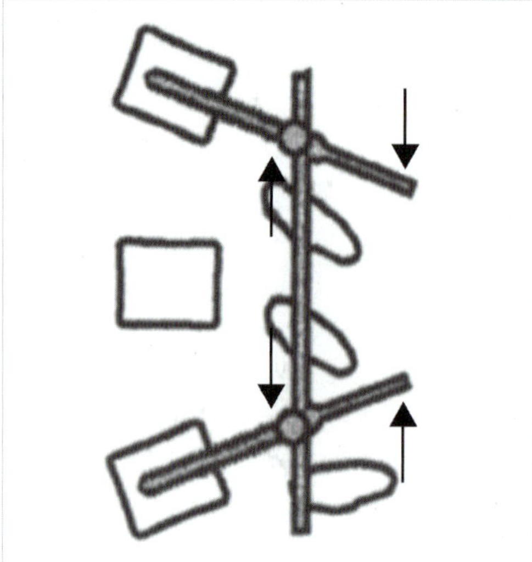

Fig. 22.4 An applied moment arm cantilever beam construct can be applied in the modes of its fixed moment arm counterpart, as well as in extension (or flexion). It is emphasized that an applied moment arm cantilever beam construct may be used to apply axial forces (distraction or compression), as well as bending moments (extension or flexion). Arrows depict applied-force vectors. (Source: Biomechanics of Spine Stabilization: Third Edition, © 2015 Thieme Medical Publishers, Inc.)

▸▸ Question 16

Three-point bending constructs are most likely to fail where?

- A. At the fulcrum
- B. At the implant–longitudinal member interface
- C. At the implant–bone interface
- D. Thoracolumbar junction
- E. At the point of maximal compression

▸▸ Question 17

Interbody spacers function more effectively in tandem with dorsally placed pedicle screw systems when placed relatively more ________.

- A. Dorsal
- B. Ventral
- C. Central
- D. Lateral
- E. Rostral

▸▸ Question 18

Cantilever beam constructs are frequently used in a multisegmental manner; the addition of intermediate screws leads to what biomechanical change to the construct?

- A. Increased strength
- B. Decreased load sharing
- C. Decreased stiffness
- D. Increased stiffness
- E. No change

▸▸ Question 19

Most modern, dorsal, multisegmental screw–rod constructs would be best categorized as ________.

- A. Dorsal distraction fixation
- B. Dorsal compression (tension-band) fixation
- C. Fixed moment arm cantilever beam fixation
- D. Nonfixed moment arm cantilever beam fixation
- E. Applied moment arm cantilever beam fixation

Answers

▸▸ Answer 1

Correct answer is E

Multisegmental instrumentation permits sharing of the load applied to the instrumentation construct with multiple vertebrae, thus substantially decreasing the chance of failure at the metal–bone interface. These pictures from the texts demonstrate several different applications of constructs utilizing Luque sublaminar wiring to a variety of Luque-type longitudinal constructs (see ▸ Fig. 22.5).

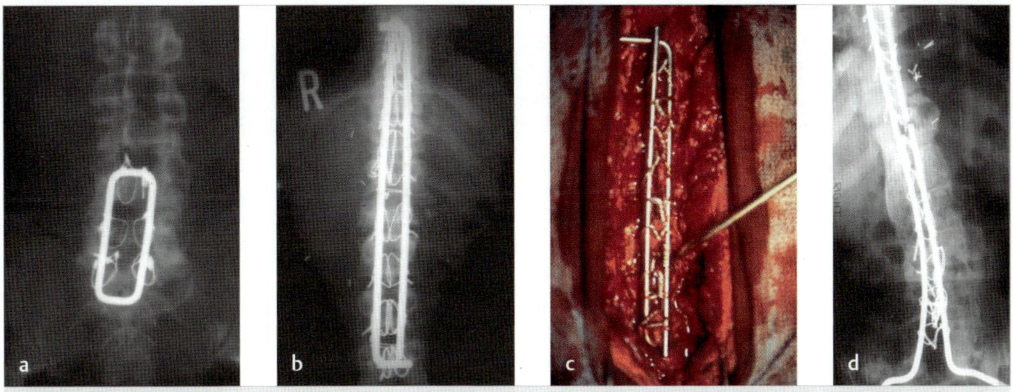

Fig. 22.5 Dorsal spine fixation devices that are of historical interest and rarely used today. **(a)** Luque loops. **(b, c)** Long Luque rod fixation, with an intraoperative photograph depicting surgical technique. **(d)** Modification of the Luque technique with "Galveston" fixation to the ilia. Note the fractured rod. (Source: Biomechanics of Spine Stabilization: Third Edition, © 2015 Thieme Medical Publishers, Inc.)

▸▸ Answer 2

Correct answer is A

Dorsal interspinous distraction systems cause force applications of distraction between the spinous processes of adjacent motion segments.

Image **c** in ▶ Fig. 22.6 is a representation of an interspinous process device.

▸▸ Answer 3

Correct answer is D

Tension-band fixation constructs function by closing the fish's mouth. To provide spinal stability, the force application requires an intact hinge serving as the IAR. Without this intact hinge, success cannot be expected.

The "hinge" of the fish's jaw is analogous to the IAR. The anatomical correlate would be the anterior and posterior ligaments. The "jaw" corresponds to dorsal elements like the spinous process or laminae.

▸▸ Answer 4

Correct answer is C

Three-point bending constructs involve instrumentation application over multiple spinal

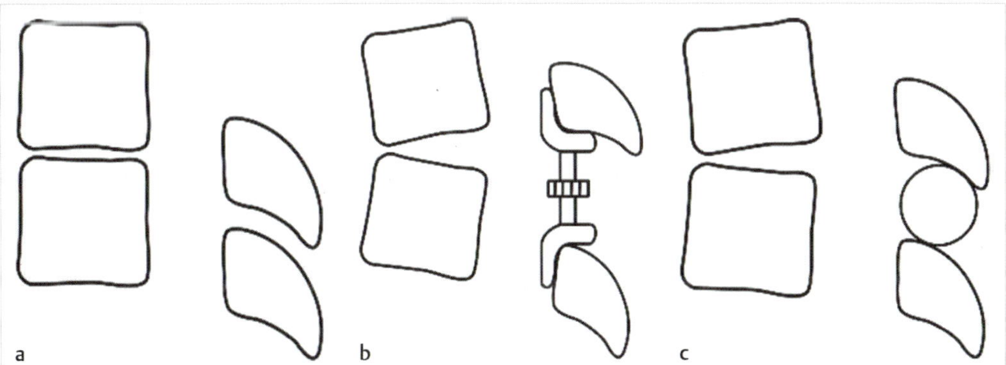

Fig. 22.6 Knodt rod application over a single motion segment. **(a, b)** Note the opening of the neuroforamina and the kyphosis created in comparison with the preoperative configuration. **(c)** Dorsal interspinous distraction systems, such as the X-Stop System (Medtronic, Minneapolis, MN), cause similar force applications. Straight arrows depict the forces applied by the implant. (Source: Biomechanics of Spine Stabilization: Third Edition, © 2015 Thieme Medical Publishers, Inc.)

segments, usually five or more, with accompanying dorsally directed forces applied at the upper and lower implant–bone interfaces and a ventrally directed force applied at the fulcrum.

Dorsal three- or four-point bending forces are commonly applied in the thoracic and lumbar regions, usually with accompanying distraction or compression forces. The Harrington distraction rod is the prototype of this type of fixation.

▸▸ Answer 5

Correct answer is B

The forces applied to the spine by a dorsal tension-band fixation construct (*solid arrows* in ▸ Fig. 22.7) are perpendicular to those applied by a three-point bending construct (*hollow arrows*).

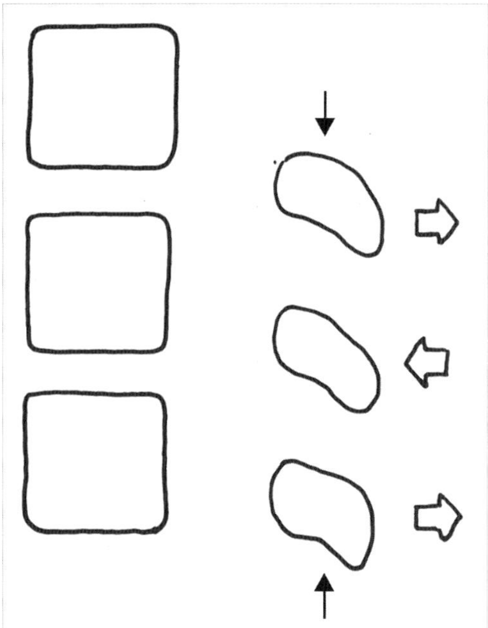

Fig. 22.7 The forces applied to the spine by a dorsal tension-band fixation construct (*solid arrows*) are perpendicular to those applied by a three-point bending construct (*hollow arrows*). (Source: Biomechanics of Spine Stabilization: Third Edition, © 2015 Thieme Medical Publishers, Inc.)

▸▸ Answer 6

Correct answer is A

To provide appropriate spinal stability, tension-band fixation requires an intact hinge serving as the IAR. In the case of the flexion deformity, as depicted, the only remaining structure that would be potentially able to serve as a hinge would be the anterior longitudinal ligament.

▸▸ Answer 7

Correct answer is E

The moment arm (d) associated with the forces applied by dorsal tension-band fixation construct (*straight arrows* in ▸ Fig. 22.8) provides resistance to flexion. *Curved arrows* depict the flexion bending moments that must be resisted.

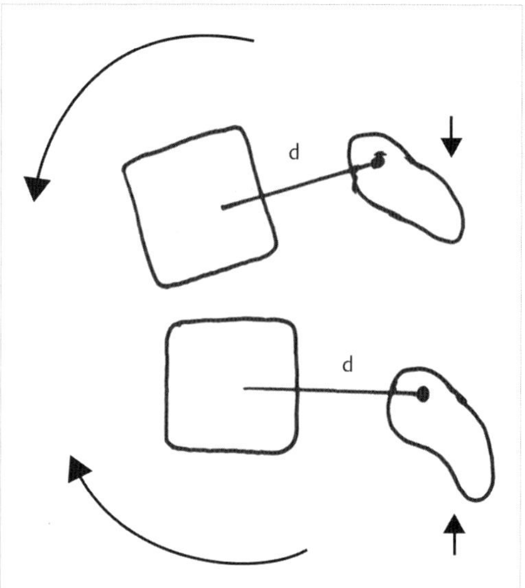

Fig. 22.8 The moment arm (*d*) associated with the forces applied by dorsal tension-band fixation construct (*straight arrows*) provides resistance to flexion. Curved arrows depict the flexion bending moments that must be resisted. (Source: Biomechanics of Spine Stabilization: Third Edition, © 2015 Thieme Medical Publishers, Inc.)

▸▸ **Answer 8**

Correct answer is C

The dorsally and ventrally directed forces (*arrows* in ▶ Fig. 22.9a,b) applied by three-point bending constructs. Sleeve application facilitates engagement of the fulcrum by the rod.

▸▸ **Answer 9**

Correct answer is B

The application of isolated dorsal spinal distraction forces may exaggerate a kyphotic deformity.

▸▸ **Answer 10**

Correct answer is D

The direction of the force applied to the spine by tension-band fixation is perpendicular to the long axis of the spine. Because of the parallel orientation of the force application and the fact that the moment arm is perpendicular to this orientation, the length of the construct does not affect the bending moment applied at the termini of the construct. Therefore, the length of the construct does not affect the efficacy of deformity correction. The only factor affecting the length of the moment arm is the distance from the IAR to the point of attachment of the construct.

▸▸ **Answer 11**

Correct answer is B

Dorsal tension-band fixation techniques for application in the subaxial cervical region have one significant advantage that similar applications in the thoracic and lumbar region do not: the orientation of the facet joints in the coronal plane. The dorsal application of tension between two vertebral segments at the lamina or spinous process level (dorsal to the IAR) positions the involved facets so that ventral translation cannot occur. The juxtaposed nature of the cervical facets results in their contribution to translation resistance by virtue of their engagement.

▸▸ **Answer 12**

Correct answer is B

Lengthening the construct increases the length of the applied moment arm (distance from fulcrum to terminus), which in turn decreases the dorsally directed forces applied at the upper implant–bone interface ($M = F \times D$). Alternatively, multiple points of pedicle screw fixation can diminish the load in comparison to a single instrumented segment.

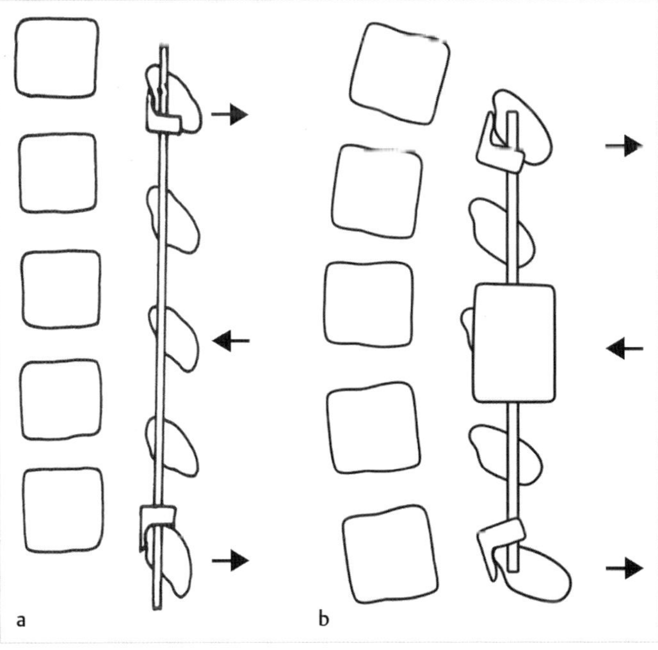

Fig. 22.9 **(a)** The dorsally and ventrally directed forces (arrows) applied by three-point bending constructs. **(b)** Sleeves may be used as spacers to provide an advantage in the form of ventrally directed force application at the fulcrum. Arrows depict the forces applied. (Source: Biomechanics of Spine Stabilization: Third Edition, © 2015 Thieme Medical Publishers, Inc.)

▸▸ Answer 13

Correct answer is A

The lower screw of a long screw rod construct may fail by fracture. This screw is loaded more than all other screws. A shorter construct (one less lumbar segment) rather than a longer construct might have prevented this. Screw fracture may occur most often at the lower screw of a long screw–rod construct. This so because of the long moment arm applied (see ▸ Fig. 22.10).

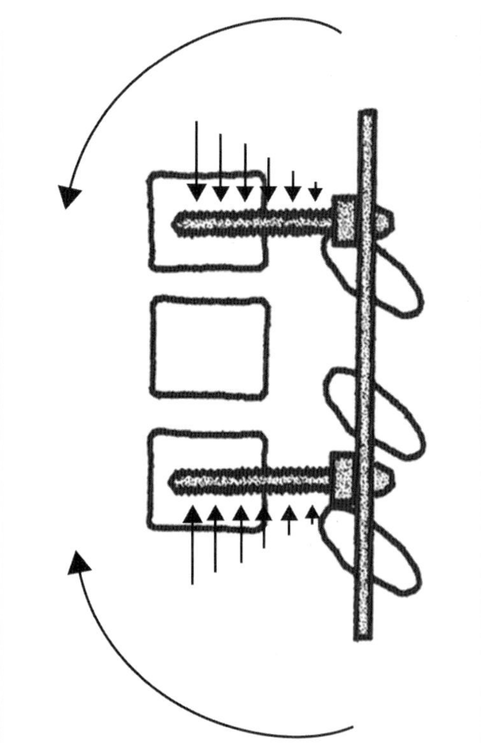

Fig. 22.10 The forces (*straight arrows*) and bending moments (*curved arrows*) resisted by rigid (fixed moment arm) cantilever beam constructs (Source: Biomechanics of Spine Stabilization: Third Edition, © 2015 Thieme Medical Publishers, Inc.)

▸▸ Answer 14

Correct answer is E

Pedicle fixation constructs may fail during axial loading because of a parallelogram-like translational deformation. A simple toe-in of the screws, rigid cross-fixation, extension of the length of the implant to incorporate an extra segmental level, or a combination of these strategies should minimize or eliminate the chance of this complication occurring.

▸▸ Answer 15

Correct answer is C

An applied moment arm cantilever beam construct can be applied in the modes of its fixed moment arm counterpart, as well as in extension (or flexion). It is emphasized that an applied moment arm cantilever beam construct may be used to apply axial forces (distraction or compression), as well as bending moments (extension or flexion).

The use of a Schanz screw technique allows the application of very complex forces at the time of surgery. These usually are either extension or flexion forces. They have been used to treat fractures of the thoracic and lumbar spine.

▸▸ Answer 16

Correct answer is C

In three-point bending constructs, shear forces are greatest at the terminal implant–bone interface; this tends to be where these constructs fail (see ▸ Fig. 22.11).

▸▸ Answer 17

Correct answer is B

A fixed moment arm cantilever beam construct resists axial loading and provides significant stabilization, but it does not completely shield the disc interspace from loading in the upright position. This notion is corroborated by the observation that ventral interbody spacers function more effectively (than dorsally placed interbody spacers) in tandem with dorsally placed pedicle screw systems.

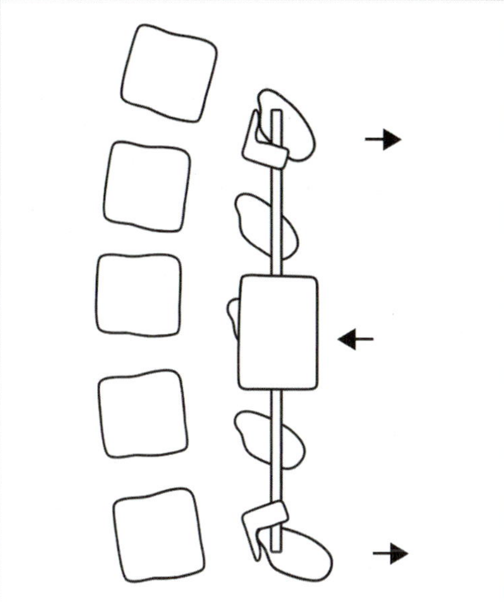

Fig. 22.11 Sleeves may be used as spacers to provide an advantage in the form of ventrally directed force application at the fulcrum. Arrows depict the forces applied. (Source: Biomechanics of Spine Stabilization: Third Edition, © 2015 Thieme Medical Publishers, Inc.)

▸▸ Answer 18

Correct answer is D

Multiple-level rigid pedicle screw fixation is biomechanically superior to terminal-level screw fixation via an augmentation of stiffness.

▸▸ Answer 19

Correct answer is C

Fixed moment arm cantilever beam fixation describes the biomechanical principles in application for most modern, dorsal, multisegmental screw-rod constructs. In this setting the typical pedicle screw is the cantilever or beam that projects from an immobile object. The construct is "fixed", because either it is a rigid pedicle screw to begin with, secured to a longitudinal member or once tightening a polyaxial screw head with associated fixation mechanism to a rod it becomes rigid.

Key Principles

- The evolution of dorsal subaxial spine constructs has led to tremendous change over time and this trend will likely continue even if at a slower rate of change. The biomechanical principles will, however, remain and need to be considered with current and future instrumentation.
- In general, modern multisegmental instrumentation constructs, when planned and applied appropriately, provide many benefits over their historical predecessors.
- Biomechanical strengths, weaknesses, and stresses change along the length of the spine relative to the region, anatomy, and pathological process, if present.
- Loads resisted or supported by dorsal constructs are not fixed and change with patient position and activity.
- Knowledge and consideration of biomechanical properties and principles can lead to more successful instrumentation with fewer complications or mechanical failures.

23 Interbody Constructs

Mohamed Macki, Praveen V. Mummaneni

Understanding interbody constructs is essential to successful spinal surgery practice. There are fundamental principles that can guide our approach to stabilizing the spinal column with an interbody graft.

Learning Objectives

- Understand the different types of interbody constructs.
- Describe the biomechanical importance of the location and placement of interbody constructs.
- Understand the clinical implications of different interbody constructs.

Questions

▸▸ Question 1

Trainees must understand which of the following in learning the basic tenets of interbody constructs?

- A. Interbody constructs provide the ability to optimally bear axial loads along the neutral axis by applying a significant bending moment to the spine
- B. Interbody constructs bear axial loads most effectively when placed in line with the neutral axis
- C. Interbody constructs enhance the chance of arthrodesis because of bone distraction forces that are "seen" during assumption of the upright posture
- D. Cantilever beams, three-point bending, or tension-band fixation implants may not be used in conjunction with interbody constructs
- E. Location of interbody constructs in the intervertebral disc space is of little relevance

▸▸ Question 2

How does the modulus of elasticity relate to nonautologous bony spacers?

- A. The elasticity of the strut should be more than that of the accepting body to prevent subsidence
- B. The cortical bone component of a graft heals faster than the cancellous component
- C. The fibula has a high ratio of cortical to cancellous bone. This diminishes the ability to rapidly heal
- D. The high modulus of elasticity of an interbody strut, relative to parent vertebral body, protects against subsidence
- E. Modulus of elasticity is not important regarding ultimate construct success

▸▸ Question 3

Which of the following biomechanical properties appropriately applies to cervical interbody constructs?

- A. The dorsal placement of the crestal portion of an iliac crest graft allows load sharing between the anterior column (interbody strut) and intact posterior column structures (e.g., the facet joints)
- B. Ventral placement of the crestal portion of an iliac crest graft may provide advantages when ventral cantilevered implants are used in conjunction
- C. The middle column of Denis and a ventrally placed implant (plate and screws) share the load during the acquisition of fusion
- D. The location of the axial load-bearing intervertebral component, with respect to ventral–dorsal end plate positioning, is more important for long dorsal constructs
- E. None of the above

▸▸ Question 4

Interbody fusion techniques, compared with dorsal onlay grafting techniques, are associated with ________.

- A. Decreased incidence of pseudarthrosis
- B. Decreased rate of fusion acquisition
- C. Decreased axial load-bearing ability
- D. Technically equal difficulty
- E. Fusion success is not related to onlay grafting

▸▸ Question 5

The chance of subsidence of an interbody bone graft into a vertebral body is inversely proportional to ________.

- A. The cross-sectional area of the interbody strut
- B. The height of the interbody strut
- C. The modulus of elasticity of the interbody strut
- D. The expansion of the interbody strut
- E. Higher bone mineral density

▸▸ Question 6

Flat-faced cages have unique properties that include ________.

- A. A shape that is round, square, or rectangular at the end plate
- B. A parallel, instead of a trapezoidal, shape in the sagittal plane
- C. Always a high modulus of elasticity
- D. Less surface area than round-faced cages
- E. Flat-faced cages do not have any unique properties

▸▸ Question 7

Which of the following must be considered with interbody constructs in the lumbar spine?

- A. Allograft performs worse than autograft in anterior lumbar interbody fusions
- B. Axial load force vectors may cause resultant translational and angular force vectors
- C. Suboptimal surface area of contact between the bone graft and the vertebral body resists the axial and resultant translational and angular force vectors
- D. The chance of subsidence of an interbody bone graft into a vertebral body is proportional to the cross-sectional area of contact
- E. Lumbar interbody constructs have a high rate of failure

▸▸ Question 8

A surgeon places the crestal portion of the cervical interbody iliac crest graft in line with the neutral axis (i.e., toward the dorsal portion of the vertebral body). The cervical interbody iliac crest graft now has which of the following properties?

- A. Axial loads are ineffectively borne
- B. Stronger bony fusion compared with dorsal placement of the crestal portion of a cervical interbody iliac crest strut graft, in combination with a ventral plate
- C. Kyphosis prevention is somewhat limited
- D. No relevance has been shown regarding the position of the cervical interbody iliac crest graft
- E. The position of the cervical interbody iliac crest graft is unrelated to the neutral axis

▸▸ Question 9

The biomechanical properties of flat-faced cages are unique in that ________.

- A. Translational and angular deformation (rocking) is much less likely with a strut with round ends than with a flat-faced cage
- B. A strut with a round end and a flat-faced cage provide equivalent degrees of resistance to rocking
- C. Excessive compression can be applied, with an alteration of angulation, by means of a ventral fixator
- D. The end plates of expandable titanium cages are round-faced
- E. Flat-faced and round-faced cages have equal biomechanical properties

▸▸ Question 10

Which of the following pertains to flat-faced cages?

- A. Compared with the trapezoidal shape, a parallel shape to the end plates is more advantageous at the lumbosacral junction
- B. Flat-faced cages present a smaller surface area of contact to the vertebral body than do round-faced cages
- C. Smaller-diameter flat-faced cages provide a greater advantage from an implant–bone interface perspective
- D. Adding an internal end ring further augments implant–bone integrity but sacrifices surface area of contact for bony fusion functions like a “toilet seat”
- E. Flat-faced cages have a high rate of failure

▸▸ Question 11

Which biomechanical and geometric factors apply to the efficacy of interbody cages?

- A. Disruption of the anterior longitudinal ligament may decrease the strength of the tension band in flexion, and disruption of the posterior longitudinal ligament may decrease the strength of the tension band in extension
- B. Use of a disc interspace spreader/retractor prevents a loss of sagittal balance that results in pain (e.g., the flat-back syndrome)
- C. Because of the lenticular shape of an end plate, the area of contact between the strut and the end plate may leave undesirable "gaps" that impair optimal fusion surfaces
- D. Devices with threads or hooks provide less resistance than ridged devices
- E. Interbody cage selection should be unrelated to end plate shape

▸▸ Question 12

When a surgeon inserts an interbody cage, which of the following must be considered for attainment of disc interspace distraction?

- A. Insertion of smaller-diameter cages may overcome the need for extensive facet removal but may not achieve sufficient distraction for stability or restoration of interbody height for foraminal decompression
- B. A round-faced cage cannot maintain a constant "region of contact" with the end plate
- C. The use of a single cage, as opposed to two parallel cages, maximizes dorsal element disruption
- D. Expandable cages are inappropriate for grade I spondylolisthesis because of the inability to tension ligaments
- E. Interspace distraction is unrelated to the insertion of an interbody cage

▸▸ Question 13

What are strategies to maintain disc interspace distraction?

- A. A repetitive, cyclical axial loading of the spine significantly contributes to the subsidence phenomenon
- B. Subsidence decreases when disc height has been elevated significantly by the surgery
- C. Although deleterious to disc height, subsidence does enhance stress shielding, according to Wolff's law
- D. Posterior lumbar interbody fusion with bone graft alone achieves less stiffness than that of the intact spine
- E. Disc space distraction is irrelevant in spine surgery

▸▸ Question 14

How must patients be counseled on long-term risk of fusions?

- A. End-fusion degenerative changes occur at a greater frequency with shorter fusion constructs
- B. End-fusion degenerative changes occur more frequently if abnormal spinal alignment (kyphosis) are created by the fusion
- C. A stiffer fusion construct may decrease the incidence of adjacent segment disease
- D. Fusion constructs terminating at the thoracolumbar junction have a lower incidence of adjacent segment disease
- E. No long-term risks are associated with spinal surgery

▸▸ Question 15

A surgeon's interbody selection should take which of the following into consideration?

- A. A higher incidence of neurologic complications was noted with dowels compared with impacted wedges
- B. Insertion of dowels via the posterior lumbar interbody fusion technique obviates substantial exposure or substantial nerve root traction
- C. Cylindrical implants are more prone to magnetic resonance imaging (MRI) artifact than more cuboidal or rectangular implants
- D. Threaded interbody fusion cages are safer and easier to remove than pedicle screw implants
- E. All interbodies are created equally

▸▸ **Question 16**

Shaping of a curved iliac crest graft for ventral cervical interbody must take which of the following into consideration?

- A. Allows for a loose fit laterally
- B. A snugly fit graft compromises the stability the fusion mass
- C. Care must be taken to maximize cortical bone removal
- D. A snugly fit graft increases the chance for vascularization at intermediate segmental levels
- E. Shaping of iliac crest graft is irrelevant in spine surgery

Answers

▸▸ **Answer 1**

Correct answer is B

Interbody constructs provide the ability to optimally bear axial loads along the neutral axis without applying a significant bending moment to the spine. This enhances the chance of achieving an arthrodesis because of bone compression–related augmentation of the bone healing–enhancing forces that are "seen" during assumption of the upright posture (see ▸ Fig. 23.1). Interbody struts bear axial loads (*arrows*) most effectively when placed in line with the neutral axis (*shaded region*).

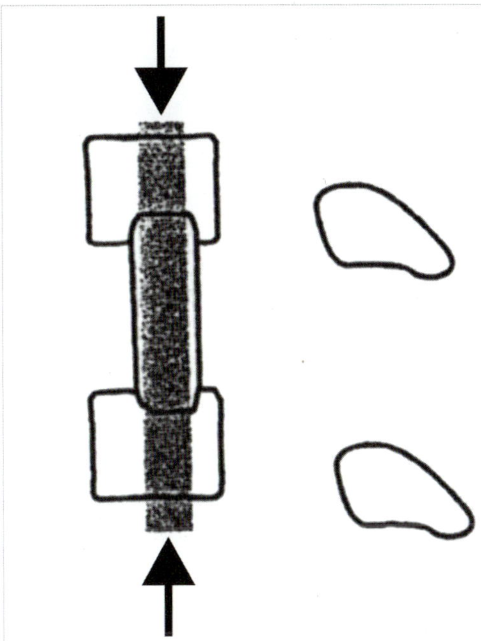

Fig. 23.1 Interbody struts bear axial loads (*arrows*) most effectively when placed in line with the neutral axis (*shaded region*). (Source: Biomechanics of Spine Stabilization: Third Edition, © 2015 Thieme Medical Publishers, Inc.)

Interbody devices consist of bone implants, implants other than bone, or a combination. They may be nonabsorbable or absorbable—with fluctuating, intermittent, and fleeting enthusiasm for the latter type shown over the years. They can be used alone or in combination with other implants (cantilever beams, three-point bending, or tension-band fixation implants) that may be applied via either a ventral or dorsal approach.

▸▸ **Answer 2**

Correct answer is C

Nonautologous bone alternatives may also be used. The most common of these is the fibula allograft strut graft. Its high modulus of elasticity relative to parent vertebral body bone may result in subsidence. Ideally, the modulus of elasticity of the strut should approximate that of the accepting body (i.e., end plate). Two factors are significant in this regard: (1) the fibula has a high ratio of cortical to cancellous bone, and (2) the cortical bone component of a graft heals very slowly. Hence, there exists a diminished ability to heal, or at least heal rapidly, when such grafts are employed. This negative attribute can be partially neutralized by the placement of autologous medullary bone in the central (medullary) region of the allograft fibula strut. This provides an enhanced bone-healing capacity component to the already present structural component of the allograft fibula.

▸▸ **Answer 3**

Correct answer is C

The ventral placement of the crestal portion of an iliac crest graft is biomechanically prudent, particularly when other implant adjuncts are not used. This allows load sharing between the anterior column (interbody strut) and intact posterior column structures (e.g., the facet joints). However, dorsal placement of the crestal portion of the graft may provide advantages when ventral cantilevered implants are used in conjunction.

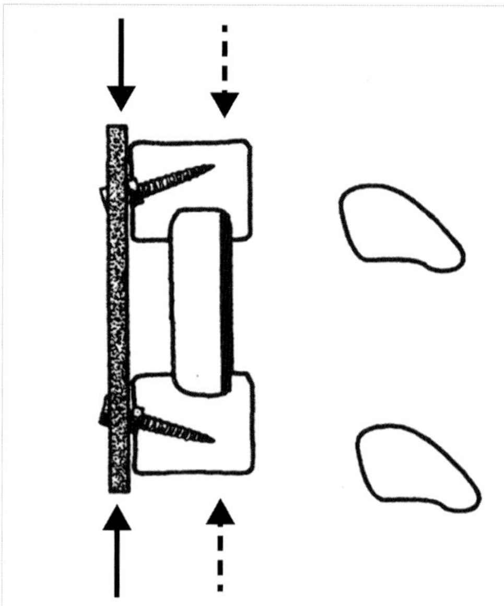

Fig. 23.2 Dorsal placement of the crestal portion of a cervical interbody iliac crest strut graft, in combination with a ventral plate, allows the axial load to be shared between the ventral implant and the dorsally placed crestal portion of the graft (*dashed arrows*). (Source: Biomechanics of Spine Stabilization: Third Edition, © 2015 Thieme Medical Publishers, Inc.)

This permits the middle column of Denis and the ventrally placed implant to share the load during the acquisition of fusion.

Dorsal placement of the crestal portion of a cervical interbody iliac crest strut graft, in combination with a ventral plate, allows the axial load to be shared between the ventral implant and the dorsally placed crestal portion of the graft (see ▶ Fig. 23.2, *dashed arrows*).

With accompanying long dorsal constructs, however, the location of the axial load-bearing intervertebral component, with respect to ventral–dorsal end plate positioning, does not appear to matter.

▸▸ Answer 4

Correct answer is A

Interbody fusion techniques provide many theoretical and proven advantages over dorsal onlay grafting techniques. These include (1) a decreased incidence of pseudarthrosis, (2) an accelerated rate of fusion acquisition, and (3) an increased axial load-bearing ability. In the lumbar spine, additional extenuating circumstances may neutralize some or all of the aforementioned advantages, not the least of which includes the technical pitfalls associated with the operative procedure: overly aggressive end plate debridement may result in the loss of integrity of the end plate with subsequent subsidence of the graft; insufficient debridement may result in the preparation of an inadequate graft bed and nonunion (pseudarthrosis).

▸▸ Answer 5

Correct answer is A

The chance of subsidence of an interbody bone graft into a vertebral body is inversely proportional to the cross-sectional area of contact. The higher the modulus of elasticity, the higher the risk of subsidence. Destruction of the end plate has been associated directly with subsidence.

▸▸ Answer 6

Correct answer is A

The flat-faced cages may be round, square, or rectangular at the end, and they may have a parallel or trapezoidal shape in the sagittal plane to conform to the shape of the disc interspace. They may have a high modulus of elasticity (e.g., stainless steel or titanium alloys), a relatively low modulus of elasticity (e.g., bone), or an intermediate modulus of elasticity (e.g., carbon fiber, polyether ether ketone [PEEK], or femoral ring allograft). Some flat-faced cages provide a greater surface area of contact with the accepting fusion bed than others, but flat-faced cages almost always provide more surface area than round-faced cages.

▸▸ Answer 7

Correct answer is B

Of interest is that allograft performs as well as, if not better than, autograft in anterior lumbar interbody fusion procedures. The loads borne by the lumbosacral region include axial loads (*vertical arrows*) and resultant translational loads (*diagonal arrows*), as well as bending moments (*curved arrows*) (see ▶ Fig. 23.3).

Suboptimal surface area of contact between the bone graft and the vertebral body *fails* to resist the axial and resultant translational and

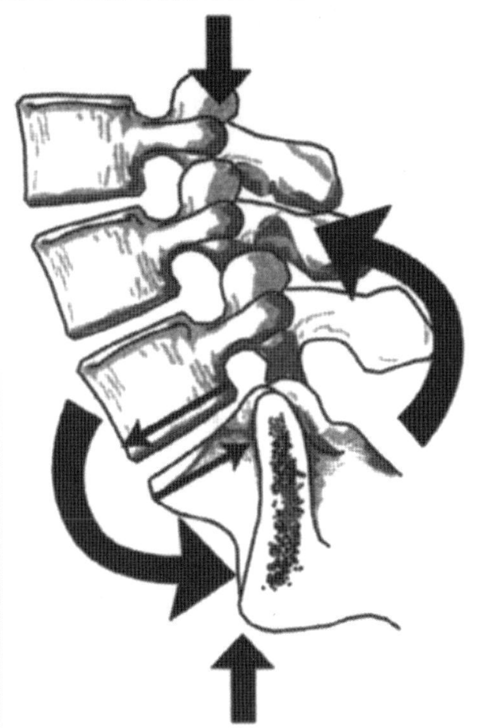

Fig. 23.3 The loads borne by the lumbosacral region include axial loads (*vertical arrows*) and resultant translational loads (*diagonal arrows*), as well as bending moments (*curved arrows*). (Source: Biomechanics of Spine Stabilization: Third Edition, © 2015 Thieme Medical Publishers, Inc.)

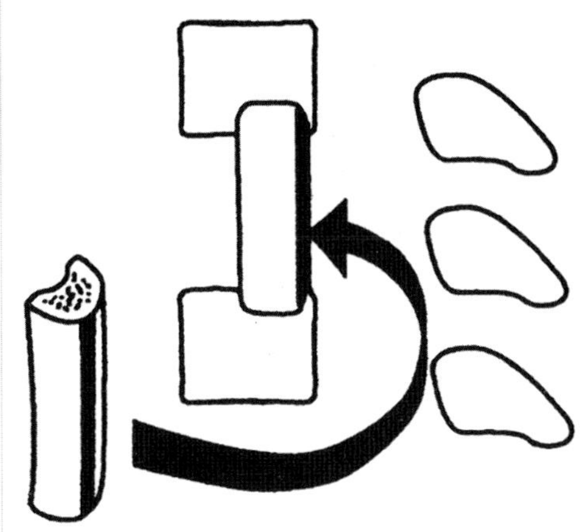

Fig. 23.4 If the crestal portion of a cervical interbody iliac crest graft is placed in line with the neutral axis (i.e., toward the dorsal portion of the vertebral body), as depicted, axial loads are effectively borne, but kyphosis prevention is somewhat limited. (Source: Biomechanics of Spine Stabilization: Third Edition, © 2015 Thieme Medical Publishers, Inc.)

angular force vectors. The chance of subsidence of an interbody bone graft into a vertebral body is *inversely* proportional to the cross-sectional area of contact.

▸▸ Answer 8

Correct answer is C

Dorsal placement of the crestal portion of a cervical interbody iliac crest strut graft, in combination with a ventral plate (see ▸ Fig. 23.4). If the crestal portion of a cervical interbody iliac crest graft is placed in line with the neutral axis (i.e., toward the dorsal portion of the vertebral body), as depicted, axial loads are effectively borne, but kyphosis prevention is somewhat limited.

▸▸ Answer 9

Correct answer is C

The end plates of expandable titanium cages are flat-faced. Translational and angular deformation (rocking) is much more likely with a strut with round ends than with a flat-faced cage. (**a**) A strut with a round end. (**b**) A flat-faced cage. Excessive compression can be applied, with the creation of a deformity, by means of a ventral fixator (see ▸ Fig. 23.5).

▸▸ Answer 10

Correct answer is D

A flat-faced cage presents (**a**) a parallel or (**b**) a trapezoidal shape to the end plates. The latter may be particularly pertinent at the lumbosacral junction, where the end plates are not parallel.

Flat-faced cages present a greater surface area of contact to the vertebral body than do round-faced cages. (**c**) Larger-diameter flat-faced cages provide a greater advantage from an implant–bone interface perspective. (**d**) Adding an internal end ring further augments implant–bone integrity but sacrifices surface area of contact for bony fusion

fixation devices provide stress shielding to one degree or another. Intimately intertwined with the concept of subsidence is the rigidity achieved by the fixation technique. Posterior lumbar interbody fusion with bone graft alone achieves less stiffness than that of the intact spine, whereas the addition of either dorsal instrumentation (e.g., pedicle screw fixation) or interbody implants increases stiffness and stability significantly, particularly during cyclical loading.

▸▸ Answer 14

Correct answer is B

End-fusion degenerative changes have been shown to occur, and at a greater frequency, with longer fusions. They also occur more frequently if abnormal spinal contours (kyphosis) are created by the fusion. Therefore, the maintenance of a relatively normal spinal alignment is prudent in this regard. Adjacent segment disease does not decrease with stiffer fusion constructs. Fusion constructs terminating at the thoracolumbar junction have a higher incidence of adjacent segment disease.

▸▸ Answer 15

Correct answer is A

A higher incidence of neurologic complications was noted with dowels when dowels were compared with impacted wedges. The substantial exposure required to insert dowels via the posterior lumbar interbody fusion technique requires substantial nerve root traction, likely explaining the high complication rate. Of final note, postoperative imaging is significantly affected by spinal implants. Implant volume, material, and shape all affect MRI artifact. Cylindrical implants are less prone to MRI artifact than more cuboidal or rectangular implants. The use of threaded interbody fusion cages has one additional drawback: the degree of difficulty and the morbidity associated with cage removal, if it is ever deemed appropriate. Pedicle screw implants can be removed with relative ease with a low risk for morbidity.

▸▸ Answer 16

Correct answer is D

Shaping a curved graft in all planes allows a close fit laterally in the case of a ventral cervical fusion. It also can minimize ventral prominence. However, care must be taken to minimize cortical bone removal (see ▸ Fig. 23.9).

An axial view of a snugly fit graft in a ventral cervical trough. This provides significant stability (*arrows*), as well as an increased chance for vascularization at intermediate segmental levels (see ▸ Fig. 23.10).

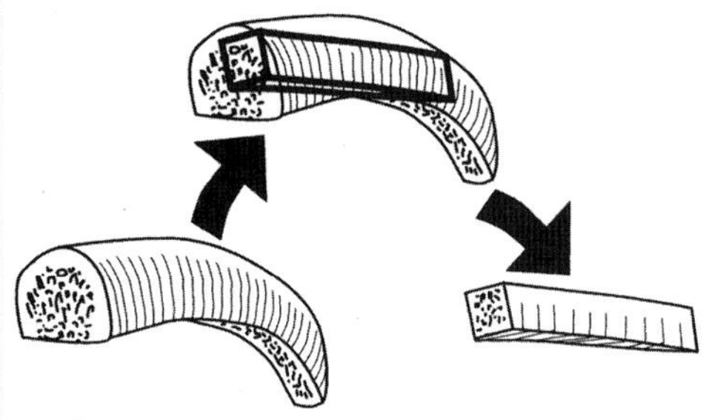

Fig. 23.9 Shaping a curved graft in all planes allows a close fit laterally in the case of a ventral cervical fusion. It also can minimize ventral prominence. However, care must be taken to minimize cortical bone removal. (Source: Biomechanics of Spine Stabilization: Third Edition, © 2015 Thieme Medical Publishers, Inc.)

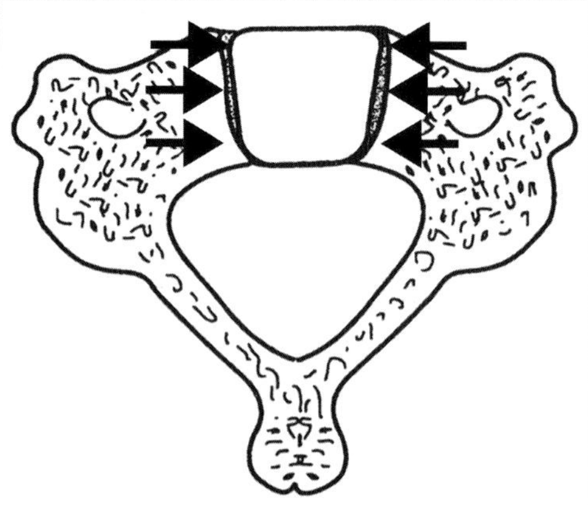

Fig. 23.10 An axial view of a snugly fit graft in a ventral cervical trough. This provides significant stability (*arrows*), as well as an increased chance for vascularization at intermediate segmental levels. (Source: Biomechanics of Spine Stabilization: Third Edition, © 2015 Thieme Medical Publishers, Inc.)

Key Principles

- The ventral positioning of the cervical interbody spacer provides a greater advantage for kyphosis prevention by positioning the load-bearing portion of the strut in line with the ventral vertebral body cortex.
- Axial load force vectors may cause resultant translational and angular force vectors with interbody constructs in the lumbar spine.
- Translational and angular deformation (rocking) is much more likely with a strut with round ends than with a flat-faced cage. Flat-faced cages present a greater surface area of contact to the vertebral body than do round-faced cages.
- Most commonly applied in the thoracic spine, interbody polymethylmethacrylate causes gaps created at the acrylic–bone juncture, which are created in part by blood present at the time of acrylic application. Care must be taken to avoid extravasation and neural element impingement and thermal injury of neural elements.

24 Lumbosacral-Pelvic Constructs

Raj Swaroop Lavadi, Thomas J. Buell, Nitin Agarwal, D. Kojo Hamilton

The lumbosacral spine and pelvis are critically important structures that support a majority of the body's weight. Awareness of lumbosacral spine and pelvis biomechanics can facilitate the optimal implantation of various constructs.

Learning Objectives

- Understand the importance of sagittal balance and identify the signs of sagittal imbalance.
- Understand how to avoid complications and lower the risks of neurological deficits during lumbosacral spine and pelvis instrumentation surgery.
- Understand how to achieve spinal stability using internal fixation.
- Understand the methods to augment lumbosacral stability.

Questions

▸▸ Question 1

Which of the following statements indicates sagittal balance/alignment?

- A. The angle between the superior end plate of the superior-most vertebrae of the curve and the inferior end plate of the inferior-most vertebrae of the curve is 20 degrees
- B. The angle between the lines passing through the superior end plate of L1 and the sacral end plate of S1 is 70 degrees
- C. The angle between a line parallel to the sacral end plate of S1 and the horizontal reference line is 50 degrees
- D. The vertical line from the midpoint of the C7 vertebral body passes through the lumbosacral junction
- E. The vertical line extending from the center of the sacrum is 6 cm from the vertical line passing through the midpoint of the C7 vertebral body

▸▸ Question 2

A 71-year-old woman presents with medically refractory lower back pain for the past 6 years. Imaging shows degenerative changes throughout the lumbar spine, as well as severe central canal stenosis and anterolisthesis of L4 on L5. She visits a spine surgeon who suggests she undergo a short-segment lumbar decompression and instrumented fusion. The patient is at risk of developing which of the following postoperative alignment changes if appropriate attention is not paid to lumbar sagittal alignment and its relation to pelvic incidence?

- A. Loss of lumbar lordosis
- B. Gain of lumbar lordosis
- C. Loss of thoracic kyphosis
- D. Increase in pelvic incidence
- E. Decrease in pelvic incidence

▸▸ Question 3

The flattening of the back is associated with two fundamental problems:

- A. Characteristic pain syndrome (flatback) and pathologic stresses and forces to the spine both in the fused and adjacent nonfused levels
- B. Improved sagittal balance and reduced disability
- C. Improved sagittal balance and worsening disability
- D. Worse lower back pain and reduced disability
- E. Improvements in sagittal balance and improvements in disability

▸▸ Question 4

Which of the following statements best describes the compensatory changes of a patient with flatback syndrome?

- A. Flexion of the neck
- B. Reduction of lumbar lordosis
- C. Increase in thoracic kyphosis
- D. Flexion of the knees
- E. Flexion of the hips

▸▸ Question 5

What is the ideal degree of hip flexion to intraoperatively restore lordosis?

- A. 30 degrees
- B. 60 degrees
- C. 0 degrees
- D. 90 degrees
- E. 65 degrees

▸▸ Question 6

A 44-year-old woman presents to the clinic with a long history of lower midline back pain, which recently increased in intensity over the past 2 weeks. Magnetic resonance imaging (MRI) showed a large, lobulated sacral mass of mixed signal intensity. An en bloc resection via a partial sacrectomy was performed. In the postoperative period, the patient complains of bowel and bladder incontinence without lower extremity weakness. Which nerve root is likely involved?

- A. L5
- B. S1
- C. S2
- D. S3
- E. S4

▸▸ Question 7

Which statement about the lumbosacral pivot point is most accurate?

- A. It is located at the ventral annulus fibrosus of the L5–S1
- B. It facilitates motion in the axial plane
- C. Fixating ventral to it reduces stability
- D. Fixating cephalad to it increases stability
- E. It is located at the dorsal annulus fibrosus of the L5–S1

▸▸ Question 8

Which of the following statements about posterior lumbar spine fixation is most accurate?

- A. Dorsal fixation most effectively reduces pelvic flexion
- B. Dorsal fixation most effectively increases pelvic extension
- C. Dorsal fixation most effectively increases twisting motion
- D. Dorsal fixation most effectively increases lateral bending
- E. Dorsal fixation preserves motion

▸▸ Question 9

A 63-year-old male patient comes in with lumbar flatback syndrome. The treating surgeon wants to perform a wedge osteotomy (Schwab grade 4) to correct the sagittal deformity. Which of the following statements about wedge osteotomy is most accurate?

- A. Wedge osteotomy should not be used in patients with intractable pain
- B. Wedge osteotomy should not be used in patients with neurologic deficit
- C. Wedge osteotomy can improve segmental and regional lordosis
- D. Wedge osteotomy achieves flexion of the lumbar spine
- E. Eggshell osteotomy (Schwab grade 3) is superior to wedge osteotomy

▸▸ Question 10

A 43-year-old woman is diagnosed with a sacral tumor and is admitted for a surgical work-up. She underwent a partial sacrectomy 6 months ago. A prosthesis was implanted after the initial surgery. The patient's albumin is 4 g/dL. The patient undergoes a redo surgery without intraoperative complications; however, the surgery extended beyond the expected duration. Postoperatively, the patient develops an infection. Which of the following factors in this patient do not present an added risk for infection?

- A. Redo surgery
- B. Albumin level
- C. Type of surgery
- D. Duration of surgery
- E. Instrumentation

▸▸ Question 11

Accurate screw placement is best assessed using which of the following imaging modalities?

- A. X-ray
- B. Ultrasound
- C. Computed tomography (CT)
- D. MRI
- E. None of the above

▸▸ Question 12

Vertebrae from which portion of the spine can be resected with minimal risk for neurologic injury?

- A. Cervical
- B. Thoracic

- C. Lumbar
- D. Sacral
- E. Coccygeal

▸▸ Question 13

Which of the following statements about an abnormal sagittal alignment is most accurate?

- A. Confers added stability
- B. Accelerates the degeneration of end plates
- C. Decreases the length of the moment arm through which forces are applied
- D. Decreases the risk of construct failure
- E. Results in a concentric loading of the discs

▸▸ Question 14

Which one of the following is not a stable technique to support the lumbosacral junction?

- A. S1 screws
- B. S2 alar-iliac screws
- C. Iliac bolts
- D. Interbody cage
- E. Transfacet screw

▸▸ Question 15

Dorsal longitudinal fixation of L5–S1 by transsacral techniques is occasionally useful for what pathology?

- A. Grade 4 spondylolisthesis
- B. L2–L3 disc herniation
- C. Facet dislocation
- D. Sacral tumor
- E. Baastrup's disease

▸▸ Question 16

Which of the following is not a consideration or technique to manage lumbosacral instability?

- A. Sagittal balance
- B. Transpsoas approach and lateral lumbar interbody fusion at L5–S1
- C. Neurologic function
- D. Acute spinal stability by means of internal fixation
- E. Long-term stability by means of bony fusion

▸▸ Question 17

Dorsal distraction of the lumbar spine produces which of the following?

- A. Increase in lordosis
- B. Decrease in kyphosis
- C. Loss of lordosis
- D. Improvement in flatback syndrome
- E. Improvement in the ability to stand erect

▸▸ Question 18

Compensatory loss of thoracic kyphosis is associated with ________.

- A. Appropriately contoured rods for lumbar fusion
- B. Improved lumbar lordosis
- C. Improved spinopelvic mismatch
- D. Flatback syndrome
- E. Appropriately planned for wedge osteotomies

▸▸ Question 19

Which of the following is not a nerve of the sacral plexus?

- A. Superior gluteal nerve
- B. Inferior gluteal nerve
- C. Sciatic nerve anterior division
- D. Sciatic nerve posterior division
- E. Coccygeal nerve

▸▸ Question 20

Which one of the following is typically not utilized in sacropelvic reconstruction?

- A. Sacral prostheses
- B. Allograft bone struts
- C. Iliac bolts
- D. Fibular bone struts
- E. Transfacet screws

Answers

▸▸ Answer 1

Correct answer is D

Sagittal balance/alignment can be measured through several parameters. Pertinent examples of spinopelvic parameters include pelvic tilt, pelvic incidence, and sacral slope. In an adult who is aligned in the sagittal plane, the vertical line from the midpoint of the C7 vertebral body (C7 plumb line) should pass through the lumbosacral junction (D). If this reference line passes anteriorly or posteriorly through this line, the patient has a more positive sagittal balance or negative sagittal balance, respectively.[1] The Cobb angle (A) is a common measurement used to determine the severity of a scoliotic curve. It can also be used to acquire information to describe sagittal alignment. Lumbar lordosis is an important sagittal parameter that is related to pelvic incidence (B).[2] Sacral slope is measured as the angle between the horizontal reference line and a line parallel to the S1 sacral end plate (C). The horizontal distance between the C7 plumb line and the central sacral vertical line is a measure of global coronal alignment/malalignment (C7–coronal vertical axis [CVA]). Many surgeons use CVA ≤ 4 cm as a target for global coronal correction since residual coronal imbalance may be associated with worse patient satisfaction and self-image (E) (see ▶ Fig. 24.1).[3]

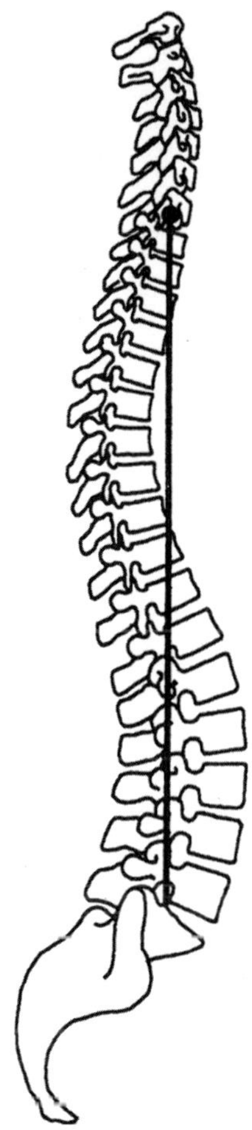

Fig. 24.1 Sagittal balance. A plumb line dropped from the C7 vertebral body in the standing position should pass through the lumbosacral junction when normal sagittal balance is present, as depicted. Source: Biomechanics of Spine Stabilization: Third Edition, © 2015 Thieme Medical Publishers, Inc.

▸▸ Answer 2

Correct answer is A

Following lumbar or lumbosacral instrumented fusion that does not match lordosis to pelvic incidence, this patient is at risk for sagittal imbalance due to a loss of lumbar lordosis (flatback deformity). Flatback syndrome often results in patients experiencing mechanical back pain and adopting a compensatory posture that commonly involves pelvic retroversion. Furthermore, improper restoration of lumbar lordosis stresses the adjacent vertebrae, leading to adjacent segment disease.[4] To counteract the loss of lordosis, surgeons may utilize appropriate interbody fusion techniques and hyperlordotic cages to manage flatback syndrome.[5,6] Thoracolumbar deformity correction is unlikely to result in loss of thoracic kyphosis (C). Pelvic incidence is generally fixed by adulthood unless sacral osteotomy is performed (D, E). ▶ Fig. 24.2 illustrates how to measure pelvic incidence.

▸▸ Answer 3

Correct answer is A

Flatback syndrome can result after lumbosacral fixation and may be a fixed sagittal deformity in patients with longer fusions. Patients with flatback syndrome have a loss of lumbar lordosis and sagittal imbalance. This pathological state may accelerate degenerative changes in the end plates of both the fused and nonfused vertebrae (A). Patients suffer from chronic, fatigue-induced pain, which results in disability (B, C, D, and E).[7]

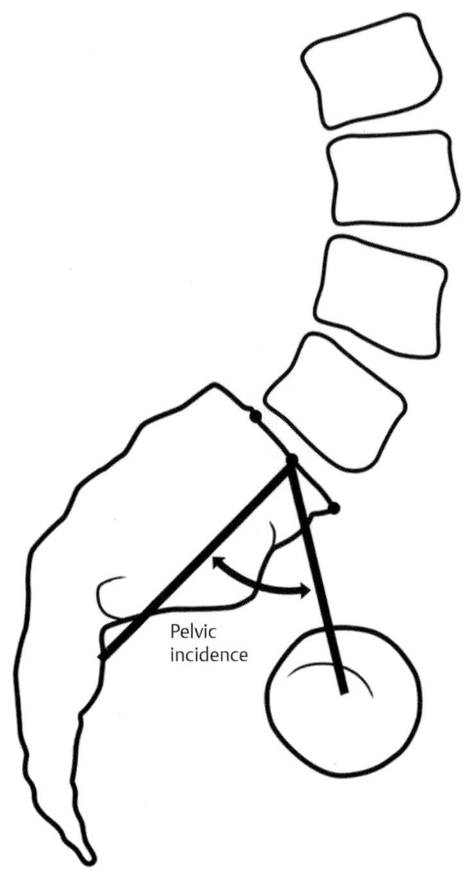

Fig. 24.2 Pelvic incidence is defined as the angle between a line joining the middle of the sacral end plate to the center of the femoral head (femoral head axis) and a line drawn perpendicular to the sacral end plate, as depicted. (Source: Biomechanics of Spine Stabilization: Third Edition, © 2015 Thieme Medical Publishers, Inc.)

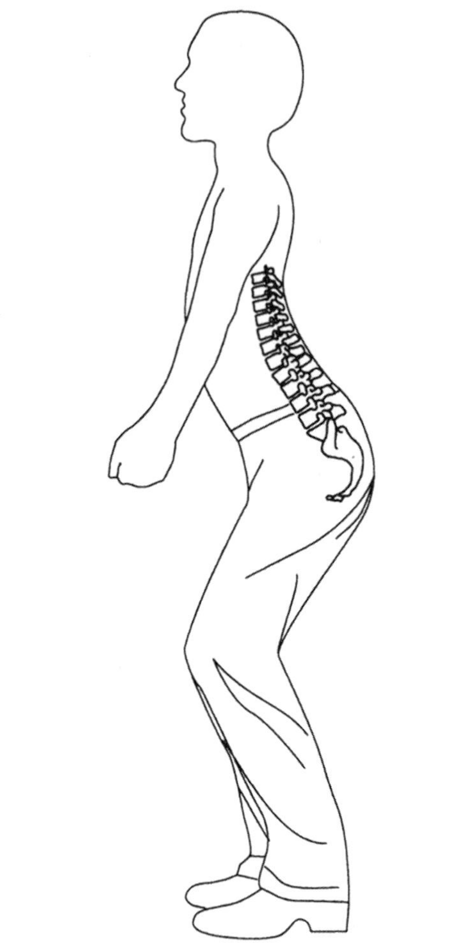

Fig. 24.3 The posture and spine configuration of a patient with the flat-back syndrome. Note the flattened lumbar spine (loss of lordosis), which is often associated with a compensatory loss of thoracic kyphosis and/or a compensatory exaggerated cervical and upper thoracic lordosis with knee flexion, as depicted. (Source: Biomechanics of Spine Stabilization: Third Edition, © 2015 Thieme Medical Publishers, Inc.)

►► Answer 4

Correct answer is D

Flatback syndrome can occur as a consequence of posterior lumbar spine instrumentation. Patients often suffer from pain, disability, reduced quality of life, and improper horizontal gaze.[8] To address the latter symptom, patients often have to retrovert their pelvis, flex their knees (D), extend their neck (A), and extend their hips (E). These patients undergo a compensatory loss in thoracic kyphosis (C). Flatback syndrome occurs as a result of loss of lordosis; the reduction itself is not a compensatory change (see ► Fig. 24.3).

►► Answer 5

Correct answer is C

Achieving a postoperative restoration of lordosis depends both on the surgery performed as well as patient positioning techniques. In preparation for a

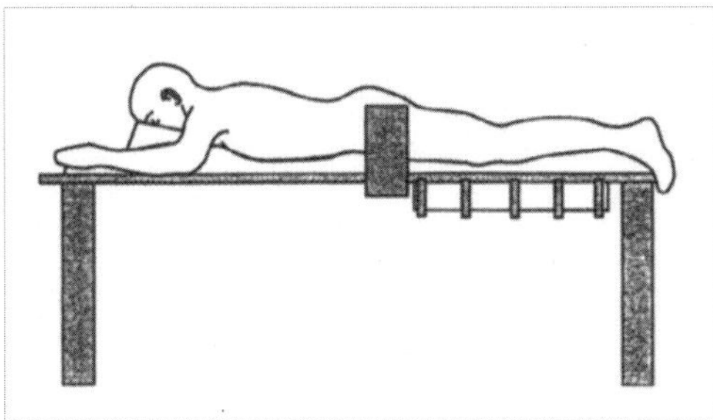

Fig. 24.4 Beds or frames that provide low back extension should be used. (Source: Biomechanics of Spine Stabilization: Third Edition, © 2015 Thieme Medical Publishers, Inc.)

lumbar fusion procedure, the patient should have their hips extended (C). Intraoperative hip flexion (A, B, D, and E) has been associated with reduced overall and segmental postoperative lordosis.[9,10] Frames that encourage extension of the lower back can also be used (see ▶ Fig. 24.4).

▸▸ Answer 6

Correct answer is D

Preserving neurologic function while addressing the regional pathology should be the goal of lumbar and sacral surgery. Occasionally, nerve roots may be sacrificed during the procedure, leading to postoperative bowel and bladder incontinence. S3 is the nerve root (D) most responsible for maintaining bowel and bladder continence. Although S1 (B) and S2 (C) contribute to this function, S3 is most responsible for this function.[11] L5 (A) and S4 (E) do not contribute to bowel and bladder continence.

▸▸ Answer 7

Correct answer is E

Lumbosacral stability can be augmented by using the lumbosacral pivot point as an anatomic landmark (McCord's point).[12] The lumbosacral pivot point is located in the dorsal annulus fibrosis of the L5–S1 (E) (A) and is responsible for the motion of the lumbosacral spine in the sagittal plane (B). The plane of the lumbosacral pivot point provides a guide for stability. To optimize the stability of lumbosacral posterior instrumentation constructs, fixation should extend further distally and ventrally past McCord's point (C, D).

▸▸ Answer 8

Correct answer is A

Posterior lumbosacral-pelvic instrumentation constructs limit pelvic flexion (A). As these are fusion procedures, they inherently limit motion (B, C, D, and E).[13]

▸▸ Answer 9

Correct answer is C

Flatback syndrome is a sagittal deformity (which can be rigid), where there is loss of lumbar lordosis. To restore harmonious lordosis or extension of the spine (C), wedge osteotomy can be performed (D is wrong). Wedge osteotomy can be performed via a dorsal approach or by a ventral and dorsal approach. It is the preferred procedure for patients with intractable pain and neurologic deficit (A, B). Eggshell osteotomy is associated with several complications and is limited in the correction that can be achieved (E). For patients with a more severe sagittal deformity, a more extensive and invasive wedge resection often needs to be performed.[14,15]

▸▸ Answer 10

Correct answer is C

Deformity corrections and tumor resections are some of the most invasive procedures in spine surgery. Several factors have been associated with infection risk. These include redo surgery (A), type of surgery and invasiveness (C), prolonged operative time (D), and utilization of implants (E). Albumin level has been associated with infection risk. Patients with an albumin level of less than 3 g/dL are at a higher risk for infection.[16]

▸▸ Answer 11

Correct answer is A

The best imaging modality to assess accurate screw placement are orthogonal X-rays (A, E) as they eliminate implant artifact.[17] Ultrasound-guided pedicle screw insertion yields promising results[18]; however, further research still needs to be performed and confirmation is still likely to be through radiographic methods (B). CT has long been used to determine screw placement but may be difficult to assess given the influence of artifact (C). MRI is not viable to assess screw placement given the concerns of MR-compatibility of the implants (D).

▸▸ Answer 12

Correct answer is E

Despite it providing structural support, the coccyx (E) may be considered a vestigial subsection of the spine given its single pair of nerve roots. The coccygeal nerve only provides sensory innervation without any sympathetic involvement. It may be resected to address coccygeal pain. The multiple nerves originating from more superior portions of the spine pose a threat and may result in neurologic injury if improper surgery is performed.

▸▸ Answer 13

Correct answer is B

When sagittal balance is lost, the normal/physiological mechanism of loading of the spine is also lost. During regular motion, the irregular intervertebral relationships can accelerate the degeneration of the end plates (B). The abnormal sagittal alignment reduces stability (A) and can lead to an increased risk of construct failure (D) postoperatively. Because axial loading does not occur in a straight line (shortest vector), the length of the moment arm through which forces are transmitted is increased (C). Normally, the transmission of force through the spine leads to a concentric loading of the discs. However, this transmission becomes eccentric in sagittal malalignment and may contribute to accelerated disc degeneration (see ▸ Fig. 24.5).

▸▸ Answer 14

Correct answer is E

There are several different fixator mechanisms to support the lumbosacral junction. S1 screws (A), S2 alar-iliac screws (B), iliac bolts (C), and interbody cages (D) can bolster the lumbosacral junction. Transfacet screws are mainly used in the thoracic and lumbar spine and are not optimal for the lumbosacral junction. However, they do present a less invasive strategy to fixate the lumbosacral junction. In combination with an interbody fusion, transfacet screws can contribute to the stability of a lumbosacral fusion construct.

▸▸ Answer 15

Correct answer is A

Dorsal translumbosacral and transsacral fixation techniques represent less invasive strategies for lumbosacral augmentation. This approach can be used for significant spondylolisthesis (A). The other pathologies mentioned are treated by different surgeries and approaches (B, C, D, and E) (see ▸ Fig. 24.6).

▸▸ Answer 16

Correct answer is B

There are several considerations to manage lumbosacral instability. Restoration/preservation of sagittal balance (A) and neurologic function (C)

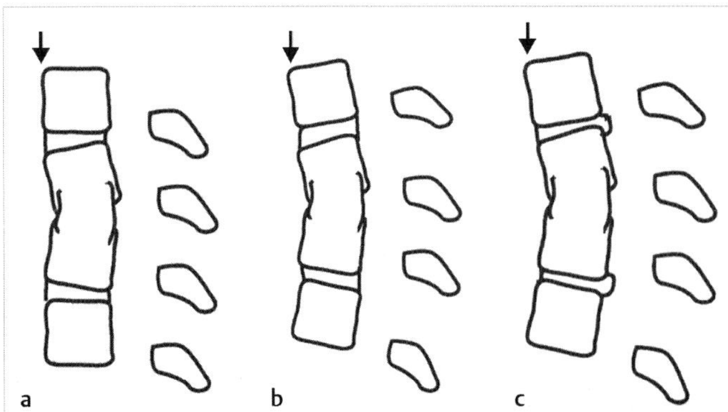

Fig. 24.5 **(a)** An alteration of normal spinal alignment increases the length of the moment arm through which forces are applied to the spine. **(b)** This causes discs to be loaded in a manner other than that to which they are "accustomed" (eccentric loading). **(c)** This can result in an acceleration of end-fusion degenerative changes. (Source: Biomechanics of Spine Stabilization: Third Edition, © 2015 Thieme Medical Publishers, Inc.)

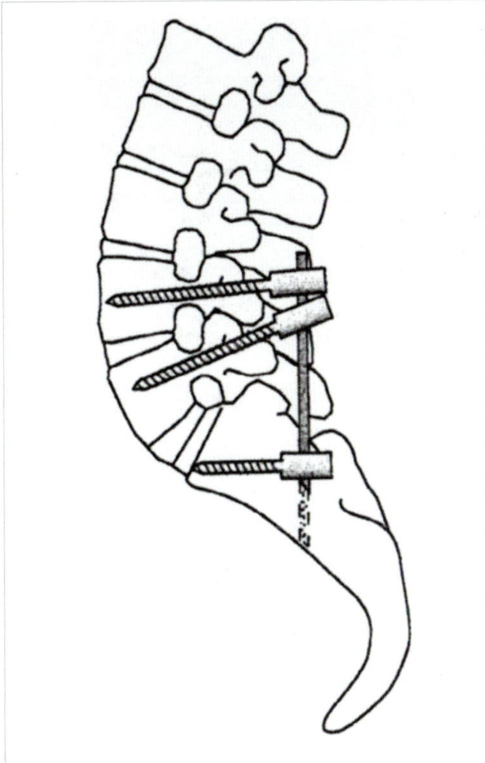

Fig. 24.6 Dorsal transsacral fixation. The rod is passed longitudinally into the sacrum. This increases the length of the moment arm caudal to the lumbosacral pivot point. (Source: Biomechanics of Spine Stabilization: Third Edition, © 2015 Thieme Medical Publishers, Inc.)

should be prioritized. Equally important is the management of acute spinal stability using internal fixation (D) and achievement of long-term stability by means of bony fusion (E). The transpsoas approach is not feasible to perform at the lumbosacral junction given the anatomic obstacle presented by the pelvic brim (B).

▸▸ **Answer 17**

Correct answer is C

Dorsal distraction as a result of instrumented fusions can result in a loss of lordosis (C, A) or kyphosis (B). This presentation can lead to flatback syndrome (D) or a fixed sagittal deformity. Such patients are not able to stand erect and depend on compensatory mechanisms to maintain a level gaze (E). Osteotomies can be performed to improve lordosis in such patients.

▸▸ **Answer 18**

Correct answer is D

Flatback syndrome (D) can occur after instrumented fusion and is associated with a compensatory loss of thoracic kyphosis. These patients have a loss of lordosis (B) and a poor spinopelvic mismatch (C). Surgical planning for such patients is a challenge (A, E).

▸▸ **Answer 19**

Correct answer is E

The coccygeal nerve (E) is not a part of the sacral plexus. The other nerves (A, B, C, and D) are a part of the sacral plexus. The single pair of coccygeal nerve roots allows for the coccyx to be resected, rarely, in patients with coccydynia. Obstacles to ventral fixation in the lumbosacral spine include the sacral plexus and the local vascular supply.

▸▸ **Answer 20**

Correct answer is E

Different types of fixators and prostheses are used in sacropelvic reconstruction, the most common of which include sacral prostheses (A), allograft bone struts (B), iliac bolts (C), and fibular bone struts (D). Translacet screws (E) are not used in sacropelvic reconstruction as their main utility is in the form of fusion procedures.

Key Principles

- Sagittal alignment is an important consideration for spine surgeons since patients with lumbar flatback (sagittal malalignment) have suboptimal outcomes.
- Maintenance of lumbar lordosis should be prioritized during patient positioning, intraoperative technique, and instrumentation. The lumbosacral pivot point (McCord's point) is an important anatomical landmark that should be exceeded ventrally or caudally to augment lumbosacral stability.
- Lumbosacral fixation may include distal fixation to the ilium for improved construct stability.

References

[1] Glassman SD, Bridwell K, Dimar JR, Horton W, Berven S, Schwab F. The impact of positive sagittal balance in adult spinal deformity. Spine (Phila Pa 1976) 2005;30(18):2024–2029

[2] Schwab FJ, Blondel B, Bess S, et al. Radiographical spinopelvic parameters and disability in the setting of adult spinal deformity: a prospective multicenter analysis. Spine (Phila Pa 1976) 2013;38(13):E803–E812

[3] Buell TJ, Smith JS, Shaffrey CI, et al. Multicenter assessment of surgical outcomes in adult spinal deformity patients with severe global coronal malalignment: determination of target coronal realignment threshold. J Neurosurg Spine 2020;34: 1–14

[4] Barrey C, Darnis A. Current strategies for the restoration of adequate lordosis during lumbar fusion. World J Orthop 2015;6(1):117–126

[5] Jagannathan J, Sansur CA, Oskouian RJ, Jr., Fu KM, Shaffrey CI. Radiographic restoration of lumbar alignment after transforaminal lumbar interbody fusion. Neurosurgery 2009;64(5):955–963; discussion 963–964

[6] Buell TJ, Shaffrey CI, Bess S, et al. Multicenter assessment of outcomes and complications associated with transforaminal versus anterior lumbar interbody fusion for fractional curve correction. J Neurosurg Spine 2021;35(6):729–742

[7] Smith JS, Singh M, Klineberg E, et al. Surgical treatment of pathological loss of lumbar lordosis (flatback) in patients with normal sagittal vertical axis achieves similar clinical improvement as surgical treatment of elevated sagittal vertical axis: clinical article. J Neurosurg Spine 2014;21(2):160–170

[8] Wiggins GC, Ondra SL, Shaffrey CI. Management of iatrogenic flat-back syndrome. Neurosurg Focus 2003;15(3):E8

[9] Miyazaki M, Ishihara T, Abe T, et al. Effect of intraoperative position in single-level transforaminal lumbar interbody fusion at the L4/5 level on segmental and overall lumbar lordosis in patients with lumbar degenerative disease. Medicine (Baltimore) 2019;98(39):e17316

[10] Harimaya K, Lenke LG, Mishiro T, Bridwell KH, Koester LA, Sides BA. Increasing lumbar lordosis of adult spinal deformity patients via intraoperative prone positioning. Spine (Phila Pa 1976) 2009;34(22):2406–2412

[11] Guo Y, Palmer JL, Shen L, et al. Bowel and bladder continence, wound healing, and functional outcomes in patients who underwent sacrectomy. J Neurosurg Spine 2005;3(2):106–110

[12] McCord DH, Cunningham BW, Shono Y, Myers JJ, McAfee PC. Biomechanical analysis of lumbosacral fixation. Spine (Phila Pa 1976) 1992;17(8 Suppl):S235–S243

[13] Bernstein J, Charette R, Sloan M, Lee GC. Spinal fusion is associated with changes in acetabular orientation and reductions in pelvic mobility. Clin Orthop Relat Res 2019;477(2): 324–330

[14] Buell TJ, Nguyen JH, Mazur MD, et al. Radiographic outcome and complications after single-level lumbar extended pedicle subtraction osteotomy for fixed sagittal malalignment: a retrospective analysis of 55 adult spinal deformity patients with a minimum 2-year follow-up. J Neurosurg Spine 2018;30(2):242–252

[15] Schwab F, Blondel B, Chay E, et al. The comprehensive anatomical spinal osteotomy classification. Neurosurgery 2014;74(1):112–120

[16] Chen KW, Yang HL, Lu J, et al. Risk factors for postoperative wound infections of sacral chordoma after surgical excision. J Spinal Disord Tech 2011;24(4):230–234

[17] Choma TJ, Denis F, Lonstein JE, et al. Stepwise methodology for plain radiographic assessment of pedicle screw placement: a comparison with computed tomography. J Spinal Disord Tech 2006;19(8):547–553

[18] Chen Z, Wu B, Zhai X, et al. Basic study for ultrasound-based navigation for pedicle screw insertion using transmission and backscattered methods. PLoS One 2015;10(4):e0122392

25 Regional Nuances

Joravar Dhaliwal, Vikram B. Chakravarthy, Ryan Khanna, Mark Bilsky

Understanding various regional nuances that impact the efficacy of a spinal implant is critical. There are regional principles that can guide the approach to stabilizing the spinal column with an implant.

Learning Objectives

- Understand regional nuances that impact the efficacy of spinal implants.
- Understand the impact of apical and neutral vertebrae when planning a long-segment fixation.
- Understand implications of instrumenting junctional segments and additional precautions that need to be exercised to minimize hardware failure.

Questions

▸▸ Question 1

What are the anatomical limitations of a low ventral cervicothoracic surgical exposure?

- A. Impedance from the right brachiocephalic vein
- B. Obstruction from the heart
- C. Hindrance from the first rib
- D. Blockage from the xiphoid of the sternum
- E. Obstruction from the right subclavian vein

▸▸ Question 2

What anatomical structure limits lateral exposure of the cervical spine from a ventral approach?

- A. Vertebral artery
- B. Common carotid artery
- C. External carotid artery
- D. Transverse cervical nerve
- E. Trapezius muscle

▸▸ Question 3

How are the craniocervical and lumbosacral regions biomechanically similar?

- A. Similar length of moment arm applied
- B. Unique rotational forces
- C. Analogous loading forces
- D. Comparable shear stresses
- E. Similar risk of translational deformity

▸▸ Question 4

What imaging finding may help determine the appropriateness of a ventral approach for a cervicothoracic junction lesion?

- A. Instrument–manubrial thoracic spine distance
- B. Thickness of manubrium
- C. Low aortic arch
- D. Cardiomegaly
- E. Distance from tracheal bifurcation to top of aortic arch

▸▸ Question 5

What imaging finding may help determine the feasibility of a ventral approach to L3–S1?

- A. Sacral slope
- B. High iliac crest
- C. Large femoral nerve
- D. Thickness of psoas muscle
- E. Narrow pelvic inlet

▸▸ Question 6

What are the limitations of posterior cervicothoracic fixation?

- A. Weakness of cervical lateral mass screws
- B. C7 pedicle too small for pedicle screw
- C. Thin cervical laminae
- D. Large spinal canal diameter in upper thoracic region
- E. Risk of vertebral artery injury with C7 lateral mass screw

▸▸ Question 7

What is a true statement about a neutral vertebra?

- A. T6
- B. Vertebra located between curves associated with the smallest angle between it and its adjacent vertebra in the curve

- C. Vertebra in a curve that is associated with the greatest angle between it and its adjacent vertebra of all the vertebrae in the curve
- D. Extending an instrumented fusion to this vertebra significantly impacts stability
- E. A large bending moment is applied to it by axial loads

▸▸ Question 8

What is the apical vertebra?

- A. Top vertebral body at the cervicothoracic junction
- B. Vertebra in a curve that is associated with the greatest angle between it and its adjacent vertebra of all the vertebrae in the curve
- C. C2
- D. Vertebra located between curves associated with the smallest angle between it and its adjacent vertebra
- E. An axial load applies a small bending moment to it

▸▸ Question 9

What are alternatives to screw-based fixation to augment the integrity of fixation at the O-C2 region?

- A. C1 posterior arch lateral mass screw
- B. C2 pars screw
- C. Sublaminar wiring
- D. C2 pedicle screw
- E. C1–C2 transarticular screw

▸▸ Question 10

What are the anatomic confines that limit a ventral exposure to the lumbosacral region?

- A. Inferior vena cava
- B. Median sacral arteries and veins
- C. External iliac vein
- D. Iliac crest
- E. Aorta

▸▸ Question 11

Why is the cervicothoracic region at high risk of hardware failure?

- A. It is a transition point from a lordotic thoracic spine to a kyphotic cervical spine
- B. It is a transition point from thoracic kyphosis to cervical lordosis
- C. It is not at risk of hardware failure
- D. Transition from a flexible thoracic spine to a rigid cervical spine
- E. Ease of ensuring alignment of the cervical and thoracic regions of the implant

▸▸ Question 12

Which of the following statements comparing endonasal endoscopic approach to the transoral approach to the odontoid is correct?

- A. Endonasal endoscopic approach is superior as it improves visualization and decreases the risk of dysphagia and airway edema
- B. The transoral approach has decreased risk of infection given the limited exposure of the wound to saliva
- C. The transoral approach is limited by the nasopalatine line
- D. Endoscopic endonasal approach provides a wider exposure

▸▸ Question 13

In the presence of narrow thoracic pedicle screws, what is the best option for fixation?

- A. In-out-in pedicle screw technique
- B. Transfacet screw
- C. Use of sublaminar wires
- D. Noninstrumented fusion
- E. Spinous process plate

▸▸ Question 14

Which of the following statements comparing iliac fixation to S2 alar-iliac (S2AI) fixation is correct?

- A. Iliac fixation is inline with lumbar and S1 pedicle screws
- B. S2AI screw fixation in adults has a significantly lower mechanical failure and complication rate than iliac fixation
- C. Iliac screws are generally lower profile than S2AI fixation
- D. Iliac screws cross four cortices along the length of screw placement
- E. Iliac screws have a lower rate of wound infection

▸▸ **Question 15**

What is the preferred location to terminate a long thoracolumbar construct to minimize the risk of complications?
- A. T12
- B. T10
- C. L1
- D. T11
- E. L5

▸▸ **Question 16**

What is an issue regarding stabilizing the lumbosacral region?
- A. The sacrum and ilium are composed of primarily cortical bone
- B. Most implant constructs are comprised of short moment arms
- C. The lumbosacral region is located at the terminus of the spine
- D. Combined dorsal and ventral fixation strategies are ineffective
- E. Shorter implant constructs are preferred

▸▸ **Question 17**

Which of the following statements comparing cervical lateral mass screws and cervical pedicle screws is correct?
- A. Cervical lateral mass screws place the exiting nerve root at greatest risk of injury
- B. Cervical pedicle screws demonstrate a significantly higher resistance to pullout forces than lateral mass screws
- C. Cervical pedicle screw malposition in the axial plane risks injury to the nerve
- D. The vertebral artery lies medial to the pedicle
- E. The trajectory of both cervical lateral mass and pedicle screws is in a sharp medial direction

▸▸ **Question 18**

What is the limiting factor for lateral approaches to the thoracic spine?
- A. Scapula
- B. Diaphragm
- C. Spleen
- D. Parietal pleura
- E. Liver

Answers

▸▸ **Answer 1**

Correct answer is A

The main barriers to a low ventral cervicothoracic surgical exposure are the midline vascular structures including either the brachiocephalic vein or artery. Brachiocephalic vein ligation can be performed when the corridor is too narrow. Either subclavian vein would be too lateral for access. The heart would be too inferior for this type of approach and the rib by itself is too lateral for our surgical corridor. The manubrium of the sternum, not the xiphoid process of the sternum, can be partially resected for appropriate surgical access.

▸▸ **Answer 2**

Correct answer is A

The most important structure limiting lateral exposure of the cervical spine from a ventral approach is the vertebral artery, which courses through the foramen transversarium. Other structures at risk also include the sympathetic chain that lies superficial to the longus colli muscle. The common and external carotid arteries can be encountered during ventral exposure of the cervical spine but can be appropriately mobilized to prevent any limitations to exposure. The transverse cervical nerve is a branch of the cervical plexus and courses over the sternocleidomastoid muscle and continues medially. It can be encountered during dissection in the anterior triangle and its sacrifice results in numbness of the skin of the anterolateral cervical region. Additionally, it too can be mobilized during initial dissection and does not prevent appropriate lateral dissection. The anterior margin of the trapezius muscle forms the posterior edge of the posterior triangle of the neck and is typically not encountered during ventral dissection and exposure of the cervical spine.

▸▸ **Answer 3**

Correct answer is A

The moment arm is the perpendicular distance between the instantaneous axis of rotation and the force vector. The terminal nature of the craniocervical and lumbosacral regions means that instrumentation constructs in this region will have similarly small moment arms. The steep angle of the lumbosacral joint means that this region is particularly vulnerable to translational deformity, although this is not the case for the craniocervical region. The unique anatomy at C1–C2 makes this the only spinal joint articulation capable of significant axial rotation. The lumbosacral spine has much higher loading forces than the craniocervical junction given its distal location in the vertebral column. There are no analogous shear stresses in the craniocervical region compared to the lumbosacral region.

▸▸ Answer 4

Correct answer is A

The instrument–manubrial thoracic spine distance on preoperative magnetic resonance imaging (MRI) has been shown to be correlated to choosing a ventral approach for a cervicothoracic junction lesion. The instrument–manubrial thoracic distance depends on distance from the suprasternal notch and the pitch of an intervertebral disc segment. Manubrial thickness is not a prohibitive factor preventing ventral cervicothoracic access, although increased time for bony resection may be required. A low aortic arch, cardiomegaly, and the distance from the tracheal bifurcation to the top of the aortic arch may change the size of the surgical corridor but neither has been shown to affect the choice of a ventral approach.[1]

▸▸ Answer 5

Correct answer is A

A high sacral slope may prevent placement of interbody instrumentation at L5–S1 from a purely ventral approach. A high iliac crest and narrow pelvic inlet make a lateral transpsoas approach to L5–S1 challenging. A large anteriorly located femoral nerve often can preclude a lateral transpsoas approach to L4–L5 as well. Psoas thickness is another factor involved in the decision making for a lateral approach to the lumbar spine.

▸▸ Answer 6

Correct answer is A

One of the main limitations of the dorsal approach to cervicothoracic fixation is weakness of the cervical lateral mass screws. Other limitations include risks from sublaminar wire or hook placement. The spinal canal diameter is in fact narrow in the upper thoracic region and this increases the risk of neural injury during placement of instrumentation. If C7 is instrumented, the pedicle is an appropriate target for fixation, providing more pullout strength than an analogous lateral mass screw. The vertebral artery enters the C7 transverse foramen in < 1% of patients, making vertebral artery injury with a C7 lateral mass screw rare.[2] Cervical laminae are not abnormally thin and can accommodate laminar screws, particularly at C2, where it is commonly used as a bailout option to more robust C2 pars or pedicle fixation.

▸▸ Answer 7

Correct answer is B

A neutral vertebra is defined as the vertebra that is located between curves (in any plane). It is associated with the smallest angle between it and its adjacent vertebra. It is usually located in line with the spinal axis, where a moment arm does not exist, minimizing the amount of bending moment axial loads apply. Extending an implant to this vertebra does not usually have an adverse effect on stability (see ▸ Fig. 25.1).

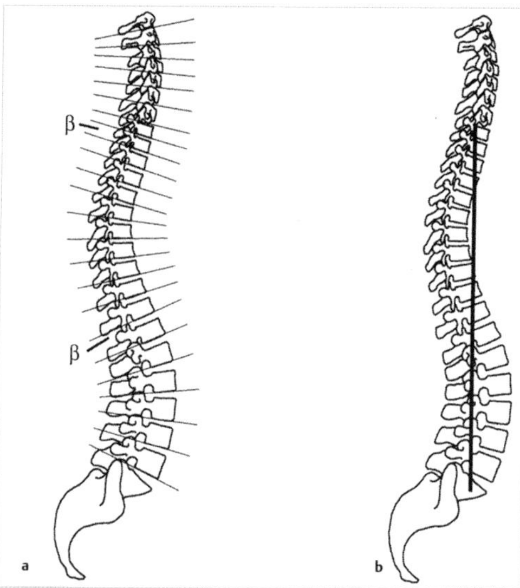

Fig. 25.1 (a) A neutral vertebra is the vertebra that is located between curves (in any plane). It is associated with the smallest angle (β) between it and its adjacent vertebrae (approximately zero). **(b)** A neutral vertebra is usually located in line with the spinal axis. Therefore, a minimal bending moment is applied by axial loads because a moment arm does not exist. Extending an implant to this vertebra does not usually adversely affect stability. (Source: Biomechanics of Spine Stabilization: Third Edition, © 2015 Thieme Medical Publishers, Inc.)

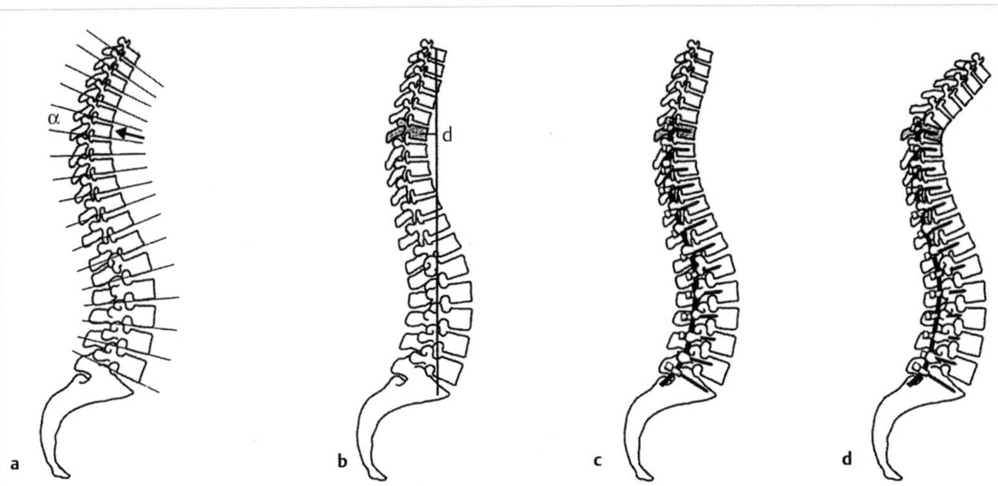

Fig. 25.2 **(a)** An apical vertebra is the vertebra in a curve (in any plane) that is associated with the greatest angle (α) between it and its adjacent vertebrae of all the vertebrae in the curve. **(b)** This vertebra and the adjacent disc interspaces are exposed to significant stresses because of the application of a bending moment (length *d*). **(c)** Extending a long construct up to, but not beyond, an apical vertebra exaggerates this effect and **(d)** causes a tendency to further deformation. (Source: Biomechanics of Spine Stabilization: Third Edition, © 2015 Thieme Medical Publishers, Inc.)

▸▸ Answer 8

Correct answer is B

An apical vertebra is the vertebra in a curve (in any plane) that is associated with the greatest angle between it and its adjacent vertebra of all the vertebra in the curve. This vertebra and the adjacent disc interspaces are exposed to significant stresses because of the application of a bending moment. Extending a long construct up to, but not beyond, an apical vertebra exaggerates that effect and causes a tendency to further deformation (see ▸ Fig. 25.2).

▸▸ Answer 9

Correct answer is C

The gold standard technique for O-C2 instrumented fusion consists of occipital plating with C2 pars or pedicle screws (skipping C1 pedicle screw for ease of rod contouring). However, in pathologies that preclude the ability for adequate placement of instrumentation, alternative methods may need to be utilized. These techniques include the use of hook, wire, or interlaminar clamp–based constructs. Initially developed by Brooks and Gallie, and later popularized by Sontag, the use of sublaminar wires with bone graft wedged between C1 and C2 laminae can be used in place of traditional screw-based fixation. Furthermore, developed in 1975, Tucker first described use of the interlaminar clamp, obviating the need for sublaminar wire passage, thus minimizing the risk of spinal cord injury.[3]

▸▸ Answer 10

Correct answer is E

Ventral exposure of the lumbosacral region is chiefly impeded by vascular rather than bony anatomy. In particular, the common iliac and the median sacral arteries and veins as well as neural structures such as the superior hypogastric plexus prevent otherwise direct access to the ventral lumbar spine The external iliac vein is usually lateral to the preferred exposure and the iliac crest impedes lateral access to the lumbosacral region rather than ventral access.

▸▸ Answer 11

Correct answer is B

The cervicothoracic region is a transition from the rigid thoracic spine with a kyphotic curvature to the flexible cervical spine with a lordotic curvature, all of which makes this region particularly vulnerable to translational deformity and, analogously, hardware failure. Other factors that increase the risk of hardware failure include the changing angle between the facet joints as well as the intervertebral joints between C6 and T1. Lastly, ensuring proper alignment of the cervical and thoracic parts of the impact is challenging.

▸▸ Answer 12

Correct answer is A

For some cases of ventral compression in the upper cervical spine, odontoidectomy is indicated. In general, transoral and endoscopic endonasal are the two primary approaches. Although technically more demanding, the endoscopic endonasal approach has less soft tissue injury and potentially has less risk of dysphonia and dysphagia. However, the transoral odontoidectomy can provide a wider exposure and is not limited by the nasopalatine line. On the other hand, the transoral odontoidectomy can provide a wider exposure and is not limited by the above bony structures.

▸▸ Answer 13

Correct answer is A

The narrowest thoracic pedicles are typically found between T4 and T6, making pedicle screw placement particularly challenging in this region. The in-out-in pedicle screw technique is a viable alternative in these cases. This technique involves starting the screw placement outside the pedicle, directing it into the pedicle, and then exiting the pedicle before re-entering, which often leads to a lateral breach. This lateral breach places the screw in the posterior mediastinum or pleural space but importantly avoids a medial breach, thereby reducing the risk of dural injury or neurological deficit.

Sublaminar wiring, while another option, carries a high risk of neurological injury in the thoracic spine and is often time-consuming, making it a less favorable option in this context.[4]

▸▸ Answer 14

Correct answer is B

Spinopelvic fixation can be used in the correction of high-grade spondylolisthesis or pelvic obliquity and after long-segment fusion procedures for pediatric or adult spinal deformity. Traditional options include iliac bolts or S2AI. Advantages of S2AI fixation compared with iliac fixation include lower profile screws and inline position with lumbar and S1 pedicle screws. Recently, a meta-analysis showed that there was a significantly lower rate of revision surgery, wound infection, and painful instrumentation in patients who received S2AI fixation compared with traditional iliac bolts.[5,6]

▸▸ Answer 15

Correct answer is B

Taking biomechanical and geometric factors into consideration, it may be prudent to avoid the termination of a long construct at C7 or T1. The extension of a thoracic construct to C5 or C6, a lumbar construct to T9 or T10, a cervical construct to T1 or T2, or a thoracic construct to L2 or L3 may diminish complications related to the termination of an implant in a transitional region.

▸▸ Answer 16

Correct answer is C

The lumbosacral region is located at the terminus of the spine. It presents significant stabilization problems for the surgeon. In addition to the factors mentioned in the section on the craniocervical and upper cervical spine, the soft character of the predominantly cancellous bone of the sacrum and ilium poses further problems for fixation security. Also, the complex forces applied to this region must be resisted by forces applied by the construct. An appropriate consideration of the biomechanics of this region should diminish the incidence of complications. Long, complex constructs may be required.

▸▸ Answer 17

Correct answer is B

For cervical fixation in the subaxial spine, lateral mass and pedicle screws are the two most common options. While cervical pedicle screws are more technically challenging with risks to the neurovascular structures, they demonstrate higher resistance to pullout forces.[7]

▸▸ **Answer 18**

Correct answer is A

Typically, approaching the thoracic spine above T5 through a lateral approach is not possible due to physical limitations from the scapula. The diaphragm can be encountered in lateral approaches in the lower region of the thoracic spine, but manipulation of this muscle can be performed in a manner that minimizes injury. The spleen and liver are intraperitoneal, and a retroperitoneal approach is typically performed for a lateral approach to the lower thoracic spine. Retropleural approaches avoid transection of the parietal pleura usually by performing blunt dissection between it and the endothoracic fascia.

Key Principles

- The stability of a spinal implant depends on approach and access of surgery, as well as construct length.
- Long constructs ending at the apical vertebra have a large moment arm, so it is important to reduce this by extending a construct to a neutral vertebra only.
- Terminating long constructs at junctional segments should be avoided due to risk of applying a moment arm to a flexible region.

References

[1] Fraser JF, Diwan AD, Peterson M, et al. Preoperative magnetic resonance imaging screening for a surgical decision regarding the approach for anterior spine fusion at the cervicothoracic junction. Spine 2002;27(7):675–681

[2] Yi X, Xie P, Zhang L, et al. Entrance and origin of the extracranial vertebral artery found on computed tomography angiography. Sci Rep 2022;12(1):15274

[3] Chen Q, Brahimaj BC, Khanna R, et al. Posterior atlantoaxial fusion: a comprehensive review of surgical techniques and relevant vascular anomalies. J Spine Surg 2020;6(1):164–180

[4] Akmese R, Us AK. Comparison of subtransverse process wiring and sublaminar wiring in the treatment of idiopathic thoracic scoliosis. J Spinal Disord Tech 2013;26(2):79–86

[5] De la Garza Ramos R, Nakhla J, Sciubba DM, Yassari R. Screw versus S2 alar-iliac screw fixation in adults: a meta-analysis. J Neurosurg Spine 2018;30(2):253–258

[6] Hasan MY, Liu G, Wong H-K, Tan J-H. Postoperative complications of S2AI versus iliac screw in spinopelvic fixation: a meta-analysis and recent trends review. Spine J 2020;20(6):964–972

[7] Jones EL, Heller JG, Silcox DH, Hutton WC. Cervical pedicle screws versus lateral mass screws. Anatomic feasibility and biomechanical comparison. Spine (Phila Pa 1976) 1997;22(9): 977–982

Part VI

Spine Instrumentation Constructs: Deformity, Management, and Prevention Strategies

VI

- D. Cross members should never be used in short-segment constructs
- E. Pliable cross members should be placed to minimize fracture

▸▸ Question 17

Which of the following is true regarding screw triangulation?

- A. Biomechanically similar to parallel screw placement
- B. Provides translational deformity prevention
- C. Biomechanically only advantageous with cross members
- D. Only should be done in cases of reduction of spondylolisthesis
- E. Provides increased stress on the rod

▸▸ Question 18

Understanding implant failure and techniques to avoid it are essential in construct planning. Screw–bone interface failure can occur via toggle, cutout, or pullout. Which of the following are methods to minimize screw toggle?

- A. Screw triangulation
- B. Minimizing plate bending
- C. Increased screw thread depth
- D. Bicortical purchase
- E. Increased screw pitch

▸▸ Question 19

Material stiffness and rod fracture are essential concepts to discern when choosing the best rod for a deformity construct. Cobalt chromium rods are thought to have what type of relationship with titanium rods when compared?

- A. CoCh rods and Ti rods have identical stiffness and rod fracture incidence
- B. CoCh rods have higher bending stiffness and higher rod fracture incidence than Ti rods
- C. CoCh rods have lower bending stiffness and higher rod fracture incidence than Ti rods
- D. CoCh rods have higher bending stiffness and lower rod fracture incidence than Ti Rods
- E. Bending stiffness does not depend on the material of the rod and only off the amount of contouring done in vivo

Answers

▸▸ Answer 1

Correct answer is B

One or a combination of two fundamental techniques can be used for deformity correction: (1) implant force and bending moment application that "brings the spine to the implant" and (2) implant force and bending moment application with in vivo implant configuration alteration techniques. A fundamental understanding of these techniques provides the surgeon with a broadened surgical latitude and allows an individualized and customized implant selection process for the patient in each case. Various techniques can be used to bring the spine to the implant. As mentioned previously, this is accomplished via the application of forces to the spine along one or a combination of the three axes of the Cartesian coordinate system. The utilization of three- or four-point bending forces is a classic strategy that "bring the spine to the implant." This can be applied to reduce subluxations. Three-point bending techniques can be employed dorsally to correct deformity by essentially "bringing the spine to the implant" (see ▸ Fig. 26.2).

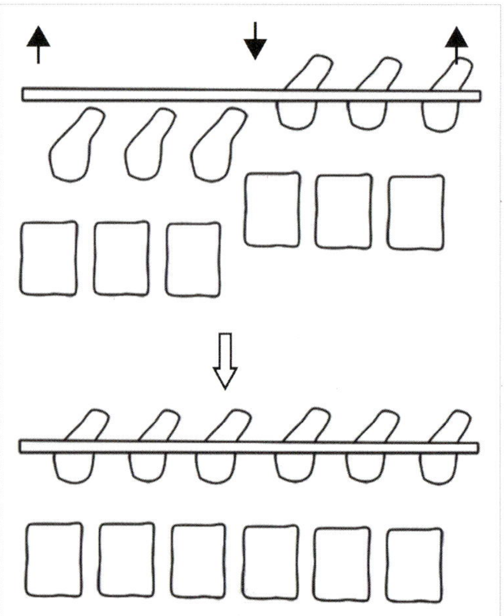

Fig. 26.2 A three-point bending construct that "brings the spine to the implant" via a dorsal approach. (Source: Biomechanics of Spine Stabilization: Third Edition, © 2015 Thieme Medical Publishers, Inc.)

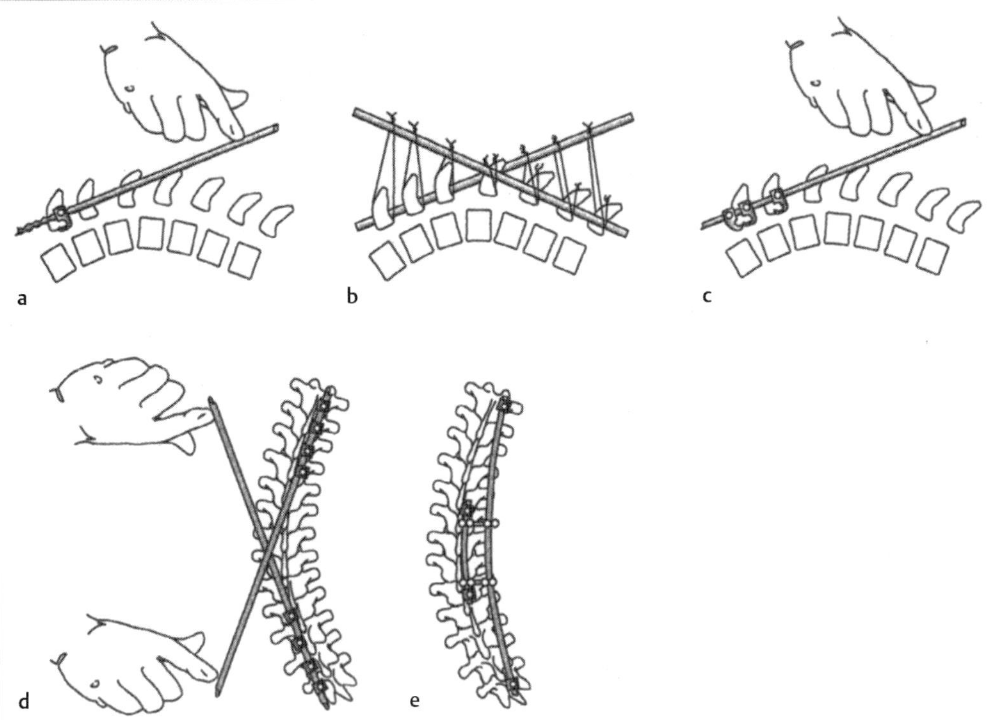

Fig. 26.3 The crossed-rod technique of thoracic and lumbar kyphotic deformity correction used with **(a)** the Harrington distraction rod, **(b)** Luque sublaminar wiring, and **(c)** universal spinal instrumentation. The latter technique is facilitated by the use of sequential hook insertion (From Benzel et al[2]). **(d)** The crossed-rod technique can be used for coronal plane (scoliotic) deformities, as well. **(e)** Two-rod translation force application strategies can similarly be used. In this situation, a small rod may be applied to the spine and brought to a longer rod that spans the concave side of the deformity, thus partially correcting the deformity. (Source: Biomechanics of Spine Stabilization: Third Edition, © 2015 Thieme Medical Publishers, Inc.)

Crossed-rod techniques can be applied in the sagittal and coronal planes. ► Fig. 26.3 illustrates the crossed-rod technique of thoracic and lumbar kyphotic deformity correction used with (**a**) the Harrington distraction rod, (**b**) Luque sublaminar wiring, and (**c**) universal spinal instrumentation. (**d**) The crossed-rod technique can be used for coronal plane (scoliotic) deformities, as well. (**e**) Two-rod translation force application strategies can similarly be used. In this situation, a small rod may be applied to the spine and brought to a longer rod that spans the concave side of the deformity, thus partially correcting the deformity. The other main fundamental techniques are implant bending force and bending moment application with in vivo implant configuration alteration techniques.

Utilizing multirod constructs might have some utility in deformity with specific indications, though it is certainly not a principle that is applied in maintaining and correcting deformity; therefore, A is false. Lateral interbodies are able to establish lumbar lordosis and theoretically have a higher chance of fusion via Wolff's law, though this does not involve the fundamentals of implant force and bending moment application; therefore, C is false. Optimal pedicle screws have maximal pitch and diameter; therefore, D is false. Cobalt chrome rods can offer some rigidity, though it is not a principle applied in all deformity cases.

►► Answer 2

Correct answer is B

For terminal three-point bending constructs to be effective in reducing translational deformation, they must be applied properly. The long arm of the construct must be placed (A) caudally with a ventral translational deformation and (B)

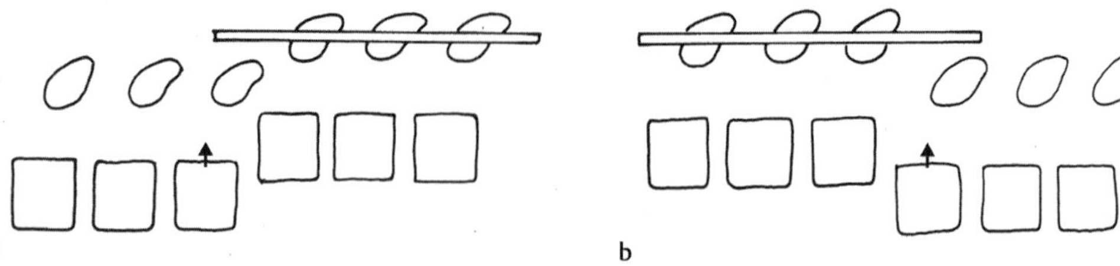

Fig. 26.4 For terminal three-point bending constructs to be effective in reducing translational deformation, they must be applied properly. The long arm of the construct must be placed **(a)** caudally with a ventral translational deformation and **(b)** rostrally with a dorsal translational deformation. (Source: Biomechanics of Spine Stabilization: Third Edition, © 2015 Thieme Medical Publishers, Inc.)

rostrally with a dorsal translational deformation (see ▶ Fig. 26.4). Therefore, C is false.

The long arm of the construct must not be symmetric in relation to the translation; therefore, A is false. Location of the long arm is dependent on the direction of translation; therefore, D is false. To maintain biomechanical stability, the location of the long arm is essential to maintain the correction; therefore, E is false.

▸▸ Answer 3

Correct answer is A

Four-point bending of the spine, as defined by White and Panjabi, involves loading a long structure (i.e., the spine) with two transverse forces on one side and two on the other. The bending moment is constant between the two intermediate points of force application if all forces are equal, whereas in three-point bending, the bending moment peaks at the intermediate point of force application (see ▶ Fig. 26.5); therefore, B and C are false. In three-point bending, the bending moment peaks at the single intermediate point of force; therefore, E is false. The closer the intermediate forces are applied to the terminus of the four-point bending construct, the greater the forces required to achieve an equivalent bending moment. If all forces are equal, the intermediate points would not be constantly varying; therefore, D is false. In the four-point bending construct depicted in the figure, all forces (F4PB) and the distance from the intermediate and terminal points of force application (1/3 × D4PB) are equal. In this situation, the maximum bending moment, which is constant between the two intermediate points of force application, is defined by the following equation: M4PB = F4PB × 1/3 D4PB. D4PB is the length of the entire construct. Because the forces (F4PB) are applied at points dividing the construct into three equal sections, the moment arm defining the bending moment is one-third of the entire construct length. In the three-point bending construct depicted, the intermediate force is applied halfway between the terminal points of force application. Therefore, the maximum bending moment occurs at the point of intermediate force application and is defined by the following equation: M3PB = 1/4 F3PB × D3PB.

▸▸ Answer 4

Correct answer is B

Three- and four-point bending implants are a classic example of the strategy that conforms the spine to the implant placed. They can be applied to reduce subluxations. Terminal three-point bending techniques can be used to "bring the spine to the implant" as well as to prevent the spine from "falling away from the implant." If the forces applied by a three- or four-point bending construct are oriented in the opposite direction, the technique is termed reversed three-point or reversed four-point bending fixation, which is typically used to reduce lumbar spondylolisthesis (see ▶ Fig. 26.6). The forces needed to reduce the spondylolisthesis are needed in the *dorsal direction* at the fulcrum; therefore, A is false. Spinal derotation is a maneuver whereby a scoliotic curvature is converted to a kyphotic curvature while the rotatory component is also corrected. This is done by rotating the rods 90 degrees, which are loosely applied to the spine via anchors. Therefore, C is false. Crossed-rod technique is a well-established method of thoracic and lumbar kyphotic deformity correction; therefore, D is false.[1,2]

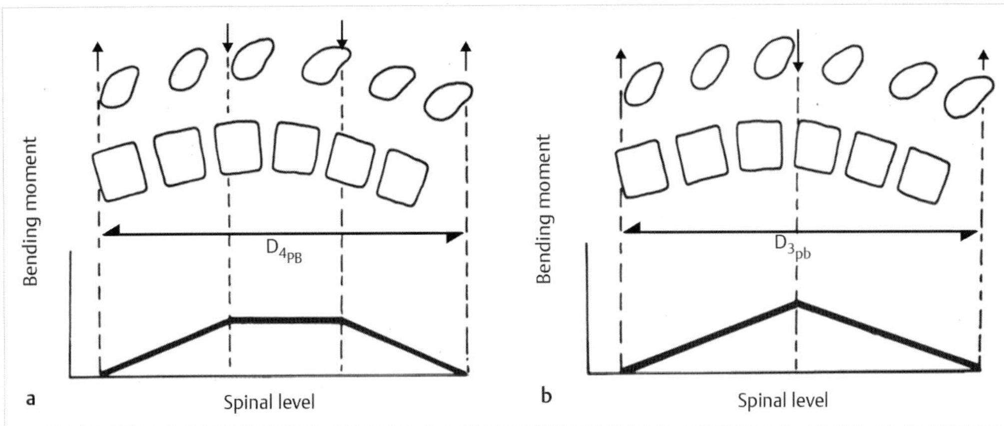

Fig. 26.5 **(a)** Four-point bending and **(b)** three-point bending construct forces and associated bending moments. In the four-point bending construct depicted here, all forces (F_{4PB}) and the distance from the intermediate and terminal points of force application ($1/3 \times D_{4PB}$) are equal. In this situation, the maximum bending moment, which is constant between the two intermediate points of force application, is defined by the following equation: $M_{4PB} = F4_{PB} \times 1/3\ D_{4PB}$. D_{4PB} is the length of the entire construct. Because the forces (F_{4PB}) are applied at points dividing the construct into three equal sections, the moment arm defining the bending moment is one-third of the entire construct length. In the three-point bending construct depicted here, the intermediate force is applied halfway between the terminal points of force application. Therefore, as demonstrated in Chapter 17, the maximum bending moment occurs at the point of intermediate force application and is defined by the following equation: $M_{3PB} = 1/4\ F_{3PB} \times D_{3PB}$. However, because F_{4PB} is the force applied at the terminal hook– bone interface and F_{3PB} is the force applied at the fulcrum, at the outset, F_{4PB} and F_{3PB} by definition vary by a factor of 2. The force applied at the terminal hook–bone interface in this example is thus $2 \times F_{3PB}$. This is defined here as $Fterminus_{3PB}$ and is equal to $2F_{3PB}$. Therefore, $M_{3PB} = 1/4 \times 2 \times Fterminus_{3PB} \times D_{3PB}$. To compare three-point and fourpoint bending constructs, the following derivation is performed. Assume that a three-point and four-point bending construct are of similar length and that the bending moments applied are equal. The following derivation, thus depicts the comparison between the constructs; because $D_{4PB} = D_{3PB}$, and $M_{4PB} = M_{3PB}$, then $F_{4PB} \times 1/3 \times D_{3PB} - 2 \times Fterminus_{3PB} \times D_{3PB}$; $F_{4PB} = 3/2 \times Fterminus_{3PB}$. The forces applied at the terminal hooks by each construct are depicted by the above equations. The closer the intermediate forces are applied to the terminus of the our-point bending construct, the greater the numerator of the right half of the equation and the greater the forces required to achieve an equivalent bending moment (compared to a three-point bending construct of similar length). Conversely, the closer the intermediate forces of a four-point bending construct are placed to the middle of the construct, the more it biomechanically approximates a three-point bending construct (i.e., $F_{4PB} = Fterminus_{3PB}$). (Source: Biomechanics of Spine Stabilization: Third Edition, © 2015 Thieme Medical Publishers, Inc.)

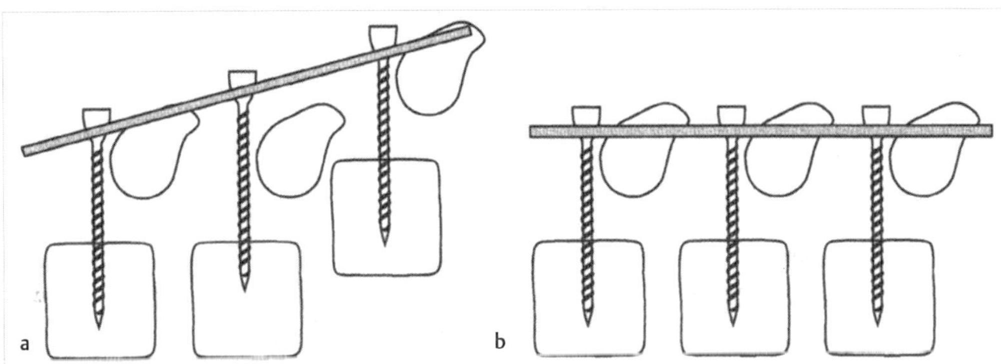

Fig. 26.6 **(a, b)** Reversed three-point bending forces (dorsally directed force at the fulcrum) can be used to reduce a spondylolisthesis. This subjects the screw to significant pullout stresses. (Source: Biomechanics of Spine Stabilization: Third Edition, © 2015 Thieme Medical Publishers, Inc.)

▸▸ Answer 5

Correct answer is B

In ▸ Fig. 26.5, assume that a three-point and four-point bending constructs are of similar length and that the bending moments applied are equal. The following derivation depicts the comparison between the constructs; because D4PB = D3PB and M4PB = M3PB, then F4PB × 1/3 × D3PB − 2 × $F_{terminus}$ 3PB × D3PB; F4PB = 3/2 × $F_{terminus}$3PB. The forces applied at the terminal hooks by each construct are depicted by the above equations. The closer the intermediate forces are applied to the terminus of the four-point bending construct, the greater the numerator of the right half of the equation and the greater the forces required to achieve an equivalent bending moment (compared with a three-point bending construct of similar length). Conversely, the closer the intermediate forces of a four-point bending construct are placed to the middle of the construct, the more it biomechanically approximates a three-point bending construct (i.e., F4PB = $F_{terminus}$3PB).

▸▸ Answer 6

Correct answer is E

Applied moment arm cantilever beam constructs are generally applied via either flexion or extension bending moments (see ▸ Fig. 26.7). They can be used with or without distraction or compression or an accompanying ventral dural sac decompression and/or interbody body. These factors are important to consider if an optimal construct design, customized to a given clinical situation, is to be used. For example, if extension and distraction, without an accompanying interbody fusion, are to be used, large screws must be employed to withstand the applied axial loads. Despite this, construct failure may result. Pedicle diameter or geometry may dictate the use of relatively small screws. In these situations, the use of distraction and extension is followed by (1) ventral decompression, (2) the placement of an interbody weight-bearing bone graft, and (3) compression of the construct onto the ventral graft and other intrinsic ventral weight-bearing spinal elements. This results in "sharing of the load" by the construct, the spinal elements, and the interbody fusion and simultaneous application of the desired extension bending moment for deformity reduction. Load bearing-to-load sharing force application permits the implant and the spine to share the load (unloading the implant). In ▸ Fig. 26.8, the spine is distracted (with or without extension or flexion bending moment application) by **(b)** the implant, followed by **(c)** bone graft placement and **(d)** compression of the implant. This causes the load to be shared between the implant and the spine. *Straight arrows* depict forces; *curved arrows* depict bending moments. Increasing screw size would increase the amount of axial load the construct would be able to withstand; therefore, A is false. Spinous process tethering, wide dorsal decompression, and posterior column osteotomies do not allow for sharing of the load ventrally or allow for application of any extension bending moment; therefore, B, C, and D are false.[3,4]

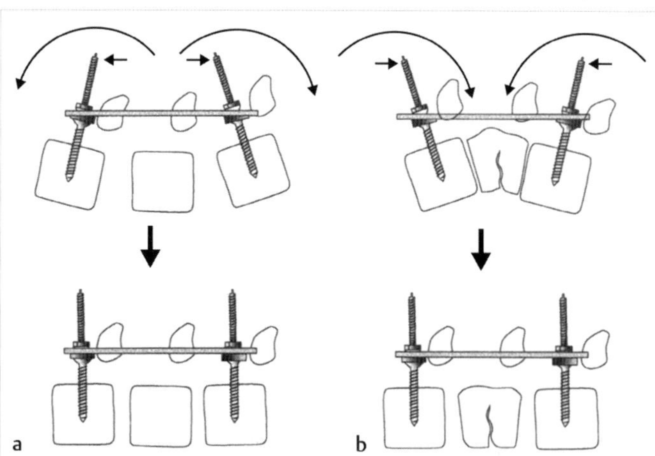

Fig. 26.7 Sagittal plane applied moment arm cantilever beam forces may be applied with either **(a)** flexion or **(b)** extension bending moments. Straight arrows depict forces; curved arrows depict bending moments. (Source: Biomechanics of Spine Stabilization: Third Edition, © 2015 Thieme Medical Publishers, Inc.)

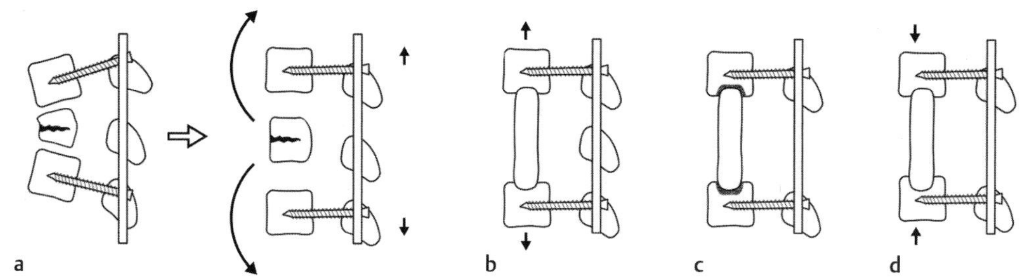

Fig. 26.8 (a) An applied moment arm cantilever beam construct that uses distraction and an extension bending moment, without an interbody fusion. This may be associated with a suboptimal success rate.5 Load bearing-to-load sharing force application may minimize this complication by permitting the implant and the spine to share the load (unloading the implant). In this case, the spine is distracted (with or without extension or flexion bending moment application) by **(b)** the implant, followed by **(c)** bone graft placement and **(d)** compression of the implant. This causes the load to be shared between the implant and the spine. Straight arrows depict forces; curved arrows depict bending moments. (Source: Biomechanics of Spine Stabilization: Third Edition, © 2015 Thieme Medical Publishers, Inc.)

▸▸ Answer 7

Correct answer is B

The forces applied to the various components of an implant must be carefully considered. For example, a screw can be exposed to significant three-point bending forces. This must be considered during the implant design decision-making process. ▶ Fig. 26.9 depicts three-point bending forces applied to a nonfixed moment arm screw that traverses potentially mobile media or media of different densities. (**a**) *Solid arrows* depict the three-point bending forces applied to the screw. (**b**) Similar forces can be applied when a screw passes across a fracture, such as a transodontoid screw used for a dens fracture. A screw fractures at the point of maximum stress (maximum bending moment if the inner diameter is constant).

The crossed-rod technique is used for kyphosis deformity correction Therefore, B is false. Reverse four-point bending forces refer to the application of two intermediate forces. In this case, there is one clear area of stress and maximal force resulting in screw failure, which would lead to three points of bending moments; therefore, A is false. Applied moment arm cantilever beams are constructs that utilize distraction and extension bending moment to attain correction. Without interbody bone graft, other methods are needed to reduce risk construct failure such as large pedicle screw diameter. Therefore, C is false. Short-segment parallelogram deformity reduction techniques are used to reduce lateral translation deformities. Rotatory and distraction forces are applied to the rods and screws to achieve rigid fixation. Therefore, E is false.

▸▸ Answer 8

Correct answer is D

A short-segment parallelogram deformity reduction is best in the lower lumbar region. It is a rigid cantilever beam pedicle fixation technique used to reduce lateral translation deformities via application of a bending moment in the coronal plane. The technique involves the application of rotatory and distraction forces to the rods and screws following by rigid cross fixation. ▶ Fig. 26.10 shows short-segment parallelogram deformity reduction. A lateral translational deformity. (**a**) Pedicle screws are placed. (**b**) The pedicle screws are connected by rods. (**c**) The rods are connected (friction–glide tightness), and a torque is applied to both rods simultaneously with rod grippers. (**d**) This technique is illustrated in a case of lateral L4–L5 dislocation. (**e**) Reduction was achieved and then maintained with rigid cross fixation. (**f**) Distraction, followed by interbody bone graft placement and finally compression, is used to secure the bone graft in place.

most commonly used in the cervical spine because of the lesser loads accepted by the implant. Therefore, C is false. Interbody placement can be helpful fashions, one of which is via the load bearing-to-load sharing technique. This does not involve placement of large transverse vertebral body screws. Therefore, D is false. Applied moment arm cantilever beam constructs involves application of either flexion or extension bending moments accompanied by ventral decompression. Placement of interbody fusion can be used; however, if not, large pedicle screws must be utilized to minimize construct failure. Therefore, E is false.[5,6]

▸▸ Answer 10

Correct answer is E

In vivo contouring (see ▸ Fig. 26.13) can be used to alter spinal alignment from a pathologic kyphotic curvature, with the rods configured to match (**a**) the curvature of the pathologic spine to (**b**) the desired alignment. It is commonly used after the implant has already been shaped to fit the spine but can raises issues because excessive in vivo contouring can cause significant stress to the spine and the screws. This can lead to rod fracture.

Derotation is a therapeutic maneuver done for complex spine deformities where a scoliotic curve is converted to a kyphotic curvature. Therefore, A is false. A deformity correction is not solely dependent on screw size. There are many factors, but screw triangulation greatly increases pullout strength. Therefore, B is false. In vivo rod contouring is also applied to all regions of the spine. Therefore, C is false. Lateral translating deformity is most often addressed with short-segment parallelogram deformity reduction. The technique involves the application of rotatory and distraction forces to the rods and screws following by rigid cross fixation. Therefore, D is false.

▸▸ Answer 11

Correct answer is B

A hook–rod instrumentation set can be used to conform to a spinal deformity, and rods can be contoured to improve overall alignment. Pedicle screws are an implant commonly utilized but not mandatory; therefore, A and E are false.

Adequate hook–bone interface is mandatory. Contouring will change the relationships of the implants to the spine. ▸ Fig. 26.14 shows (**a**) during rod contouring, implant–bone interface relationships must be observed closely. Some hooks may overdistract, although others may loosen. (**b**) Impingement of a sublaminar hook on the dural sac, and (**c**) lateral or medial migration of pedicle hooks or (**d**) transverse process hooks are all possibilities. Hooks can loosen or tighten, migrate, and cause spinal canal compromise; therefore, answer C is false. Contouring affects the relationship of all the implants to the spine; therefore, answer D is false.[7]

▸▸ Answer 12

Correct answer is C

▸ Fig. 26.15 illustrates spinal derotation technique. Spinal derotation is accomplished by careful simultaneous rotation of two rods that have been attached to the spine in its deformed scoliotic state. The rotation of the rods by 90 degrees converts (**a**) a scoliosis to (**b**) a kyphosis. If the resultant kyphotic deformity is unacceptable, it may be corrected by rod contouring. (**c**, **d**) This strategy can be applied to biconcave curves. This is done by rotating the rods 90 degrees, which are loosely applied to the spine via anchors. If the resulting

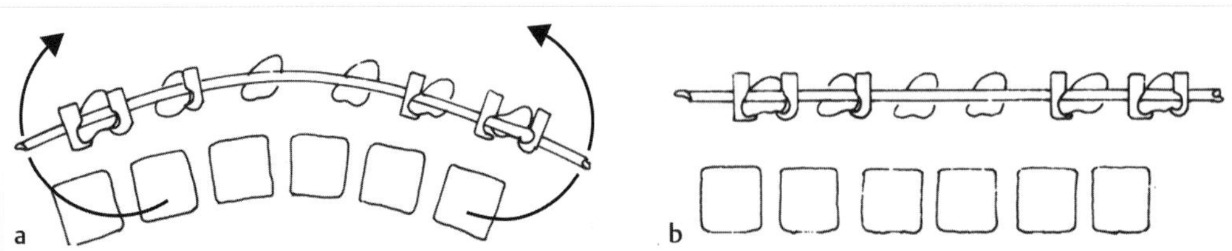

Fig. 26.13 Rod contouring can be used to alter spinal alignment from a pathologic kyphotic curvature, with the rods configured to match **(a)** the curvature of the pathologic spine to **(b)** the desired alignment (Source: Biomechanics of Spine Stabilization: Third Edition, © 2015 Thieme Medical Publishers, Inc.)

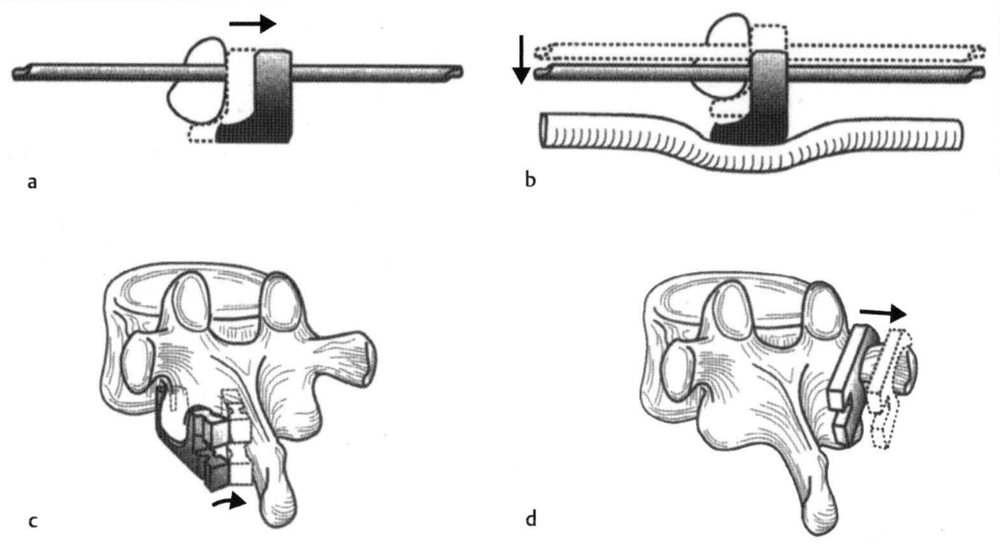

Fig. 26.14 **(a)** During rod contouring, implant–bone interface relationships must be observed closely. Some hooks may overdistract, although others may loosen. **(b)** Impingement of a sublaminar hook on the dural sac, and **(c)** lateral or medial migration of pedicle hooks or **(d)** transverse process hooks, may also occur. (Source: Biomechanics of Spine Stabilization: Third Edition, © 2015 Thieme Medical Publishers, Inc.)

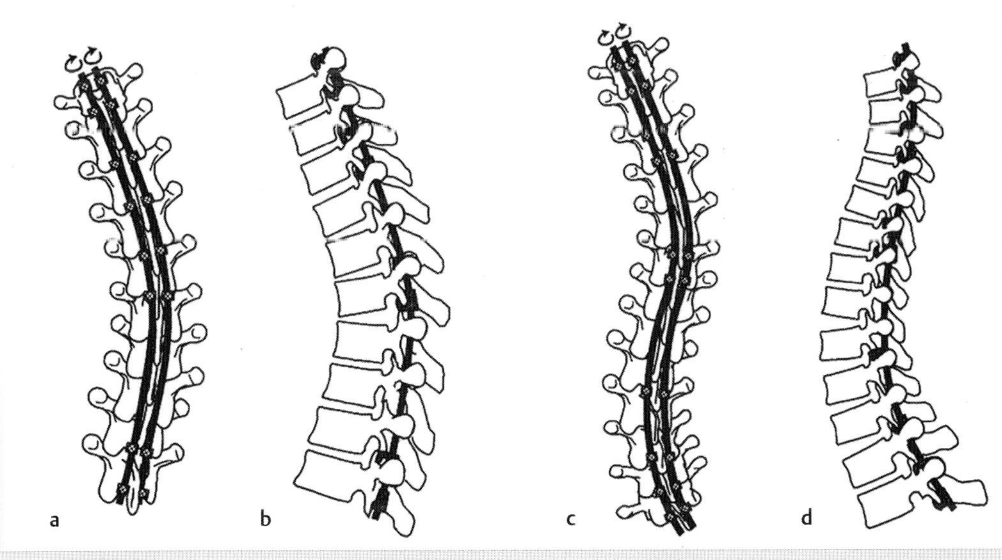

Fig. 26.15 **(a)** Spinal derotation is accomplished by careful simultaneous rotation of two rods that have been attached to the spine in its deformed scoliotic state. The rotation of the rods by 90 degrees converts **(a)** a scoliosis to **(b)** a kyphosis. If the resultant kyphotic deformity is unacceptable, it may be corrected by rod contouring. **(c, d)** This strategy can be applied to biconcave curves. (Source: Biomechanics of Spine Stabilization: Third Edition, © 2015 Thieme Medical Publishers, Inc.)

kyphotic curve is not desirable, it is then corrected with rod contouring.

▸▸ Answer 13

Correct answer is E

Intrinsic implant bending moment application in the sagittal or coronal plane is usually used to achieve the reduction of a scoliosis or kyphosis (see ▶ Fig. 26.16). This force complex can be applied in either the sagittal or the coronal plane. Intrinsic implant bending moment application is commonly used to reduce a one-segment or two-segment scoliotic deformation. This is mainly in the lumbar spine for degenerative pathologies. In order to do this, pedicle screws are placed at the levels of interest. Then, the screws on the concave side of the curve are distracted and the screws on the convex side are compressed by similar degrees.

Cross fixation is used for maintenance of the correction, and often should be used to maintain a correction of coronal scoliosis after applying an intrinsic implant bending moment. However, cross fixation in itself does not correct the deformity; therefore, A is false. In vivo implant contouring can be used to alter segmental relationships, though this can cause the relationships of the implant to change with the spine and can cause the screws to be overstressed or fatigued. In one-level pathology, it would be prudent to attempt intrinsic implant bending moment application first. Therefore, B is false. Crossed-screw fixation is used in the lateral extracavitary approach as an alternative to other short-segment fixation techniques and uses two large vertebral body screws and two small pedicle screw to attain reduction; therefore, C is false. Spinal derotation is a maneuver whereby a scoliotic curvature is converted to a kyphotic curvature while the rotatory component is also corrected. This is done by rotating the rods 90 degrees, which are loosely applied to the spine via anchors. Therefore, D is false.

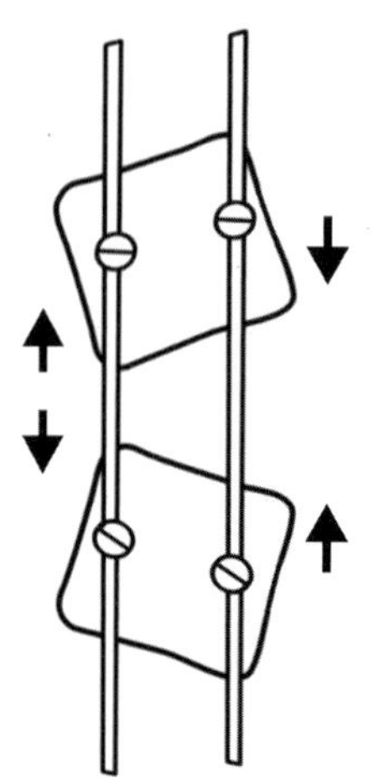

Fig. 26.16 Intrinsic implant bending moment application. (A) In this case, simple distraction of the concave side of the curvature and compression of the convex side achieves the reduction of a scoliotic deformity. (Source: Biomechanics of Spine Stabilization: Third Edition, © 2015 Thieme Medical Publishers, Inc.)

▸▸ Answer 14

Correct answer is A

With distraction or compression of screws, the relationship of the screw to the rod must be carefully monitored to avoid untoward screw–rod relationships—for example, flexion of the screw on the rod. The surgeon should carefully consider the type of screw–rod interface employed (e.g., variable-angle vs fixed-angle). The application of distraction forces to fixed-angle screws results in simple distraction with minimal or no application of a bending moment to the spine. If, however, a variable-angle screw is used, simple distraction may result in screw angulation at the screw–rod interface, thus causing a bending moment to be applied to the spine. These concepts regarding the different forces applied with different screws can be employed in fracture reduction and deformity based on the vector of forced needed. ▶ Fig. 26.17 illustrates how screw flexion may occur during distraction if the screw–rod interface is of a variable-angle type. This untoward occurrence can be avoided by taking care to achieve friction–glide tightness at the interface before distraction so that the angular relationship of the screws with the rod is maintained during distraction. *Arrows* depict distraction forces applied by the distractor. Resistance to distraction is exerted at the tip of the screw by the spinal elements (or, in this case, fingers).

▸▸ Answer 15

Correct answer is A

The connection of bilaterally placed rods can increase the biomechanical strength of the construct.

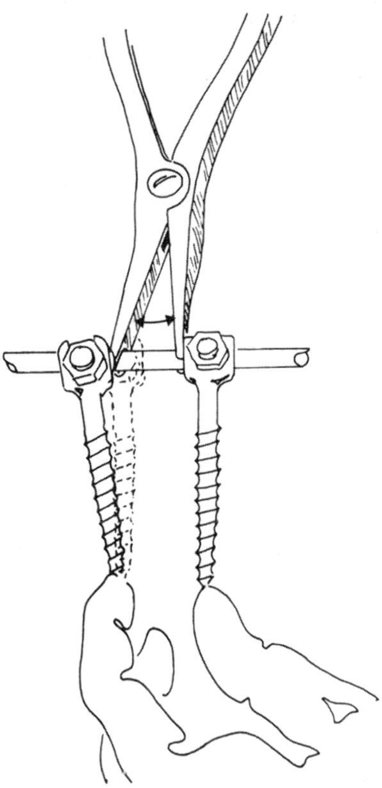

Fig. 26.17 Screw flexion may occur during distraction if the screw–rod interface is of a variable-angle type. This untoward occurrence can be avoided by taking care to achieve friction glide tightness at the interface before distraction so that the angular relationship of the screws with the rod is maintained during distraction. Arrows depict distraction forces applied by the distractor. Resistance to distraction is exerted at the tip of the screw by the spinal elements (or, in this case, fingers). (Source: Biomechanics of Spine Stabilization: Third Edition, © 2015 Thieme Medical Publishers, Inc.)

Most short-segment constructs do not benefit from this, but long-segment constructs can benefit greatly. Cross fixation in conjunction with screw triangulation can be used to maximally resist screw pullout. Cross fixation also provides a quadrilateral frame construct stabilizing the rotatory movement and increasing the integrity of implant–bone interfaces. With this, multiple metal–bone interfaces must fail simultaneously for implant failure to occur. Bilateral pedicle screw placement and triangulation provide increased stability; therefore, B and C are false. Interbody placement and spinous process tethering do not provide quadrilateral frame stability; therefore, D and E are false. ► Fig. 26.18 illustrates intrinsic implant bending moment application. (**a**) In this case, laterally placed transverse vertebral body screws are manipulated (distracted and compressed; *arrows*) to reduce a kyphotic deformity. Compression of the two most dorsal screws and distraction of the two most ventral screws achieves reduction of this deformity. (**b**) Cross fixation is usually used to assist in maintaining the reduction.

►► Answer 16

Correct answer is C

When cross members are used in short-segment deformity cases, very rigid members should be used because of the large bending moments that are often applied at the cross member–rod interface. Only cross members with substantial torsional resistance capabilities can resist these stresses. They are able to resist translational deformity.

Typically, in long constructs, the cross members are placed at the top and bottom of the middle third of the construct; therefore, A is false. Cross members should be considered irrespective of the screw placement; therefore, B is false. They can also be used within reason in short-segment deformity; therefore, D is false. Pliable cross members should never be used because they risk failure; therefore, E is false. ► Fig. 26.19 shows rigid cross members are useful with short-segment deformity reduction. The stresses placed at the cross member–rod junction are often associated with a large bending moment. Only cross members with substantial torsional resistance capabilities can resist these stresses. In this case, the cross member maintains the reduction of a translational deformity (**a**) by applying (or resisting) (**b**) a torque.

►► Answer 17

Correct answer is B

Triangulation is essential in prevention of lateral translation deformation. It provides increased screw pullout strength, translational deformity prevention, and construct security. Cross fixation can provide increased pullout and translation resistance.

Triangulation is biomechanically stronger than parallel placed screws; therefore, A is false.

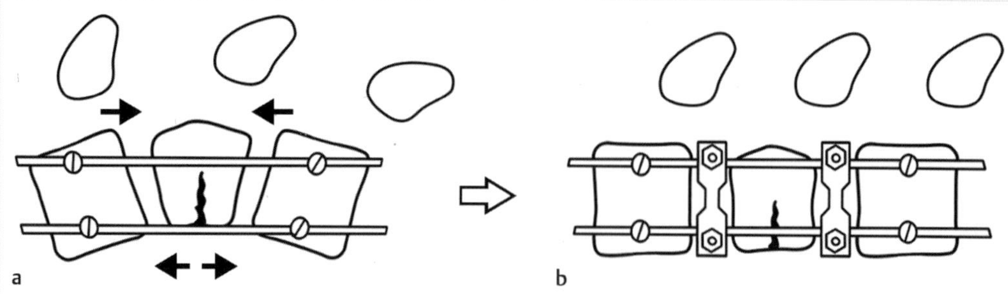

Fig. 26.18 Intrinsic implant bending moment application. **(a)** In this case, laterally placed transverse vertebral body screws are manipulated (distracted and compressed; *arrows*) to reduce a kyphotic deformity. Compression of the two most dorsal screws and distraction of the two most ventral screws achieves reduction of this deformity. **(b)** Cross fixation is usually used to assist in maintaining the reduction. (Source: Biomechanics of Spine Stabilization: Third Edition, © 2015 Thieme Medical Publishers, Inc.)

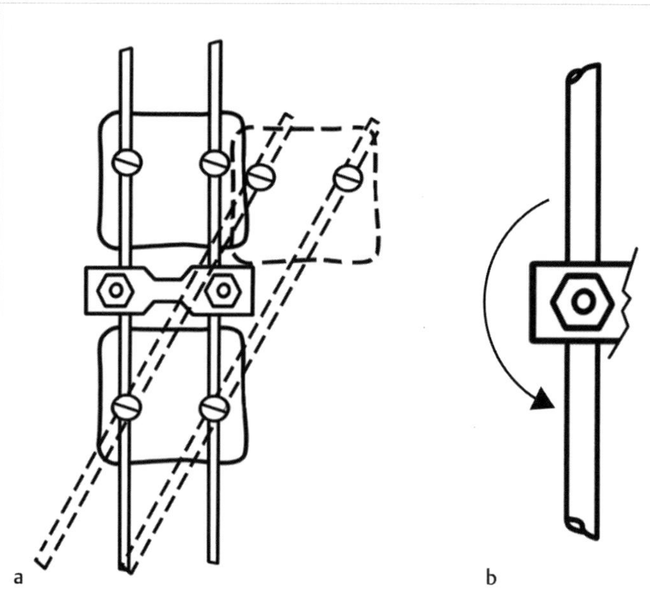

Fig. 26.19 Rigid cross members are useful with short-segment deformity reduction. The stresses placed at the cross member–rod junction are often associated with a large bending moment. Only cross members with substantial torsional resistance capabilities can resist these stresses. In this case, the cross member maintains the reduction of a translational deformity **(a)** by applying (or resisting) **(b)** a torque (Source: Biomechanics of Spine Stabilization: Third Edition, © 2015 Thieme Medical Publishers, Inc.)

Although cross members can increase construct security, they are not mutually exclusive and not needed in all cases; therefore, C is false. Reduction of spondylolisthesis can be achieved many ways and triangulation is not needed only in these cases; therefore, D is false. Biomechanically, triangulation does not augment biomechanical stress on the rod; therefore, E is false. ▶ Fig. 26.20 shows screw toe-in results in much greater pullout resistance, translational deformity prevention, and construct security. (**a**) Parallel screws cannot resist translation and resist pullout poorly. (**b**) Moderate toe-in provides moderate security in this regard. (**c**) Significant toe-in results in even greater security. (**d**) Cross fixation plus significant screw toe-in provides optimal pullout resistance and translational deformation resistance. This concept is applied in the crossed-screw fixation technique described previously. With this configuration, pivoting of the bone about a screw is prevented by its toed-in counterpart. (**e**) Finally, adding a level of screw fixation (in this case, an undetermined point of fixation) provides three-point bending characteristics that assist translation resistance in all planes.[8]

▸▸ Answer 18

Correct answer is D

▸ Fig. 26.21 shows screw–bone interface failure can occur via (**a**) toggle, (**b**) cutout, or (**c**) pullout. Screw toggle can be minimized by bicortical screw purchase and adhering to load sharing principles such as applied moment arm cantilever construct techniques. Plate or rod fracture occurs at the point of maximum bending moment application at a weak point of the implant. This occurs from excess implant contouring; therefore, B is false. Screw triangulation is essential in prevention of lateral translation deformation. Therefore, A is false. Increased screw thread depth and pitch minimize screw pullout; therefore, C and E are false.[9]

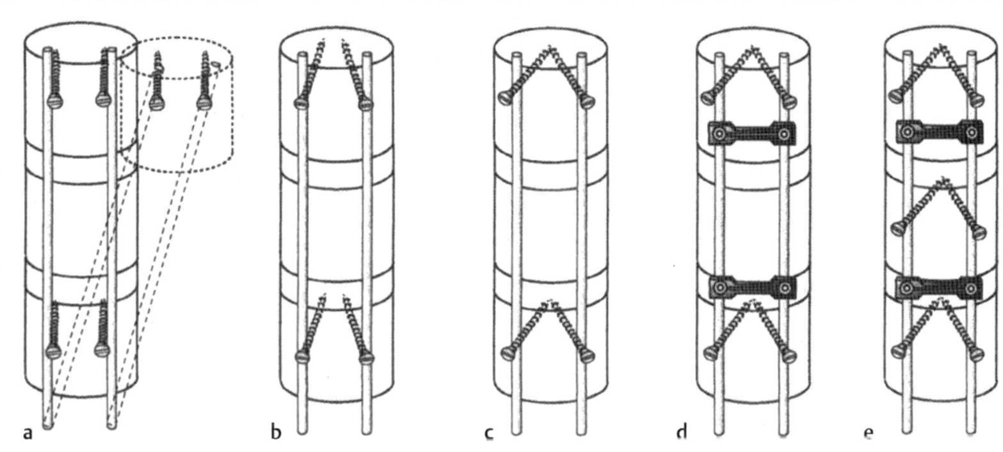

Fig. 26.20 Screw toe-in results in much greater pullout resistance, translational deformity prevention, and construct security. **(a)** Parallel screws cannot resist translation and resist pullout poorly **(b)** Moderate toe-in provides moderate security in this regard. **(c)** Significant toe-in results in even greater security. **(d)** Cross fixation plus significant screw toe-in provides optimal pullout resistance and translational deformation resistance. This concept is applied in the crossed-screw fixation technique (see ▸ Fig. 26.14 and ▸ Fig. 26.15). With this configuration, pivoting of the bone about a screw is prevented by its toed-in counterpart. **(e)** Finally, adding a level of screw fixation (in this case, an undetermined point of fixation) provides three-point bending characteristics that assist translation resistance in all planes. (Source: Biomechanics of Spine Stabilization: Third Edition, © 2015 Thieme Medical Publishers, Inc.)

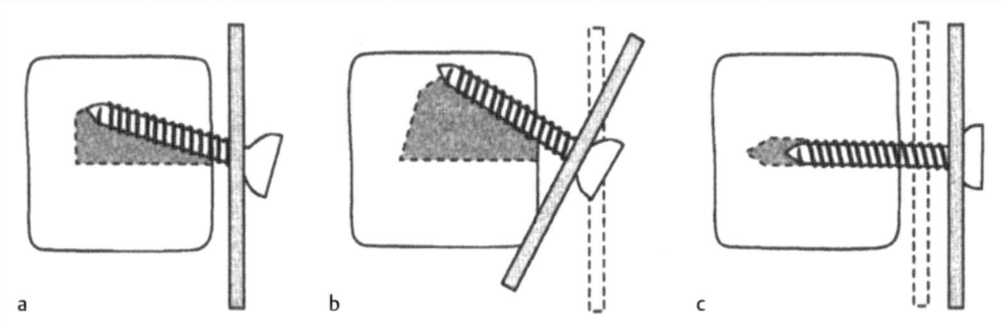

Fig. 26.21 Screw–bone interface failure can occur via **(a)** toggle, **(b)** cutout, or **(c)** pullout. Plate (or rod) fracture occurs at the point of maximum stress application—that is, maximum bending moment application at a weak point in the plate (low section modulus). (Source: Biomechanics of Spine Stabilization: Third Edition, © 2015 Thieme Medical Publishers, Inc.)

▸▸ **Answer 19**

Correct answer is D

Several factors influence the effectiveness of rods used in spine instrumentation. Rod diameter, body mass index of the patient, amount of bending and rod contouring, bending angle needed, bender type used, and biomechanical properties of the rod all play an essential role in how effective the rod is in maintaining correction. All play important roles in reducing implant failure. Therefore, E is false. Cobalt chrome is being used more commonly in deformity for its increased mechanical strength and resistance to loss of sagittal correction. Noshchenko and Demura et al demonstrated that cobalt chromium rods had higher bending stiffness than the titanium rods; therefore, C is false.

Shega et al and Han et al also demonstrated that the incidence of rod fracture is lower in cobalt chromium compared with titanium rods. Therefore, A and B are false.[10,11,12]

Key Principles

- In three-point bending, the bending moment peaks at the single intermediate point of force.
- The closer the intermediate forces are applied to the terminus of the four-point bending construct, the greater the forces required to achieve an equivalent bending moment.
- Screw triangulation is essential in prevention of lateral translation deformation. It provides increased screw pullout strength, translational deformity prevention, and construct security.
- Cross fixation can provide increased pullout and translation resistance.
- In vivo implant contouring is used to alter segmental relationships for deformity reduction.
- Short-segment parallelogram deformity reduction is a rigid cantilever beam pedicle fixation technique used to reduce lateral translation deformities via application of a bending moment in the coronal plane.

References

[1] Benzel EC. Luque rod segmental spinal instrumentation. In: Rengachary SS, Wilkins R, eds. Neurosurgical Operative Atlas. Park Ridge, IL: American Association of Neurological Surgeons; 1992:433–438

[2] Benzel EC, Ball PA, Baldwin NG, Marchand EP. The sequential hook insertion technique for universal spine instrumentation application. Technical note. J Neurosurg 1993;79:608–611

[3] Dick W. The "fixateur interne" as a versatile implant for spine surgery. Spine 1987;12:882–900

[4] Krag MH, Beynnon BD, Pope MH, Frymoyer JW, Haugh LD, Weaver DL. An internal fixator for posterior application to short segments of the thoracic, lumbar, or lumbosacral spine. Design and testing. Clin Orthop Relat Res 1986;203:75–98

[5] Cagli S, Crawford NR, Sonntag VK, Dickman CA. Biomechanics of grade I degenerative lumbar spondylolisthesis. Part 2: treatment with threaded interbody cages/dowels and pedicle screws. J Neurosurg 2001;94(Suppl):51–60

[6] Crawford NR, Cagli S, Sonntag VK, Dickman CA. Biomechanics of grade I degenerative lumbar spondylolisthesis. Part 1: in vitro model. J Neurosurg 2001;94(Suppl):45–50

[7] Cheung KM, Luk KD, Leong JC. Radiographic assessment of pedicle hook placement. Spine 1997;22:2106–2111

[8] Benzel EC, Baldwin NG. Crossed-screw fixation of the unstable thoracic and lumbar spine. J Neurosurg 1995;82: 11–16

[9] Steffee AD, Biscup RS, Sitkowski DJ. Segmental spine plates with pedicle screw fixation. A new internal fixation device for disorders of the lumbar and thoracolumbar spine. Clin Orthop Relat Res 1986;203:45–53

[10] Shega FD, Zhang H, Manini DR, Tang M, Liu S. Comparison of effectiveness between cobalt chromium rods versus titanium rods for treatment of patients with spinal deformity: a systematic review and meta-analysis. Adv Orthop 2020;2020: 8475910

[11] Noshchenko A, Xianfeng Y, Armour GA, et al. Evaluation of spinal instrumentation rod bending characteristics for in-situ contouring. J Biomed Mater Res B Appl Biomater 2011;98(1): 192–200

[12] Han S, Hyun SJ, Kim KJ, Jahng TA, Kim HJ. Comparative study between cobalt chrome and titanium alloy rods for multilevel spinal fusion: proximal junctional kyphosis more frequently occurred in patients having cobalt chrome rods. World Neurosurg 2017;103:404–409

27 Deformity Prevention and Correction: Complex Clinical Strategies

Joseph S. Hudson, Thomas J. Buell, David O. Okonkwo

Spinal deformity encompasses a broad array of pathologies that can precipitate pain and disability. Successful management, surgical and nonsurgical, of spinal deformity requires an understanding biomechanical principles, indications for surgery, and reconstructive techniques.

Learning Objectives

- Understand the different load-bearing properties in patients with spinal deformity.
- Understand and apply the terminology/ classifications used to describe spinal deformity.
- Understand spinopelvic measurements and their associated impact on patients with spinal deformity.
- Understand strategies for correction of cervical spine subluxation.
- Understand the biomechanical principles associated with anterior versus posterior approaches for spinal deformity correction.

Questions

▸▸ **Question 1**

A degenerative rotatory lumbar kyphoscoliosis shifts the primary load-bearing axis of the spine toward which of the following?

- A. Facet joints on the convexity
- B. Facet joints on the concavity
- C. Midline
- D. Lateral disc space of the convexity
- E. Posterior tension band

▸▸ **Question 2**

The region of the spine that bears the most significant portion of the axial load shifts where during a flexion and lateral bending?

- A. Does not shift
- B. Dorsal
- C. Dorsal and lateral toward the direction of lateral bend
- D. Ventral and lateral toward the direction of lateral bend
- E. Ventral

▸▸ **Question 3**

A spine in physiologic sagittal balance is characterized by which of the following?

- A. A sagittal vertical axis (SVA) that is significantly positive
- B. An SVA that approximates the lumbosacral pivot point
- C. A relatively kyphotic lumbosacral angle
- D. An upper thoracic vertebra bisected by the central sacral line
- E. Loss of lumbar lordosis

▸▸ **Question 4**

Which of the following statements is true when tasked with analyzing a scoliotic curve prior to complex spinal reconstruction?

- A. The apical vertebra is associated with the smallest segmental angulation at its rostral and caudal disc spaces
- B. The apical and neutral vertebrae should be defined only in the sagittal plane
- C. A fusion construct should extend to a neutral and stable vertebra
- D. The neutral vertebra is located at the midportion of the scoliotic curve
- E. The apical vertebra is bisected most closely by the central sacral line

▸▸ **Question 5**

Based on the Scoliosis Research Society terminology definitions, what best defines sacral obliquity?

- A. The angle between the line along the posterior border of S1 and the vertical lateral edge of a standing radiograph (or perpendiculars to these lines)
- B. The rotation of the pelvis in the transverse plane around the vertical axis of the body
- C. An angle between the line from the top of the sacrum to the top of the pubis and a horizontal line perpendicular to the lateral edge of the standing radiograph
- D. Angulation of the pelvis in the coronal plane with respect to a horizontal line

- E. An angulation of the sacrum with respect to a line drawn between the two femoral heads on a supine radiograph

▸▸ Question 6

Which of the following is true with respect to global sagittal alignment?

- A. Complete global sagittal alignment correction is typically not needed if health-related quality-of-life optimization is the goal
- B. As the C7 SVA shifts anterior, associated patient-reported disability increases and quality of life decreases
- C. The vast majority of asymptomatic adults do not maintain their sagittal alignment as they age
- D. The tilt of the pelvis is unrelated to global sagittal alignment
- E. Correction of sagittal balance typically does not result in changes in cervical alignment

▸▸ Question 7

Which of the following is true with respect to spinopelvic parameters?

- A. Pelvic tilt is not affected by patient position
- B. A small pelvic tilt is associated with a large pelvic incidence
- C. The normal sacral slope is 30 to 50 degrees
- D. Pelvic tilt = pelvic incidence + sacral slope
- E. Patients with a large pelvic incidence have a reduction in adjacent level degeneration

▸▸ Question 8

Which of the following is correct with respect to the King and Lenke classifications of coronal plane deformity in pediatric and adolescent scoliosis?

- A Lenke lumbar modifier A curve describes a curve in which the central sacral line is between the pedicles up to the stable vertebrae with minimal or no lumbar scoliosis
- B. A Lenke lumbar modifier C curve is one in which the central sacral line touches the apical vertebrae
- C. A King type I curve is a double (lumbar and thoracic) concave curve in which the thoracic curve is more rigid
- D. A King type V curve is a single thoracic curve
- E. A King type II curve is one in which the central sacral line touches the apical vertebrae

▸▸ Question 9

Which of the following is true with respect to anterior approaches to kyphotic cervical deformity?

- A. Screw pullout strength is greater with ventral instrumentation
- B. Anterior approaches inadequately address neural element compression and the developing kyphotic deformity
- C. Convergently angulated divergently directed Caspar pins can be used to facilitate extension to correct a focal kyphosis
- D. Kyphotic deformity in the cervical spine typically begins in the vertebral body
- E. As a cervical kyphotic deformity progresses over time, the moment arm applied by axial loading becomes smaller

▸▸ Question 10

Which is the correct pairing of Schwab or Aebi deformity classification schemes?

- A. Aebi type I: progressive idiopathic scoliosis of the lumbar or thoracolumbar spine
- B. Aebi type III(b): primary degenerative scoliosis of the thoracolumbar spine with a curve apex most frequently at L2–L4
- C. Schwab type T curves: associated with pelvic incidence as the sagittal modifier
- D. Schwab type L curves: associated with an SVA sagittal modifier
- E. Schwab type D curves: associated with pelvic incidence–lumbar lordosis (PI-LL) sagittal modifier

▸▸ Question 11

Which of the following is true pertaining to the management of cervical spine subluxation (i.e., locked facets)?

- A. Dorsal open reduction does not typically require full facet osteotomies
- B. Dorsal open reduction techniques often require additional rod/screw fixation above and below the pathologic level
- C. Ventral open techniques often do not require a discectomy

- D. There is often an inability to generate a mechanical advantage sufficient for reduction when employing ventral or closed strategies
- E. A potential risk associated with ventral open approach (compared with dorsal open approach) for cervical facet reduction is inadvertent disc material being displaced into the spinal canal

▸▸ Question 12

Which of the following is true regarding thoracic deformity correction?

- A. Ventral screw rod fixation techniques require longer constructs
- B. Ventral approaches require a thoracotomy
- C. Dorsal crossed-rod bending strategies or ventral interbody distraction can be used to correct sagittal plane deformity
- D. Shorter dorsal constructs provide a longer moment arm to resist sagittal plane deformity
- E. Rod diameter is unrelated to rod fracture rates

▸▸ Question 13

Which of the following is *not* associated with increased risk of disease progression in adult degenerative rotatory scoliosis?

- A. Osteoporosis
- B. Degree of lateral spondylolisthesis of the apical vertebrae
- C. Passage of the intercrest line through L4
- D. A large Harrington factor (Cobb angle divided by the number of vertebrae in a curve)
- E. Increased disc wedging within the curve (disc index)

▸▸ Question 14

For patients with sagittal plane deformities of the lumbar spine, which of the following is true?

- A. Operative beds/frame adjuncts that minimize lordosis should be employed
- B. Unilateral pedicle screw fixation is frequently used
- C. In patients with flatback deformity with positive sagittal imbalance, the SVA should be brought near the dorsal aspect of the L5–S1 disc space on standing long-cassette films
- D. They are typically not associated with coronal plane deformities
- E. Hip flexion during positioning is critical in most cases

▸▸ Question 15

When considering a lumbopelvic fixation procedure, which of the following is correct?

- A. Bony density in the sacrum is higher than in more rostral segments
- B. S1 screws directed toward the apex of the sacral promontory provide a reduced mechanical advantage
- C. Standing flexion–extension long-cassette plain films cannot help determine the degree of instability at a level of isthmic spondylolisthesis
- D. The length of the construct (longer construct) typically does provide a geometric advantage
- E. Lateral decubitus flexion extension plain films increase pain/guarding during image acquisition

▸▸ Question 16

Select the correct spinopelvic parameter relationship in the setting of isthmic spondylolisthesis.

- A. Pelvic incidence is reduced
- B. Thoracic kyphosis tends to decrease as the slip progresses
- C. The greater the sacral slope, the lesser the lumbar lordosis
- D. Thoracic and cervical alignment is typically not affected
- E. The restoration of lumbar lordosis has minimal to no effect on SVA

▸▸ Question 17

In which spinal procedure is the axis of rotation for kyphotic deformity correction situated dorsally (in the spinal canal)?

- A. Anterior cervical discectomy and fusion with interbody grafting
- B. Pedicle subtraction osteotomy
- C. Smith-Petersen or Ponte osteotomy
- D. Egg shell osteotomy
- E. Spondylectomy

▸▸ Question 18

Which of the following is true?
- A. The lumbosacral (McCord) pivot point is located 2 to 4 cm anterior to the sacral promontory
- B. The apical disc is located closest to the vertical axis of the patient (i.e., central sacral line)
- C. The inflection vertebrae is the point at which a curve changes from convex to concave (and vice versa)
- D. Vertebral tilt is measured in the sagittal plane on standing radiographs
- E. Pelvic inclination is measured as the angle between a line drawn from the pubis to the midsacrum

▸▸ Question 19

What is not a goal of spinal reconstructive surgery?
- A. Correct global spinal deformity
- B. Prevent further deformation
- C. Restore physiologic sagittal and coronal global balance
- D. Achieve an improved cosmesis/restore and preserve neurologic function
- E. Achieve a full correction of segmental and regional deformities

▸▸ Question 20

Choose the correct statement.
- A. Scoliosis produces deformity in the sagittal and coronal but not axial plane
- B. A longer implant length does not result in a larger bending moment applied to the deformed spine
- C. Implant length has little impact on the degree of stress placed on the adjacent uninstrumented vertebrae
- D. Concave distraction and convex compression can be used on screw rod constructs only in the lumbar spine
- E. The patient's degree of associated disability should be the primary variable when offering spinal reconstructive surgery

Answers

▸▸ Answer 1

Correct answer is B

The off-axis deformation of a degenerative rotatory scoliosis shifts the normal midline load-bearing axis of the spine in its nonscoliotic configuration laterally toward the facet joints on the concavity of the curve. It is postulated that loss of disc space height over time and accompanying coronal plane wedging of the vertebral bodies are responsible for this axis shift laterally, which leads to a loss of lordosis and rotation laterally. ▸ Fig. 27.1 demonstrates how displacement of a vertebral segment to this new "off axis and dorsal" ▸ Fig. 27.1(**a, b**) position results in a rotatory deformity ▸ Fig. 27.1(**c, d**). Rotatory degenerative kyphoscoliosis is a manifestation of the coupling phenomenon in which a deformation in one Cartesian axis causes motion about another axis. A scoliotic lumbar deformity causes a shift of the weight-bearing axis of the spine (neutral axis) toward the concave facet joints, which are excessively loaded along the new neutral axis (*shaded region*). This creates a new axis that is off the midline axis (off axis), which causes the rotated lumbar vertebral bodies to move (**b**) dorsally and (**c**) laterally while rotation occurs. The result is a straightening of the spine in a lateral view (loss of lumbar lordosis; **b**). (**d**) This complex deformation is akin to the swinging of a bucket handle. Note that the bucket handle grip (analogous to an apical vertebra) rotates with the handle from the down (normal lordosis) position to the scoliotic (lateral) position.

▸▸ Answer 2

Correct answer is D

The load-bearing axis of the spine is generally considered to be centered in the middle column of Denis. In flexion, this axis is shifted ventrally and in extension dorsally, and is ipsilateral toward the direction of lateral bending.

▸▸ Answer 3

Correct answer is B

A spine in appropriate physiologic sagittal alignment should have a plumb line that is dropped from

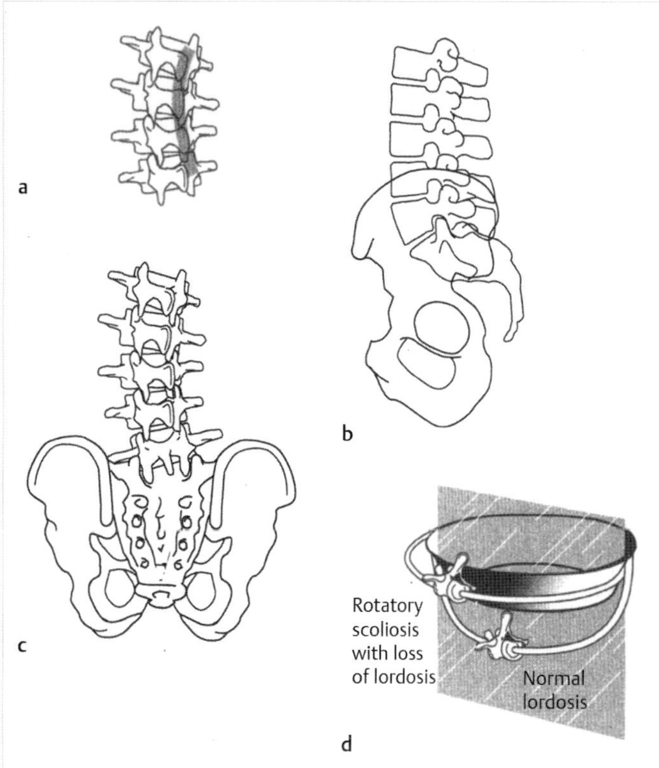

Fig. 27.1 (a) A scoliotic lumbar deformity causes a shift of the weight-bearing axis of the spine (neutral axis) toward the concave facet joints, which are excessively loaded along the new neutral axis (*shaded region*). This creates a new axis that is off the midline axis (off axis), which causes the rotated lumbar vertebral bodies to move **(b)** dorsally and **(c)** laterally while rotation occurs. The result is a straightening of the spine in a lateral view (loss of lumbar lordosis; B). **(d)** This complex deformation is akin to the swinging of a bucket handle. Note that the bucket handle grip (analogous to an apical vertebra) rotates with the handle from the down (normal lordosis) position to the scoliotic (lateral) position. (Source: Biomechanics of Spine Stabilization: Third Edition, © 2015 Thieme Medical Publishers, Inc.)

the midpoint of the vertebral body in the standing position. C7 SVA should approximate the dorsal L5–S1 annulus (interspace; see ▶ Fig. 27.2a, b). Loss of lumbar lordosis (progressive kyphosis during aging) can displace the SVA anteriorly ▶ Fig. 27.2(c, d). The presence of an isthmic spondylolisthesis and/or kyphotic deformity at the lumbosacral junction can displace the SVA anteriorly. The central sacral line is used to measure imbalance in the coronal plane. The lumbosacral point is important as placing instrumentation ventral and caudal to this point allows for maximal resistance against angular deformation and lumbosacral pseudarthrosis.[1]

▸▸ Answer 4

Correct answer is C

Ideally, a fusion construct should extend to a stable vertebral level, defined as a vertebral level rostral or caudal to the scoliotic curve that is most closely bisected by the central sacral line. The neutral level is the vertebrae defined as having the smallest segmental angulation at its rostral and caudal disc spaces and is located above or below the scoliotic curve. The apical and neutral vertebral levels should be defined in both the coronal and sagittal planes.

▸▸ Answer 5

Correct answer is E

Answer D is the definition of pelvic obliquity. Answer C is the definition of pelvic inclination. Answer B is the definition of pelvic axial rotation. Answer A defines sacral inclination.

▸▸ Answer 6

Correct answer is B

Advancing age is often associated with increased spinal kyphosis. The loss of lumbar lordosis is the most common manifestation of this problem. As we age, sagittal balance is disrupted and shifted anterior (i.e., positive sagittal imbalance); as a result, disability increases and quality of life decreases.[2,3] Correction of sagittal imbalance with pedicle subtraction

and horizontal gaze. The rest are indeed goals of spinal reconstructive surgery.

▸▸ Answer 20

Correct answer is E

When offering a patient surgery (of any variety), a surgeon must take into consideration the clinical presentation, social circumstances, medical comorbidities, and the patient's ability to tolerate a large operation. In many cases, these variables must be managed, modified, or "prehabilitated" to allow a patient to become a surgical candidate. These variables also must be discussed in detail and in the presence of the patient for informed consent. Deformities often have components in multiple planes, and scoliosis, specifically, always involves rotation in the axial plane. The length of instrumentation should be long enough to apply the appropriate bending moment but not long enough to create an excessive rigid lever arm at the junction with the uninstrumented vertebrae. Distraction and compression on their respective concavity or convexity are appropriate throughout the spine for deformity correction in the coronal plane.

Key Principles

- Global alignment should be considered prior to any spinal procedure.
- Spinal deformities often have components in multiple planes.
- Spinal deformity begets deformity.

References

[1] McCord DH, Cunningham BW, Shono Y, Myers JJ, McAfee PC. Biomechanical analysis of lumbosacral fixation. Spine (Phila Pa 1976) 1992;17(8 Suppl):S235–S243

[2] Glassman SD, Bridwell K, Dimar JR, Horton W, Berven S, Schwab F. The impact of positive sagittal balance in adult spinal deformity. Spine (Phila Pa 1976) 2005;30(18):2024–2029

[3] Glassman SD, Berven S, Bridwell K, Horton W, Dimar JR. Correlation of radiographic parameters and clinical symptoms in adult scoliosis. Spine (Phila Pa 1976) 2005;30(6):682–688

[4] Smith JS, Shaffrey CI, Lafage V, et al.; International Spine Study Group. Spontaneous improvement of cervical alignment after correction of global sagittal balance following pedicle subtraction osteotomy. J Neurosurg Spine 2012;17(4):300–307

[5] D'Andrea LP, Bets RR, Lenke LG, et al. Do radiographic parameters correlate with clinical outcomes in adolescent idiopathic scoliosis? Spine 2000;25:1795–1802

[6] Aebi M. The adult scoliosis. Eur Spine J 2005;14(10):925–948

[7] Pritchett JW, Bortel DT. Degenerative symptomatic lumbar scoliosis. Spine 1993;18(6):700-3.

28 Complex Instrumentation Constructs and Force Applications

Shawn W. Adams, Brett Rocos

The healthy spine allows for complex movements and supports complex loading. Successful, durable instrumentation of the spine must account for multiple and complex force applications. It is easy to be caught in the trap of thinking about the main force resisting potential of implants, but the demands of life are not simple, and we must be aware that implants function differently under different loading conditions. This chapter covers the complex nature of instrumented fixation of the normally mobile spine. Due to the variations in regional anatomy, different techniques and considerations are required throughout the spine.

Learning Objectives

- Regional anatomic morphological, functional, and pathological differences as well as unique instrumentation techniques for each region:
  - Craniocervical region.
  - High cervical region.
  - Subaxial cervical region.
  - Thoracic and lumbar regions.
  - Low lumbar and lumbosacral regions.
- Application of the biomechanical principles to complex construct design.
- Identification and prevention of construct failures.

Questions

▸▸ Question 1

Regarding cable–rod occipitocervical fixation construct, what is a possible complication related specifically to the technique?

- A. Cerebrospinal fluid leak
- B. Malalignment
- C. Neurologic injury
- D. Rod fracture
- E. Wire or cable cut-through

▸▸ Question 2

Fixation across the occiput–C1 segment should be designed in such a way to be biomechanically advantageous to resist which movement?

- A. Compression
- B. Distraction
- C. Flexion/extension
- D. Lateral bending
- E. Rotation

▸▸ Question 3

The C1–C2 joint has a primary rotation functional movement. What is a secondary function of this joint complex?

- A. Axial rotation
- B. Circumduction
- C. Coronal bending
- D. Horizontal translation
- E. Sagittal flexion and extension

▸▸ Question 4

Where is the thickest bone of the occiput that is commonly utilized for occipital fixation?

- A. Around the foramen magnum
- B. Midline
- C. Overlying the venous sinus
- D. Paramedian
- E. The occipital condyles

▸▸ Question 5

Given the complex movements of the occipital cervical region, constructs should be designed to resist several different forces or movements. What has become a commonly used technique to resist rotation in fixation to the occiput?

- A. Addition of laterally placed occipital screw(s)
- B. Anterior odontoid screw(s)

- C. Full-thickness midline screw(s)
- D. Midline fixation without occipital plate to reduce soft tissue dissection
- E. Multiple midline screws

▸▸ Question 6

A weakness of all C1–C2 fixation by wires or cables with or without interposed graft techniques is resisting which deformation?

- A. Coronal bending
- B. Extension
- C. Flexion
- D. Rotational
- E. Sagittal translation

▸▸ Question 7

In a three-point bending screw technique, the forces resisted are primarily oriented in which manner?

- A. Compression
- B. Distraction
- C. Parallel to the screw
- D. Perpendicular to the screw
- E. Perpendicular to the longitudinal member

▸▸ Question 8

The strength, *Z*, of a noncannulated screw is related to its inner diameter, *D*, in which way?

- A. Linearly, as D increases, Z increases equally
- B. Geometrically, proportional to two times the inner diameter
- C. Geometrically, proportional to three times the inner diameter
- D. Exponentially, proportional to the square of the inner diameter
- E. Exponentially, proportional to the cube of the inner diameter

▸▸ Question 9

The subaxial spine is defined as the entire spine below what?

- A. Occiput
- B. C1
- C. C2
- D. C3
- E. C7

▸▸ Question 10

▸ Fig. 28.1 shows a C1–C2 transarticular screw fixation technique and the *arrows* represent the forces resisted. What biomechanical technique does this represent?

- A. Cantilever beam fixation
- B. Dorsal distraction fixation
- C. Multisegmental fixation
- D. Tension-band fixation
- E. Three-point bending screw fixation

▸▸ Question 11

A long ventral implant for multilevel cervical corpectomy, as pictured in ▸ Fig. 28.2, has a weakness that may lead to failure in resisting which deformation?

- A. Compression
- B. Distraction
- C. Extension
- D. Flexion
- E. Translation

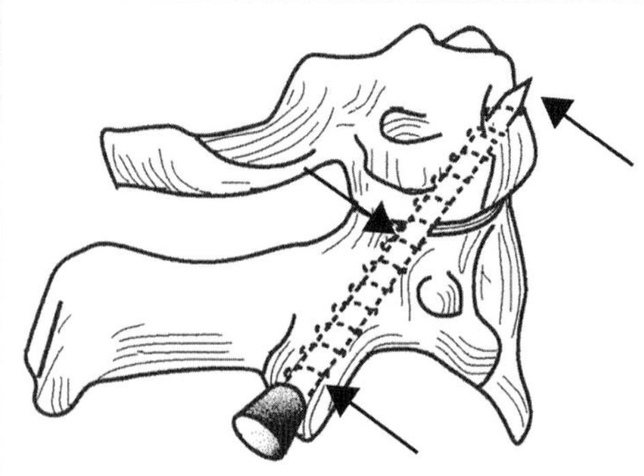

Fig. 28.1 Three-point bending screw technique with the use of C1–C2 transarticular screw fixation. Arrows indicate typical forces (loads) applied or resisted by the implant (three-point bending). (Source: Biomechanics of Spine Stabilization: Third Edition, © 2015 Thieme Medical Publishers, Inc.)

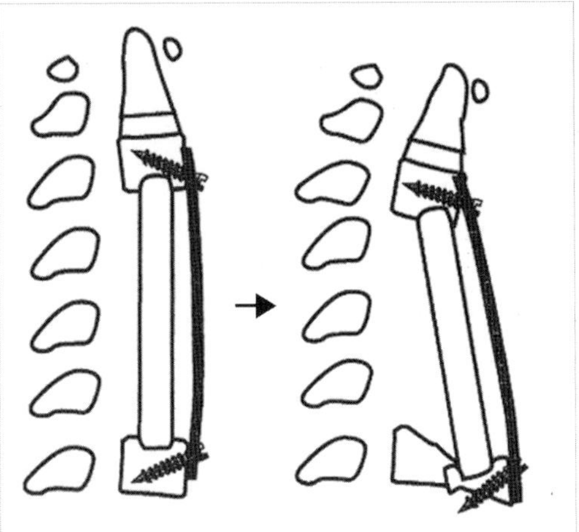

Fig. 28.2 Mechanisms of ventral cervical implant failure. Subsidence-related kickout. (Source: Biomechanics of Spine Stabilization: Third Edition, © 2015 Thieme Medical Publishers, Inc.)

▸▸ Question 12

Cross fixators can be utilized to augment a construct for various purposes. Cross fixators can significantly alter attributes of a construct in which way?

- A. Increase axial load bearing
- B. Increase three-point bending forces
- C. Increase pullout resistance of triangulated pedicle screws
- D. Decreased torsional stiffness
- E. Decreased stress shielding

▸▸ Question 13

In general, to maximize implant–bone interface for sacral screws, the screws should be oriented in which fashion from the S1 start point?

- A. Ventral and parallel to the sacroiliac joint
- B. Ventrolateral
- C. Ventromedial
- D. Ventrocaudal
- E. Ventral with minimal medial/lateral angulation

▸▸ Question 14

The lumbosacral pivot point has been described by McCord. Optimal biomechanical stabilization regarding flexion/extension about this point, iliac, and/or sacral fixation should have what orientation with respect to this point?

- A. Caudal
- B. Caudal with multipoints of fixation
- C. Caudal and dorsal
- D. Caudal and ventral
- E. Screws should pass through it

▸▸ Question 15

The interference screw fixation technique can be used to do what?

- A. Improve pedicle screw pullout resistance
- B. Enhance screw triangulation
- C. Increase shear strength of a screw
- D. Enhance bone graft security
- E. Provide a fulcrum for three-point bending

▸▸ Question 16

Which of the following is an example of interference screw fixation?

- A. Threaded interbody fusion cage
- B. C1–C2 transarticular screw
- C. Translaminar facet fixation
- D. Combining ventral and dorsal screw fixation
- E. Dorsal transsacral fixation

▸▸ Question 17

The depicted occipitocervical fixation construct functionally resists which force (see ▸ Fig. 28.3)?

- A. Axial loading
- B. Coronal bending
- C. Flexion
- D. Rotation
- E. Depends on the loading conditions

▸▸ Question 18

A multilevel cervical corpectomy with interbody graft and anterior plate may be susceptible to repeated deformations leading to nonunion and instrumentation failure. Which technique would be most helpful to resist translational deformation (see ▸ Fig. 28.4)?

- A. Larger diameter screws for plate fixation

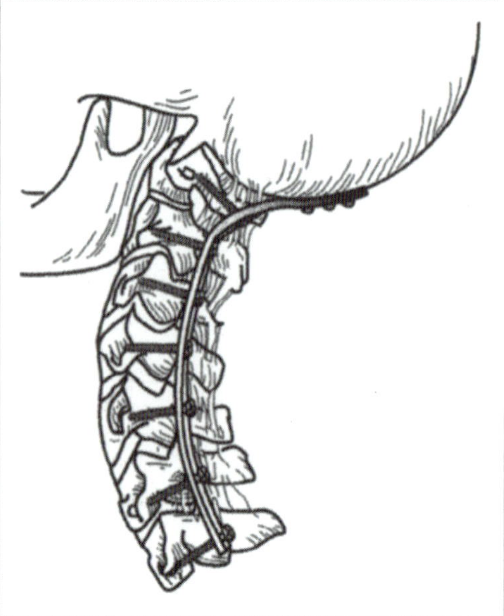

Fig. 28.3 The subaxial component of an occipitocervical screw–plate technique may fail. (Source: Biomechanics of Spine Stabilization: Third Edition, © 2015 Thieme Medical Publishers, Inc.)

- B. Intermediate fixation
- C. Thicker plate
- D. Use of a dynamic plate
- E. Use of a nonfixed moment arm construct

▸▸ Question 19

In occiput to subaxial cervical fixation, one of the complex forces that should be considered and ideally stabilized is rotary deformation. Which of the following is *not* a technique that would resist rotatory deformation at C1–C2?

- A. Ventral C2 (dens) screw
- B. C1–C2 transarticular screws
- C. C1–C2 wire or cable fixation
- D. C1–C2 pars/pedicle screw fixation to rod
- E. Halo orthosis fixation

▸▸ Question 20

Fixed moment arm cantilever beam constructs, especially in the thoracolumbar spine, are placed such that repetitive loading may lead to instrumentation failure. A modification to limit screw fracture could be which of the following, when possible?

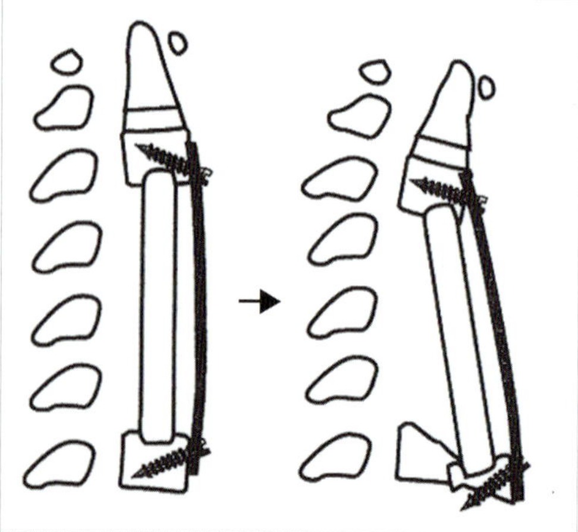

Fig. 28.4 Mechanisms of ventral cervical implant failure. Subsidence-related kickout. (Source: Biomechanics of Spine Stabilization: Third Edition, © 2015 Thieme Medical Publishers, Inc.)

- A. Cannulated screws
- B. Increased screw diameter
- C. Increased screw thread depth (with constant major diameter)
- D. Lengthen construct
- E. Longer screws

Answers

▸▸ Answer 1

Correct answer is E

In cable–rod occipitocervical fixation construct, some motion occurs at the metal–bone interface. Wire or cable cut-through can be problematic with this technique.

▸▸ Answer 2

Correct answer is C

At the occiput–C1 segment, flexion occurs with very little rotation or lateral bending.

▸▸ Answer 3

Correct answer is E

C1–C2 joint functions primarily in rotation and secondarily in flexion and extension (see ▸ Fig. 28.5).

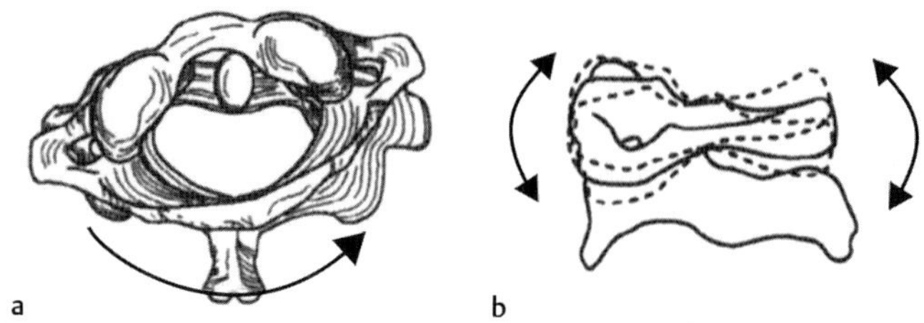

Fig. 28.5 (a) the C1–C2 joint functions predominantly in rotation and (b) secondarily in flexion and extension. (Source: Biomechanics of Spine Stabilization: Third Edition, © 2015 Thieme Medical Publishers, Inc.)

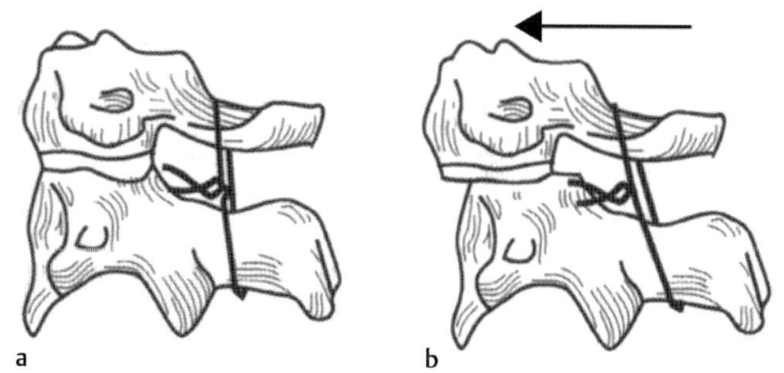

Fig. 28.6 Dorsal upper cervical wire fixation techniques may inadequately resist parallelogram-type sagittal plane deformation. This is particularly so if the facet joints are incompetent or axially oriented. (a,b) The latter is the case at C1–C2. (Source: Biomechanics of Spine Stabilization: Third Edition, © 2015 Thieme Medical Publishers, Inc.)

▸▸ Answer 4

Correct answer is B

The occiput provides several options for implant fixation. However, the depth of bone to which screws can be anchored is short, except in the midline.

▸▸ Answer 5

Correct answer is A

Laterally placed occipital screws may be used to minimize the rotatory tendency. A plate that is fixed to the occiput by midline (and lateral) screws and that securely abuts the occipital bone laterally on both sides perhaps provides the optimal occipital bone fixation and minimizes the rotational instability associated with motion about the long axis of the spine.

▸▸ Answer 6

Correct answer is E

The Gallie, Brooks, and combination techniques have been used for C1–C2 fusions for decades. All (especially the Gallie technique) minimally resist sagittal plane translation deformation. This deformation occurs in a parallelogram-like manner. Because the C1–C2 facet joints are axially oriented with respect to each other in the sagittal plane, they minimally contribute to parallelogram deformation resistance (see ▸ Fig. 28.6).

▸▸ Answer 7

Correct answer is D

It is emphasized that these implants are usually placed in a neutral mode at the time of surgery. However, they are required to resist three-point bending forces during the activities of daily living. These forces are oriented perpendicular to the long axis of the screw.

▸▸ Answer 8

Correct answer is E

The strength of a screw, and its ability to resist fracture, is proportional to the cube of its inner diameter, D^3.

▸▸ Answer 9

Correct answer is C

The subaxial spine is defined as the entire spine below the axis (C2).

all regions of the spine considering the inherent anatomical demands and any changes due to various pathologies.

- The occipital bone is thickest in the midline keel, but the addition of lateral fixation, especially with a plate, greatly increases rotational stability.
- Approximately 50% of cervical flexion occurs at the occipital–C1 joint.
- Approximately 50% of cervical rotation occurs at the C1–C2 joint.
- Intermediate fixation can be considered in long cervical corpectomies to add translational stability and potentially reduce the need for additional posterior fixation.
- C1–C2 wiring techniques provide good tension band but lack translational stability.
- The addition of an interposed graft to C1–C2 wiring increases stability by resisting extension and provides substrate for arthrodesis.
- The three-point bending screw technique can be used to cross a joint or a fracture. The forces on the screw are sheer and oriented perpendicular to its long axis.
- Screw strength is related to inner diameter to the third power. Cannulated screws are weaker than solid screws.
- Thoracic and lumbar constructs, in general, have to be able to resist higher axial loading forces.
- Instrumentation spanning the lumbosacral joints should extend caudal and ventral to the lumbosacral pivot point for optimal stabilization of flexion and extension at this level.
- S1 screws should be directed toward and into the sacral promontory.
- Interference screws and wiring have been used to enhance bone graft security.
- Tripod geometry of implants for sacropelvic fixation provides improved implant–bone interface security.

Part VII

Iatrogenic Pathologies and New Spine Surgery Techniques and Technologies

VII

29 Subsidence and Dynamic Spine Stabilization

Benjamin Motley, Owoicho Adogwa, Juan C. Mejia, Joseph Cheng

Life is a kyphosing event. The spine deforms with age due to loads placed while weight bearing. The spine also deforms around implants used during surgery. The spine is a dynamic structure and many of the implants utilized during spine surgery allow for controlled movement. Understanding subsidence, dynamic stabilization, and the dynamic implants at your disposal are essential to achieving a satisfactory outcome.

Learning Objectives

- Understand the processes leading to subsidence and steps taken to combat these processes.
- Understand dynamism and its relationship with subsidence.
- Understand Wolff's law and its relationship to subsidence and dynamism.
- Understand the different types of implants used to achieve dynamic stabilization.
- Understand mechanisms of construct failure and implant fracture.
- Understand negative effects of stress shielding.

Questions

▸▸ Question 1

Subsidence is an important concept to understand when choosing spinal implants. Which of the following is the most likely to reduce subsidence in a spinal construct?

- A. System that allows for toggling of screws
- B. Slotted/collapsible anterior cervical plating system
- C. Use of a fixed moment arm cantilever beam screw and plate system
- D. Use of tension band fixation devices
- E. Increasing axial load on system

▸▸ Question 2

Spine surgeons have known for years that interbody fusions can be complicated by "pistoning" of the interbody graft into the vertebral body, contributing to kyphosis. Which of the following would reduce the likelihood of developing cervical kyphosis?

- A. Use of allograft rather than autograft for interbody fusion
- B. Decreasing the end plate–graft contact area
- C. Performing cervical corpectomy rather than interbody fusion
- D. Decreasing the vertebral body bone density
- E. Increasing footprint of an interbody graft

▸▸ Question 3

Wolff's law is an important principle of spinal biomechanics. Which of the following best characterizes Wolff's law as applied to the ventral spine?

- A. Bone heals optimally with distracting loads
- B. Bone heals optimally when immobilized
- C. Bone heals optimally with compressive loads
- D. Bone heals optimally when non–weight bearing
- E. Bone heals optimally with dynamic stabilization

▸▸ Question 4

The term "dynamism" refers to an implant that allows the spine to deform. Dynamism can be achieved via two fundamental mechanisms: (1) the use of absorbable implants or (2) the use of implants that themselves deform. Which of the following is false regarding dynamic implants?

- A. Absorbable implants permit early deformation within a few days of placement
- B. Deformable implants allow spine deformation immediately
- C. Absorbable implants allow deformity only after the integrity of the implant is lost
- D. Deformable implants allow either angular deformation, axial deformation, or both
- E. A collapsible cervical plate is an example of a deformable implant

▸▸ **Answer 10**

Correct answer is B

Use of the margin of the vertebral body takes advantage of the "boundary effect" where there is an enhanced ability to support axial loads by the apophyseal ring as compared with the softer cancellous bone of the inner body.

▸▸ **Answer 11**

Correct answer is A

Thoracic and lumbar dynamic implants, although not as commonly employed as in the cervical spine, have nevertheless found utility. In the thoracic and lumbar spine, the loads are greater and the advantages of dynamic implants are less than in the cervical spine. Therefore, the risk–benefit ratio for the use of dynamic implants in the thoracic and lumbar spine is not optimal.[6]

▸▸ **Answer 12**

Correct answer is D

Failure to permit subsidence in cervical implants can cause construct failure due to (1) kick-out of the construct (implant, vertebrae, graft), (2) failure of the implant (screw fracture or plate fracture), or (3) failure of the implant to permit bone–graft vertebral junction to see adequate compression, resulting in stress reduction osteoporosis or nonunion (stress shielding).

▸▸ **Answer 13**

Correct answer is D

Failure of implant–bone and interbody strut–vertebral body interface failure has led some surgeons to adopt a philosophy of dorsal multisegmental instrumentation in addition to ventral fusion in order to resist translational and rotational stresses by using a three-point bending mechanism of fixation and stabilization.

▸▸ **Answer 14**

Correct answer is A

Subsidence is obligatory to one degree or another, even in the setting of rigid fixation. Subsidence can proceed to the point where an implant can no longer resist it, resulting in either construct or implant failure.

▸▸ **Answer 15**

Correct answer is D

Stress shielding is defined as "an implant-induced reduction of bone healing–enhancing stresses and loads applied to the spine to such a degree that stress reduction osteoporosis, or nonunion, may result." Bone heals best under compression via the bone healing–enhancing forces according to Wolff's law. Doh and colleagues evaluated four ventral cervical strategies: (1) strut graft plus halo, (2) ventral cervical plate plus strut graft, (3) ventral strut graft plus dorsal instrumentation and fusion, and (4) ventral strut graft plus kick plate. They observed lowest pseudarthrosis rates in the ventral strut graft and dorsal instrumentation techniques. Of note, uninstrumented fusion in this series was very efficacious, a finding that has been observed by others. Addition of dorsal instrumentation has been seen to prevent excessive settling and promote fusion. Kick plates can also allow for graft subsidence but have the negative features of possible angular deformation with risks of catastrophic graft kick-out.

▸▸ **Answer 16**

Correct answer is D

Good carpentry is very important for optimization of outcomes in spine surgery. The three factors that most affect the incidence and extent of subsidence in this regard are (1) the closeness of fit of the bone graft in the vertebral body mortise, (2) the surface area of contact between the bone graft and vertebral body, and (3) the character or quality of the contact surfaces.

Failure to optimize closeness fit, or fit a round peg in a square hole, will lead to either (1) nonunion due to inadequate surface area contact or (2) excessive subsidence caused by concentration of stresses and loads at the points of contact, leading to excessive subsidence and degradation of the end plate contact (A).

Surface area of contact is inversely proportional to the extent of subsidence. Larger the surface area of contact, the less the subsidence (B).

Quality of contact surfaces is primarily related to (1) extent of preservation of the end plate of the vertebral body and (2) proximity of the point of contact to the edge of the vertebral body. Use of the margin of the vertebral body takes advantage of the "boundary effect" (C) where there is an

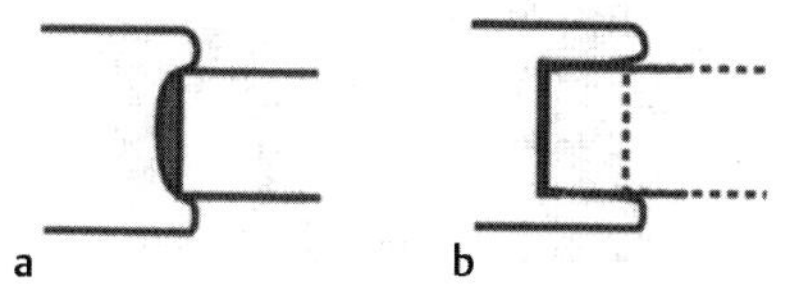

Fig. 29.2 **(a)** A bone graft with a square end (flat) does not "fit well" into a rounded vertebral body mortise. Nonunion may occur as a result of an inadequate surface area of contact (*shaded area*). **(b)** Alternatively, excessive subsidence, which may not be desirable, may occur because of the inability of the vertebral body mortise to prevent "penetration" by the ill-fitted strut graft. **(c)** Maximizing the surface area of contact and the closeness of fit between the bone graft and the vertebral body minimizes the concentration of stress and the chance of nonunion or excessive subsidence. (Source: Biomechanics of Spine Stabilization: Third Edition, © 2015 Thieme Medical Publishers, Inc.)

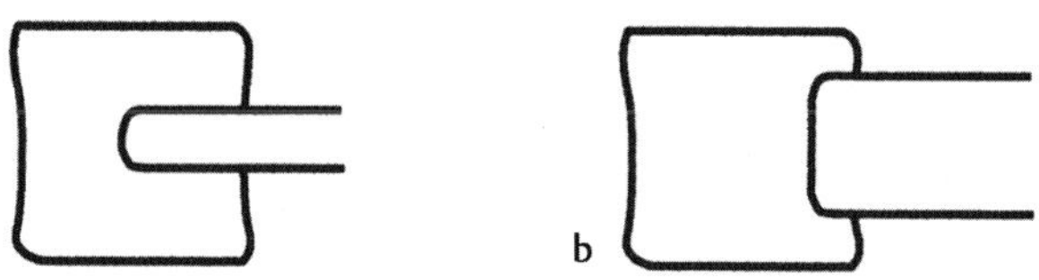

Fig. 29.3 The surface area of contact between the bone graft and the accepting bone (vertebral body mortise) is inversely proportional to the extent of penetration (subsidence) of the bone graft. **(a)** A smaller surface area of contact resists penetration less well than **(b)** a larger surface area of contact. (Source: Biomechanics of Spine Stabilization: Third Edition, © 2015 Thieme Medical Publishers, Inc.)

enhanced ability to support axial loads by the apophyseal ring as compared with the softer cancellous bone of the inner body. Sculpting the bone graft and end plate region to optimize fit should reduce subsidence (see ▶ Fig. 29.2, ▶ Fig. 29.3, ▶ Fig. 29.4).

▸▸ Answer 17

Correct answer is C

Doh and colleagues evaluated their clinical experience with four ventral cervical strategies. The authors observed that pseudarthrosis rates for ventral strut graft plus halo, ventral cervical plate plus strut graft, ventral strut graft plus dorsal instrumentation and fusion, and ventral strut graft plus kick plate were 20%, 40%, 0%, and 7%, respectively.[7]

▸▸ Answer 18

Correct answer is B

While subsidence is common in the thoracic and lumbar spine, dynamic implants have not been as commonly employed due to greater loads in the thoracic and lumbar spine leading to a less favorable risk–benefit ratio.

▸▸ Answer 19

Correct answer is C

Rigid implants have been routinely employed in the cervical spine. Although rigidity is often desirable, it is, in and of itself, a potential cause of construct failure. The failure to permit subsidence with the use of cervical implants can in fact result in three mechanisms of construct failure: (1) the construct (implant, vertebrae, and graft) may fail (e.g., kick-out); (2) the implant itself may fail (e.g., via screw fracture or plate fracture); and (3) failure of the implant to permit the bone graft–vertebral body junction to "see" adequate compression (bone healing–enhancing forces) results in nonunion. Variable-angle screw toggling is a form of dynamic instrumentation and not an example of construct failure.

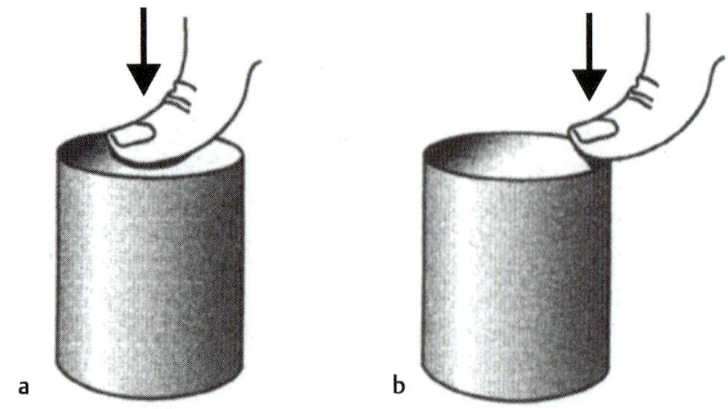

Fig. 29.4 A depiction of the "boundary effect." **(a)** When a thumb applies force to the center of the end of a tin can, the extent of depression is greater than **(b)** when the thumb applies a similar force to the edge of the can. This is analogous to applying a force to the center of an end plate as opposed to the vertebral body–end plate region along the vertebral body cortex wall. The integrity of the vertebral body, regarding its ability to bear axial loads, is relatively increased at the edge of the vertebral body. This phenomenon is known as the "boundary effect." The cortical margin along the ventral surface of the vertebral body is a very effective buttress where the "boundary effect" can be used to a clinical advantage (Source: Biomechanics of Spine Stabilization: Third Edition, © 2015 Thieme Medical Publishers, Inc.)

Key Principles

- Subsidence is a natural part of the aging process.
- Multiple surgical techniques and implants have been designed to prevent excess subsidence and progressive kyphosis in the cervical spine.
- Bone has piezoelectric properties. Wolff's law states that bone heals optimally with compressive loads.
- Dynamic implants allow for acceptable spinal deformation while preventing undesirable spinal deformation.
- Although rigidity is often desirable in a construct, failure to allow for subsidence can result in construct failure, graft failure, or nonunion.
- Appropriate fitting of bone components is key for the optimization of outcomes.

References

[1] Hughes SS, Pringle T, Phillips FM, Bohlman H, Emery SE. Multilevel cervical corpectomy and fibular strut grafting. Paper presented at: 23rd Annual Meeting of the Cervical Spine Research Society; Santa Fe, NM; November 29–December 2, 1995.

[2] Bishop RC, Moore KA, Hadley MN. Anterior cervical interbody fusion using autogeneic and allogeneic bone graft substrate: a prospective comparative analysis. J Neurosurg 1996;85:206–210

[3] Yasuda I, Noguchi K, Sata T. Dynamic callus and electric callus J Bone Joint Surg 1955;37A:1292–1293

[4] Steinmetz MP, Warbel A, Whitfield M, Bingaman W. Preliminary experience with the DOC dynamic cervical implant for the treatment of multilevel cervical spondylosis. J Neurosurg 2002;97(Suppl):330–336

[5] Bose B. Anterior cervical arthrodesis using DOC dynamic stabilization implant for improvement in sagittal angulation and controlled settling. J Neurosurg 2003;98(Suppl):8–13

[6] Mageswaran P, Techy F, Colbrunn RW, Bonner TF, McLain RF. Hybrid dynamic stabilization: a biomechanical assessment of adjacent and supraadjacent levels of the lumbar spine. J Neurosurg Spine 2012;17:232–242

[7] Doh ES, Heller JG. Multi-level anterior cervical reconstructions: comparison of surgical techniques and results. Paper No. 5 presented at: 26th Annual Meeting of the Cervical Spine Research Society; Atlanta, GA; December 3–5,1998:28–29

30 Vertebral Augmentation

Shawn W. Adams

Vertebral augmentation has been employed by a variety of different techniques for multiple different indications with several different biomaterials. This variety combined with varying research methodologies has made it difficult to develop strong evidence regarding application, technique, indications, and outcomes. It is therefore imperative to understand the biomechanics involved, as it is important to provide a knowledge base from which to critically review the, at times, conflicting reports of efficacy.

Learning Objectives

- Understand the basic biomechanics of vertebroplasty and kyphoplasty.
- Consider the regional effects on adjacent levels.
- Review the biomaterials used and understand how they compare to bone and each other.

Questions

▸▸ Question 1

Buchbinder et al performed a multicenter, randomized, double-blinded, placebo-controlled trial of vertebroplasty for painful osteoporotic vertebral fractures. They found ________.

- A. No beneficial effect of vertebroplasty compared with placebo control
- B. Clinically significant pain reduction in the vertebroplasty group
- C. A high complication rate associated with the procedure versus placebo
- D. Clinically significant outcomes in the kyphoplasty group
- E. Equal pain outcomes but increased ambulation in the vertebroplasty group

▸▸ Question 2

Choose the name of the described procedure: stand-alone vertebral body filler techniques.

- A. Cranioplasty
- B. Foraminoplasty
- C. Kyphoplasty
- D. Laminoplasty
- E. Vertebroplasty

▸▸ Question 3

Choose the name of the described procedure: vertebral body expansion and filler techniques.

- A. Cranioplasty
- B. Foraminoplasty
- C. Kyphoplasty
- D. Laminoplasty
- E. Vertebroplasty

▸▸ Question 4

Which of the following statements is suggested by the literature?

- A. Vertebroplasty is superior to kyphoplasty in deformity correction
- B. Kyphoplasty is superior to vertebroplasty for pain outcomes
- C. Vertebral augmentation is an experimental technique with theoretical benefit but is untested
- D. The evidence regarding vertebral augmentation strategies as a treatment for vertebral compression fractures is not strong, but it does support their use
- E. The evidence regarding vertebral augmentation strategies as a treatment for vertebral compression fractures is strong and considered to be a "gold standard" treatment if not otherwise contraindicated

▸▸ Question 5

Which condition could be considered a relative contraindication for vertebral augmentation with injectable cement?

- A. Ventral wedge compression
- B. Lateral wedge compression
- C. Burst fractures
- D. Pathologic fractures
- E. Osteoporotic fractures

▸▸ **Question 6**

Which setting would be most liable for decreased success in correcting a fracture-related deformity by kyphoplasty techniques?

- A. Acute fracture (days)
- B. Subacute fracture (weeks)
- C. Chronic fracture (months)
- D. Multiple fractures
- E. Osteoporosis

▸▸ **Question 7**

Adjacent-level fractures following vertebral augmentation procedures are ________.

- A. Related to overcorrection of deformity
- B. Related to higher than recommended injectate volumes
- C. Quite rare
- D. Related to which injectate material was used
- E. Relatively common

▸▸ **Question 8**

For which tumor histology is vertebral augmentation most often performed?

- A. Aneurysmal bone cyst
- B. Breast
- C. Lung
- D. Multiple myeloma
- E. Prostate

▸▸ **Question 9**

Which substance is commonly used to increase the radiopacity of the injectate material in vertebral augmentation?

- A. Barium sulfate
- B. Cobalt chromium
- C. Titanium oxide
- D. Onyx
- E. Colloidal silver

▸▸ **Question 10**

Which category of bone "cement" does PMMA belong to?

- A. Calcium phosphate cements
- B. Acrylic cements
- C. Calcium sulfate cements
- D. Composite cements
- E. Biocompliant injectates

▸▸ **Question 11**

What is the most commonly used bone "cement" for vertebral augmentation?

- A. Biocompliant injectates
- B. Calcium phosphate cements
- C. Calcium sulfate cements
- D. Composite cements
- E. PMMA

▸▸ **Question 12**

Compared with cancellous bone, PMMA bone cement ________.

- A. Has a lower modulus of elasticity
- B. Has an equivalent stress/strain profile
- C. Has an equivalent modulus of elasticity
- D. Has less stiffness
- E. Has a higher modulus of elasticity

▸▸ **Question 13**

Which of the following is *not* a factor believed to be related to the development of adjacent-level fractures following vertebral augmentation?

- A. Natural progression of osteoporosis
- B. Increased kyphosis causing load amplification
- C. Increased stiffness of the treated segment transmitting more force to the adjacent segment(s)
- D. Acceleration of osteoporosis due to injection of nonbiocompatible materials
- E. The patient and their bone are susceptible because of structural and load-bearing characteristics.

▸▸ **Question 14**

When considering properties of injectable bone cement, high ________ would be less desirable due to possibility of complication when used for vertebral augmentation of osteoporotic fractures.

- A. Radiopacity
- B. Curing temperature
- C. Osteconductivity
- D. Osteoinductivity
- E. Biocompatibility

Answers

▸▸ Answer 1

Correct answer is A

Buchbinder et al performed a multicenter, randomized, double-blinded, placebo-controlled trial of vertebroplasty for painful osteoporotic vertebral fractures. They found no beneficial effect of vertebroplasty compared with placebo control.

▸▸ Answer 2

Correct answer is E

Vertebral augmentation procedures can be categorized into two groups: (1) stand-alone vertebral body filler techniques (i.e., vertebroplasty) and (2) vertebral body expansion and filler techniques (i.e., kyphoplasty and related techniques) (see ▸ Fig. 30.1). (**a**) Vertebroplasty involves the placement of a large-bore needle into the substance of the vertebral body. (**b**) This is followed by the injection of a semiliquid injectate under pressure. (**c**) The injection needle is then removed.

▸▸ Answer 3

Correct answer is C

Vertebral augmentation procedures can be categorized into two groups: (1) stand-alone vertebral body filler techniques (i.e., vertebroplasty) and (2) vertebral body expansion and filler techniques (i.e., kyphoplasty and related techniques) (see ▸ Fig. 30.2). (**a**) Kyphoplasty involves the placement of a large-bore needle into the substance of the vertebral body. (**b**) Then a balloon is expanded, creating a cavity in the vertebral body. (**c**) The cavity is filled with semiliquid injectate, usually under less pressure than that used in vertebroplasty. (**d**) The needle is then removed.

▸▸ Answer 4

Correct answer is D

The evidence regarding vertebral augmentation strategies as a treatment for vertebral compression fractures is not strong, but it does support their use. Again, conflicting reports do exist. Vertebroplasty would not be expected to significantly increase vertebral body height or correct deformity (e.g., kyphosis). Vertebral augmentation is not experimental, although conflicting reports on outcomes exist and it cannot be considered the "gold standard" for treatment.

▸▸ Answer 5

Correct answer is C

Of concern with all vertebral techniques is the potential for leakage of liquid acrylic into the extravertebral spaces, particularly the spinal canal. This may be most commonly expected when breaches of the dorsal vertebral cortex are present.

Burst fractures, by definition, have breaches of the dorsal vertebral cortex.

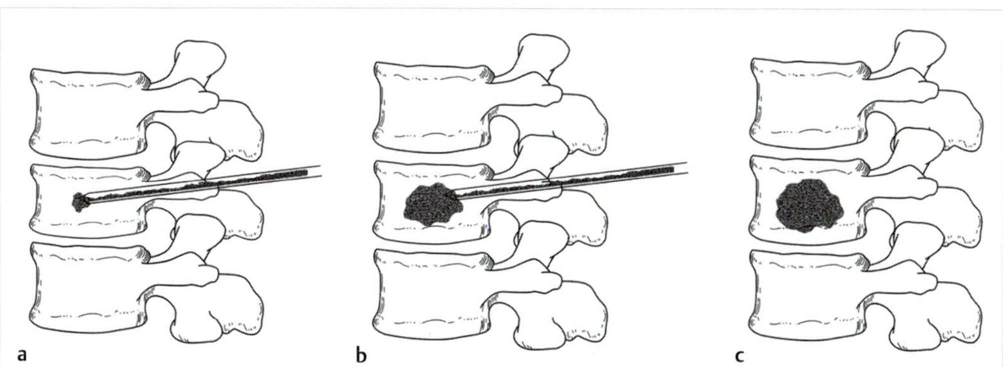

Fig. 30.1 **(a)** Vertebroplasty involves the placement of a large-bore needle into the substance of the vertebral body. **(b)** This is followed by the injection of a semiliquid injectate under pressure. **(c)** The injection needle is then removed. (Source: Biomechanics of Spine Stabilization: Third Edition, © 2015 Thieme Medical Publishers, Inc.)

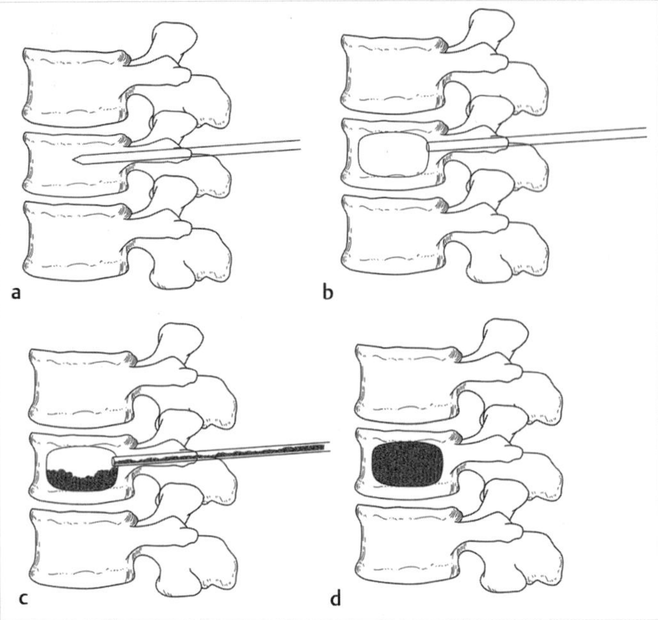

Fig. 30.2 (a) Kyphoplasty involves the placement of a large-bore needle into the substance of the vertebral body. (b) Then a balloon is expanded, creating a cavity in the vertebral body. (c) The cavity is filled with semiliquid injectate, usually under less pressure than that used in vertebroplasty. (d) The needle is then removed. (Source: Biomechanics of Spine Stabilization: Third Edition, © 2015 Thieme Medical Publishers, Inc.)

▸▸ Answer 6

Correct answer is C

The stiffness of a vertebra increases rapidly following fracture. Hence, a delay of weeks to months following fracture radically affects the chance for correcting a fracture-related deformity.

▸▸ Answer 7

Correct answer is E

Adjacent-level fractures following vertebral augmentation procedures are relatively common. This phenomenon is related to several factors. First, the patient and the patient's bone are susceptible because of structural and load-bearing characteristics. Second, if a kyphotic deformity exists, excessive stresses are applied to adjacent levels. Third, the vertebral augmentation procedure itself stiffens the treated segment and in turn causes greater forces to be applied to adjacent segments. Overcorrection of deformity is not really possible with these techniques. Adjacent-level fractures following vertebral augmentation procedures are relatively common. The link to adjacent-level fracture is multifactorial and as of yet there is no direct link to injectate volume or material.

▸▸ Answer 8

Correct answer is D

The tumor for which vertebral augmentation is most often performed is multiple myeloma, although other cancers may be amenable to such treatment.

▸▸ Answer 9

Correct answer is A

Polymethylmethacrylate (PMMA) can be manipulated by varying the amount of radiopaque material. Barium sulfate in varying proportions can be used to both opacify and alter structural characteristics. Iodine-containing compounds may also be used.

▸▸ Answer 10

Correct answer is B

PMMA is an acrylic formulation that reacts in an exothermic fashion to polymerize methylmethacrylate polymers to make PMMA.

▸▸ Answer 11

Correct answer is E

PMMA has been the mainstay injectate for vertebral augmentation procedures, in large part because the material has been approved for other orthopaedic and neurosurgical applications for years, resulting in familiarity with its characteristics. PMMA and other acrylic-based injectates polymerized by exothermic reaction and are not true cements. A true cement will harden and adhere to other surrounding material to bind them; PMMA does not bond to tissues.

▸▸ **Answer 12**

Correct answer is E

PMMA is very hard and brittle. It has a high modulus of elasticity, quite unlike that of bone. Such a mismatch fosters bone erosion and halo formation around the acrylic. PMMA and bone have quite divergent stress/strain (i.e., stiffness) profiles. It seems prudent to consider such stiffness characteristics in the decision-making process, particularly as additional materials become available clinically.

▸▸ **Answer 13**

Correct answer is D

Adjacent-level fractures following vertebral augmentation procedures is related to several factors. First, the patient and the patient's bone are susceptible because of structural and load-bearing characteristics. Second, if a kyphotic deformity exists, excessive stresses are applied to adjacent levels. Third, the vertebral augmentation procedure itself stiffens the treated segment and in turn causes greater forces to be applied to adjacent segments. Regardless, controversy also prevails in this arena, with conflicting reports refuting the aforementioned notion that stiffness augmentation transmits increased loads to adjacent segments.

▸▸ **Answer 14**

Correct answer is B

The exothermic polymerization process associated with acrylic cements can negatively impact bone and neural tissue.

Key Principles

Despite the intuitive biomechanical benefits, there is some controversy regarding multiple factors of vertebral augmentation for osteoporotic or pathologic fractures due to tumor. A few to consider:

- Optimal timing.
- Efficacy for pain control.
- Relation to adjacent segment fractures.

While this may be considered a "minimally invasive" technique from the perspective of its percutaneous application, it is not without risks. Potential complications include injuries related to inability to safely cannulate diseased pedicles, leakage of injectate causing epidural compression of neural elements or embolization of vasculature, and potential for thermal injury with materials that react exothermically.

Not all materials available for augmentation have the same properties; differences should be noted and considered when selecting.

Judicious application through careful patient selection and excellent technique is warranted.

Reference

[1] Buchbinder R, Osborne RH, Ebeling PR et al. A randomized trial of vertebroplasty for painful osteoporotic vertebral fractures. N Engl J Med 2009; 361:557–568

31 Adjacent Segment Degeneration and Disease

Nikhil Jain

There are important differences between "older" pre-total disc arthroplasty (pre-TDA) and modern literature influenced by the TDA era. Given discrepancy in literature between pre-TDA and TDA era, it appears spinal posture and sagittal balance are major factors affecting adjacent segment stresses and the risk of adjacent segment degeneration and disease.

Learning Objectives

- Understanding the difference between adjacent segment degeneration and adjacent segment disease.
- Understand the reported rate of adjacent segment disease from historical literature.
- Understand how "older" pre-TDA literature differs from modern literature of the TDA era.
- Understand change in motion and loads at same level and adjacent levels between native disc, cervical fusion, and TDA.
- Understand the influence of posture and sagittal balance on adjacent segment degeneration and adjacent segment disease.

Questions

▸▸ Question 1

There is a clear difference between adjacent segment degeneration and adjacent segment disease. Which of the following is a true statement regarding this difference?

- A. The radiographic and imaging characteristics are different
- B. Magnetic resonance imaging is highly sensitive to distinguish between them
- C. Adjacent segment degeneration is asymptomatic, whereas adjacent segment disease is symptomatic
- D. The presence of adjacent segment degeneration is typically defined on objective criteria
- E. Although different, these terms can be used interchangeably

▸▸ Question 2

The annual incidence of adjacent segment disease has been reported to vary between 1.5% and 4.5% (Hilibrand et al, Lunsford et al, and Henderson et al). What is the true statement regarding adjacent segment disease from this historical literature?

- A. Hilibrand et al observed a notable difference in incidence of adjacent segment disease after anterior cervical discectomy and fusion (ACDF) from natural unoperated history of disease
- B. Observations by Lunsford et al suggest that ventral cervical spine intervention or fusion significantly alters the adjacent segment mechanics in a clinically meaningful way
- C. Henderson et al observed a much lower incidence of adjacent segment disease than others in their study of over 800 patients undergoing posterior laminoforaminotomy, as it is a motion preservation procedure
- D. The incidence of adjacent segment disease appears to be related to factors other than fusion and it occurs independently of surgery
- E. Modern literature by Clarke et al from the TDA era corresponds to historical findings by Henderson et al

▸▸ Question 3

Hilibrand et al published a large series of 409 patients undergoing ACDF in 1999. What is the true statement based on their study?

- A. They observed a higher rate of adjacent segment disease than natural history
- B. The incidence of adjacent segment disease was less with multiple-level fusions than with single-level fusions
- C. A longer moment arm from longer fusion is associated with greater stresses at adjacent levels and hence greater incidence of adjacent segment disease after ACDF
- D. Majority of ACDFs are performed at relatively degeneration-resistant levels, resulting in adjacent

levels that are prone to degeneration and higher incidence of adjacent segment disease
- E. A longer moment arm from longer fusion supersedes the effect of sagittal alignment and restoration of normal posture in development of adjacent segment disease

▸▸ Question 4

Would you consider a "skip fusion construct" for two noncontiguous cervical disc herniations?
- A. No, the intermediate level strain results in high rate of adjacent segment degeneration
- B. No, due to longer fusion length (moment arm) at intermediate level and its relation to higher adjacent segment degeneration
- C. Yes, a study by Finn at al observed that retention of a motion segment between two noncontiguous cervical fusions resulted in less adjacent segment and intermediate segment strain
- D. Yes, two-level fusion is better than three-level fusion
- E. No, this has not been studied

▸▸ Question 5

What is the true statement regarding modern literature on adjacent segment disease from TDA studies?
- A. Initial biomechanical studies do not corroborate with early clinical studies of TDA regarding range of motion at operated and adjacent levels
- B. In a cadaveric study by Puttlitz et al, direct measurement at adjacent levels between native disc and TDA at C4–C5 was performed to conclude that motion at adjacent levels was replicated by TDA
- C. With respect to range of motion between TDA and native disc at operated and adjacent levels, DiAngelo et al found no difference and Chang et al found increased range of motion at operated level and decreased range of motion at adjacent level
- D. Dmitriev et al showed similar intradiscal pressures at rostral adjacent level on comparison of TDA and arthrodesis constructs
- E. Recent clinical literature described by Harrod et al, Nunley et al, Cho and Riew, and Boselie at al correlated with findings of cadaveric studies and found a significant difference in adjacent segment disease between fusion and TDA

▸▸ Question 6

Which is the true statement regarding adjacent-level intradiscal pressure from findings in a cadaver model comparing arthroplasty versus native versus arthrodesis constructs in cervical spine?
- A. Adjacent-level intradiscal pressures were higher in arthroplasty versus native spine
- B. Adjacent-level intradiscal pressures were lower in arthroplasty versus native spine
- C. Adjacent-level intradiscal pressures were lower in arthrodesis constructs versus native spine
- D. Adjacent-level intradiscal pressures were similar in arthroplasty versus native spine
- E. Adjacent-level intradiscal pressures were similar in arthrodesis versus native spine

▸▸ Question 7

What is the true statement regarding sagittal alignment and adjacent segment disease?
- A. Postoperative spinal malalignment is not a major contributor of motion segment stressors and degeneration
- B. Adjacent segment disease is caused by motion segment fusion alone
- C. The end-fusion alignment is not related to adjacent segment degeneration
- D. The postoperative spinopelvic parameters are independent to the risk of adjacent segment degeneration and disease
- E. Sagittal balance appears to be the major contributor to adjacent segment degeneration and disease based on observations from literature, and have cast a doubt on the previously established rationales for the effect of TDA and adjacent segment degenerative pathology

▸▸ Question 8

How are postoperative spinal alignment parameters related to adjacent segment stresses and degenerative changes?
- A. Large pelvic incidence and small lumbar lordosis are associated with lower risk

- B. Large pelvic incidence and large lumbar lordosis are associated with greater risk
- C. Pelvic incidence and lumbar lordosis are not as crucial
- D. Maintenance of lumbar lordotic angle following fusion results in similar risk as compared with kyphotic spine
- E. Large pelvic incidence and small lumbar lordosis are associated with greater risk

▸▸ Question 9

In addition to fusion of motion segment, which is the correct statement regarding risk for adjacent segment disease?

- A. Fusion alone is the major risk factor
- B. Long dorsal fusions ending at T1 are always associated with junctional destabilization
- C. Preservation of osteoligamentous integrity is protective against junctional destabilization, even in long dorsal fusions ending at T1
- D. End-fusion alignment is not as crucial
- E. Rationales for TDA hold true and are most protective against adjacent segment degenerative pathology

▸▸ Question 10

What is true regarding the effect of length of fusion on adjacent segment degenerative pathology based on published studies?

- A. Multilevel fusion in cervical spine has higher incidence than single-level fusion
- B. Multilevel fusion of levels prone to natural degeneration (i.e., C5–C6 and C6–C7) leaves degeneration-resistant levels, resulting in a lower incidence of adjacent segment disease
- C. Multilevel fusion of levels prone to natural degeneration in the lumbar spine (i.e., L4–L5 and L5–S1) leaves degeneration-resistant levels and resultant lower incidence of adjacent segment disease
- D. Length of fusion is the most important risk factor for adjacent segment disease due to longer moment arm length
- E. Minimizing length of fusion and moment arm is more important than restoration of sagittal alignment and posture

Answers

▸▸ Answer 1

Correct answer is C

The difference between adjacent segment degeneration and adjacent segment disease should be clearly delineated. The two terms are (inappropriately) occasionally used interchangeably. To be clear, adjacent segment degeneration is asymptomatic, whereas adjacent segment disease is symptomatic. This makes option C correct and option E incorrect. Despite such clinical differences, their radiographic and imaging characteristics can be identical. Therefore, option A is incorrect. Magnetic resonance imaging can be used to identify adjacent segment degeneration, but with a very high sensitivity. One should, hence, be cautious when determining the presence or absence of adjacent segment degeneration (option B is incorrect). The actual definition of the presence of adjacent segment degeneration, it is emphasized, is relatively subjective. This makes option D incorrect.

▸▸ Answer 2

Correct answer is D

The annual incidence of de novo adjacent segment disease varies from 1.5% to 4.5%.[1,2,3] In a compilation of three studies, Hilibrand et al[4] corroborated the low incidence of adjacent segment disease (1.5–4.5%) following ACDF. They, in fact, observed that the incidence of adjacent segment disease did not differ from the natural unoperated history of the "disease": "There appears to be an incidence of adjacent segment degeneration and disease after arthrodesis that may be related to natural degeneration of the adjacent fusion" (therefore, option A is incorrect). Lunsford et al[5] also observed an annual incidence of adjacent segment disease of 2.5% in a study examining ACD with and without fusion. In addition, the authors observed no difference between the incidence rates of adjacent segment disease in the fusion and no-fusion groups. This observation suggests that neither ventral cervical spine intervention nor fusion significantly alters adjacent segment mechanics to a clinically relevant extent (this makes option B incorrect). In a particularly revealing study from the 1980s, Henderson et al[6] demonstrated an annual incidence of adjacent segment

disease of 3% in more than 800 patients undergoing posterior laminoforaminotomy. Posterior laminoforaminotomy is, strictly speaking, a motion preservation procedure. To observe a consistent 3% incidence of adjacent segment disease following such a procedure strongly suggests that the incidence of adjacent segment disease is related to factors other than fusion and that it occurs independently of surgery (this makes option C incorrect and option D correct). In a somewhat controversial recent paper, Clarke et al[7] observed an annual incidence of adjacent segment disease significantly lower than that observed by Henderson et al. Their methodology was, however, challenged by McCormick. It is emphasized that the study of Clarke et al is modern and the methodology and results were influenced by the TDA era (therefore, option E is incorrect).

▸▸ Answer 3

Correct answer is B

Hilibrand et al published their large series of patients undergoing ACDF (409 patients) in 1999.[8] They observed an annual incidence of adjacent segment disease of 3% following ACDF. This, again, does not differ from the incidence associated with the natural history (this makes option A incorrect). Furthermore, they observed that the incidence of adjacent segment disease was less with multiple-level fusions than with single-level fusions (therefore, option B is correct). This counterintuitive observation truly deemphasizes and in fact negates the association between fusion and adjacent segment disease. From a biomechanical perspective, this finding is counterintuitive because of the notion that a longer fusion (and, hence, moment arm) should be associated with greater stresses at adjacent motion segments. This, in turn, should be associated with a greater incidence of adjacent segment disease—not a lesser incidence, as indeed was observed (this makes option C incorrect). The explanations for the observation by Hilibrand et al are at least twofold. First, the majority of ACDFs are performed at the levels most prone to degeneration (C5–C6 and C6–C7). Hence, a two-level ACDF most likely would involve both C5–C6 and C6–C7. This leaves only relatively degeneration-resistant levels—in which the incidence of degenerative changes following surgery, or occurring naturally, is diminished. This makes option D incorrect. Second, it is also probable that fusion length (moment arm length) is not a significant factor regarding the development of adjacent segment disease. Other factors, such as sagittal alignment and the restoration of normal posture at the index surgery level(s), may far supersede moment arm length regarding relevance (this makes option E incorrect). Others, however, have biomechanically refuted these findings.

▸▸ Answer 4

Correct answer is C

Hilibrand et al published their large series of patients undergoing ACDF (409 patients) in 1999.[9] They observed that the incidence of adjacent segment disease was less with multiple-level fusions than with single-level fusions. This counterintuitive observation truly deemphasizes and in fact negates the association between fusion and adjacent segment disease. From a biomechanical perspective, this finding is counterintuitive because of the notion that a longer fusion (and, hence, moment arm) should be associated with greater stresses at adjacent motion segments. This, in turn, should be associated with a greater incidence of adjacent segment disease—not a lesser incidence, as indeed was observed. The explanations for the observation by Hilibrand et al are at least twofold. First, the majority of ACDFs are performed at the levels most prone to degeneration (C5–C6 and C6–C7). Hence, a two-level ACDF most likely would involve both C5–C6 and C6–C7. This leaves only relatively degeneration-resistant levels—in which the incidence of degenerative changes following surgery, or occurring naturally, is diminished. Second, it is also probable that fusion length (moment arm length) is not a significant factor regarding the development of adjacent segment disease (option B is incorrect). Other factors, such as sagittal alignment and the restoration of normal posture at the index surgery level(s), may far supersede moment arm length regarding relevance. Others, however, have biomechanically refuted these findings.

To add to the fray, Finn et al observed that the retention of a motion segment between two noncontiguous cervical fusions resulted in less adjacent segment and intermediate segment strain. This "skip fusion construct" study suggests that it might be appropriate to consider noncontiguous fusions instead of three-level fusions in selected situations (therefore option C is correct and options A, D, and E are incorrect). As expected, controversy prevails.[10]

▸▸ Answer 5

Correct answer is C

Initial biomechanical studies of TDA kinematics in cadaveric models supported the hypothesis that TDA retained native range of motion at the operated and adjacent levels. This is quite unlike ACDF, which decreases range of motion at the operated level and, as a consequence, increases motion and stresses at adjacent levels. Early clinical studies also corroborated such findings.[11,12,13,14] Therefore, option A is incorrect. Puttlitz et al compared ProDisc-C (Synthes, West Chester, PA) arthroplasty with the native intervertebral disc at C4–C5 in a cadaveric model. Using a pure moment bending methodology, they observed no difference between TDA and the native disc. They concluded, without direct measurement, that motion at adjacent levels was replicated by TDA.[15] The conclusion regarding motion at adjacent levels is, however, not based on fact and may be overstated (this makes option B incorrect).

DiAngelo et al compared the Bristol cervical disc (Medtronic Sofamor Danek, Memphis, TN), which is similar to the Prestige cervical disc (Medtronic Sofamor Danek)—metal on metal; native disc; and graft with plate at C5–C6 in a cadaver model. They found no difference between arthroplasty and native disc at the operated and adjacent levels, whereas they found decreased range of motion at the operated level and increased motion at adjacent levels with graft and plate.[16] Of significant note here is the fact that they did not control for sagittal alignment at the index level(s). This is a major methodologic deficiency. Chang et al compared ProDisc-C (metal on polymer), Prestige (metal on metal), ACDF, and native disc at C6–C7 in a cadaveric model. They observed that ACDF decreased range of motion at the operated level and increased range of motion at the adjacent levels.[17] Again, the conclusion regarding motion at adjacent levels was based on a study in which there was no control for sagittal alignment at the index level(s). Chang et al also observed an increased range of motion at the operated level in the arthroplasty group compared with the native spine and a decreased range of motion at adjacent levels in the arthroplasty group (this makes option C correct). Dmitriev et al compared arthroplasty versus native versus allograft dowel versus allograft dowel and plate regarding index level range of motion in all modes and adjacent level intradiscal pressure at C5–C6 in cadaver model. They observed no differences in range of motion at the index level in a comparison of arthroplasty and native spine. Adjacent-level intradiscal pressures were unchanged in arthroplasty versus native spine, whereas these were increased at the rostral adjacent level and trended toward increased at the caudal adjacent level in the arthrodesis constructs.[18] Hence, option D is incorrect. The aforementioned data, on the surface, appear convincing. However, more recent studies and analyses provide conflicting views. Harrod et al, for example, published their systematic review of adjacent segment pathology following cervical motion-sparing procedures compared with fusion. They observed a paucity of high-quality literature in this arena. Regardless, they found no significant difference in the development of adjacent segment degeneration or disease when they compared arthroplasty and fusion.[19] Nunley et al confirmed these findings in a clinical assessment. No conclusions regarding the superiority of either management strategy could be made.[20] Cho and Riew[21] and Boselie et al[22] recently provided reviews that are in agreement with that of Harrod et al and that demonstrated no difference in adjacent segment disease between fusion and TDA. This makes option E incorrect.

▸▸ Answer 6

Correct answer is D

Dmitriev et al compared arthroplasty versus native versus allograft dowel versus allograft dowel and plate regarding index level range of motion in all modes and adjacent-level intradiscal pressure at C5–C6 in cadaver model. They observed no differences in range of motion at the index level in a comparison of arthroplasty and native spine. Adjacent-level intradiscal pressures were unchanged in arthroplasty versus native spine, whereas these were increased at the rostral adjacent level and trended toward increased at the caudal adjacent level in the arthrodesis constructs.[23] Hence, option D is correct and options A, B, C, and E are incorrect.

▸▸ Answer 7

Correct answer is E

Postoperative spinal malalignment is a major contributor to motion segment stressors, and it is perhaps the major contributor to adjacent segment degeneration and adjacent segment disease in both the cervical and lumbar spine. Hence, option A is incorrect and option E is correct. Certain postoperative spinal pelvic parameters, most notably a large pelvic incidence and a small lumbar lordotic angle, are associated with a greater risk for adjacent segment stresses and degenerative changes. Specifically, regarding the lumbar lordotic angle, the maintenance of lumbar lordosis following fusion results in a diminished incidence of adjacent segment stresses and instability, in comparison with a kyphotic spine (this makes option D incorrect). To be sure, sagittal alignment is strongly related to segmental mobility and disc degeneration. Adjacent segment disease is not caused by motion segment fusion alone (option B is incorrect). Even with long dorsal thoracic fusions ending at T1, junctional destabilization is infrequent if the ligamentous integrity of the junctional segment is preserved. Fusion plus the presence of abnormal end-fusion alignment (usually kyphosis) appears to be the major factor affecting end-fusion stresses that result in adjacent segment degeneration and adjacent segment disease (therefore, option C is incorrect). This observation and conclusion, based on the data presented in this chapter, cast further doubt on previously established rationales for TDA, at least on the basis of the effect of TDA and adjacent segment degenerative pathology (making option E correct).

▸▸ Answer 8

Correct answer is E

Certain postoperative spinal pelvic parameters, most notably a large pelvic incidence and a small lumbar lordotic angle, are associated with a greater risk for adjacent segment stresses and degenerative changes. Specifically regarding the lumbar lordotic angle, the maintenance of lumbar lordosis following fusion results in a diminished incidence of adjacent segment stresses and instability, in comparison with a kyphotic spine (this makes option E correct and options A, B, C, and D incorrect).

▸▸ Answer 9

Correct answer is C

Adjacent segment disease is not caused by motion segment fusion alone (option A is incorrect). Even with long dorsal thoracic fusions ending at T1, junctional destabilization is infrequent if the ligamentous integrity of the junctional segment is preserved (making Option B incorrect and option C correct). Fusion plus the presence of abnormal end-fusion alignment (usually kyphosis) appears to be the major factor affecting end-fusion stresses that result in adjacent segment degeneration and adjacent segment disease (therefore, option D is incorrect). This observation and conclusion, based on the data presented in this chapter, cast further doubt on previously established rationales for TDA, at least on the basis of the effect of TDA and adjacent segment degenerative pathology (making option E incorrect).

▸▸ Answer 10

Correct answer is B

Hilibrand et al published their large series of patients undergoing ACDF (409 patients) in 1999.[24] They observed that the incidence of adjacent segment disease was less with multiple-level fusions than with single-level fusions (option A is incorrect). This counterintuitive observation truly deemphasizes and in fact negates the association between fusion and adjacent segment disease. From a biomechanical perspective, this finding is counterintuitive because of the notion that a longer fusion (and, hence, moment arm) should be associated with greater stresses at adjacent motion segments. This, in turn, should be associated with a greater incidence of adjacent segment disease—not a lesser incidence, as indeed was observed. The explanations for the observation by Hilibrand et al are at least twofold. First, the majority of ACDFs are performed at the levels most prone to degeneration (C5–C6 and C6–C7). Hence, a two-level ACDF most likely would involve both C5–C6 and C6–C7. This leaves only relatively degeneration-resistant levels—in which the incidence of degenerative changes following surgery, or occurring naturally, is diminished (option B is correct). This concept has not been borne out in the lumbar spine (therefore, option C is incorrect). Second, it is also probable that fusion length (moment arm length) is not a significant factor regarding the development of adjacent segment disease (option D is incorrect). Other factors, such as sagittal alignment and the restoration of normal posture at the index surgery level(s), may far supersede moment arm length regarding relevance (making option E incorrect).

Key Principles

- Although radiographic and imaging features can be identical, the key difference is that adjacent segment degeneration is asymptomatic, whereas adjacent segment disease is symptomatic.
- The annual incidence of de novo adjacent segment disease from historical literature varies from 1.5% to 4.5%.
- Multilevel anterior cervical fusions leave relatively degeneration-resistant levels and show low incidence of adjacent segment disease as compared with single-level fusion, thereby challenging fusion length (moment arm) as the significant factor in development of adjacent segment disease.
- There are discrepancies in literature on adjacent segment disease between historical and modern TDA era literature.
- Adjacent segment disease is not caused by motion segment fusion alone, and suboptimal sagittal alignment, balance, and posture appear to be major contributors.

References

[1] Bohlman HH, Emery SE, Goodfellow DB, Jones PK. Robinson anterior cervical discectomy and arthrodesis for cervical radiculopathy. Long-term follow-up of one hundred and twenty-two patients. J Bone Joint Surg Am 1993;75:1298–1307

[2] Cauthen JC, Kinard RE, Vogler JB, et al. Outcome analysis of noninstrumented anterior cervical discectomy and interbody fusion in 348 patients. Spine 1998;23:188–192

[3] Gore DR, Sepic SB. Anterior discectomy and fusion for painful cervical disc disease. A report of 50 patients with an average follow-up of 21 years. Spine 1998;23:2047–2051

[4] Hilibrand AS, Robbins M. Adjacent segment degeneration and adjacent segment disease: the consequences of spinal fusion? Spine J 2004;4(Suppl):190S–194S

[5] Lunsford LD, Bissonette DJ, Jannetta PJ, Sheptak PE, Zorub DS. Anterior surgery for cervical disc disease. Part 1: treatment of lateral cervical disc herniation in 253 cases. J Neurosurg 1980;53:1–11

[6] Henderson CM, Hennessy RG, Shuey HM, Shackelford EG. Posterior-lateral foraminotomy as an exclusive operative technique for cervical radiculopathy: a review of 846 consecutively operated cases. Neurosurgery 1983;13:504–512

[7] Clarke MJ, Ecker RD, Krauss WE, McClelland RL, Dekutoski MB. Same-segment and adjacent-segment disease following posterior cervical foraminotomy. J Neurosurg Spine 2007;6:5–9

[8] Hilibrand AS, Carlson GD, Palumbo MA, Jones PK, Bohlman HH. Radiculopathy and myelopathy at segments adjacent to the site of a previous anterior cervical arthrodesis. J Bone Joint Surg Am 1999;81:519–528

[9] Hilibrand AS, Carlson GD, Palumbo MA, Jones PK, Bohlman HH. Radiculopathy and myelopathy at segments adjacent to the site of a previous anterior cervical arthrodesis. J Bone Joint Surg Am 1999;81:519–528

[10] Finn MA, Samuelson MM, Bishop F, Bachus KN, Brodke DS. Two-level noncontiguous versus three-level anterior cervical discectomy and fusion: a biomechanical comparison. Spine 2011;36:448–453

[11] Tharin S, Benzel EC. Cervical spine arthroplasty: fact or fiction: the absence of need for arthroplasty. Clin Neurosurg 2012;59:82–90

[12] Sasso RC, Best NM. Cervical kinematics after fusion and bryan disc arthroplasty. J Spinal Disord Tech 2008;21:19–22

[13] Wigfield C, Gill S, Nelson R, Langdon I, Metcalf N, Robertson J. Influence of an artificial cervical joint compared with fusion on adjacent-level motion in the treatment of degenerative cervical disc disease. J Neurosurg 2002;96(Suppl):17–21

[14] Robertson JT, Papadopoulos SM, Traynelis VC. Assessment of adjacent-segment disease in patients treated with cervical fusion or arthroplasty: a prospective 2-year study. J Neurosurg Spine 2005;3:417–423

[15] Puttlitz CM, Rousseau MA, Xu Z, Hu S, Tay BK, Lotz JC. Intervertebral disc replacement maintains cervical spine kinetics. Spine 2004;29:2809–2814

[16] DiAngelo DJ, Roberston JT, Metcalf NH, McVay BJ, Davis RC. Biomechanical testing of an artificial cervical joint and an anterior cervical plate. J Spinal Disord Tech 2003;16:314–323

[17] Chang UK, Kim DH, Lee MC, Willenberg R, Kim SH, Lim J. Range of motion change after cervical arthroplasty with ProDisc-C and prestige artificial discs compared with anterior cervical discectomy and fusion. J Neurosurg Spine 2007;7:40–46

[18] Dmitriev AE, Cunningham BW, Hu N, Sell G, Vigna F, McAfee PC. Adjacent level intradiscal pressure and segmental kinematics following a cervical total disc arthroplasty: an in vitro human cadaveric model. Spine 2005;30:1165–1172

[19] Harrod CC, Hilibrand AS, Fischer DJ, Skelly AC. Adjacent segment pathology following cervical motion-sparing procedures or devices compared with fusion surgery: a systematic review. Spine 2012;37(Suppl):S96–S112

[20] Nunley PD, Jawahar A, Cavanaugh DA, Gordon CR, Kerr EJ, Utter PA. Symptomatic adjacent segment disease after cervical total disc replacement: re-examining the clinical and radiological evidence with established criteria. Spine J 2013;13:5–12

[21] Cho SK, Riew KD. Adjacent segment disease following cervical spine surgery. J Am Acad Orthop Surg 2013;21:3–11

[22] Boselie TFM, Willems PC, van Mameren H, de Bie R, Benzel EC, van Santbrink H. Arthroplasty versus fusion in single-level cervical degenerative disc disease. Cochrane Database Syst Rev 2012;9:CD009173

[23] Dmitriev AE, Cunningham BW, Hu N, Sell G, Vigna F, McAfee PC. Adjacent level intradiscal pressure and segmental kinematics following a cervical total disc arthroplasty: an in vitro human cadaveric model. Spine 2005;30:1165–1172

[24] Hilibrand AS, Carlson GD, Palumbo MA, Jones PK, Bohlman HH. Radiculopathy and myelopathy at segments adjacent to the site of a previous anterior cervical arthrodesis. J Bone Joint Surg Am 1999;81:519–528

32 Motion Preservation Technologies

Daniel Farivar, Christopher A. Sy, Terrence T. Kim

Learning Objectives

- Understand the spectrum of motion preservation technologies.
- Understand the biomechanical properties of total disc arthroplasty (TDA) devices.
- Understand the complications reported for TDA devices.

Questions

▸▸ Question 1

When counseling patients on motion preservation options, it is important to discuss what important concept?

- A. All procedures involving an implant/device (interspinous spacers, dynamic stabilization, nucleus replacement devices, TDA) are equally efficacious and selection largely depends on the patient's anatomy
- B. Neural element decompression without fusion is preferred because there are no foreign implants/devices and there is no risk of destabilization
- C. Clinical outcomes using motion preservation techniques have given mixed results and thus patients should be encouraged to pursue spinal fusion when discussing surgery for mechanical back pain
- D. Nearly all invasive procedures alter spinal motion by increasing and/or decreasing overall stability; thus, avoidance of surgery may be the best motion preservation strategy
- E. Motion preservation techniques are the future of spine surgery and TDA will likely become the "gold standard" procedure for mechanical back pain instead of spinal fusion

▸▸ Question 2

Stiffness of biological tissues is defined by what equation?

- A. Stiffness = bending moment/section modulus
- B. Stiffness = stress/torque
- C. Stiffness = stress/load
- D. Stiffness = momentum/strain
- E. Stiffness = stress/strain

▸▸ Question 3

Select the best statement regarding TDAs.

- A. TDAs are manufactured such that they match the aging of native intervertebral discs
- B. Subsequent clinical trials have matched the early enthusiasm for TDAs
- C. TDAs are able to accurately replicate the native instantaneous axis of rotation (IAR)
- D. Adjacent segment degeneration and disease are concerns for patients undergoing fusion procedures, but not TDA
- E. In addition to the motion preservation provided by TDAs, posture and sagittal alignment also impact the onset of adjacent segment degeneration and disease

▸▸ Question 4

Stress/strain curves are a helpful way to visualize and compare spinal motion segments as well as prospective spinal devices. What is true regarding use of stress/strain curves?

- A. Stiffness is determined by calculating the slope of the elastic zone
- B. Solid fusion can be portrayed as a straight horizontal line on a stress/strain curve
- C. Failure is depicted by the transition from the neutral zone to the elastic zone
- D. Unconstrained segments are represented by the plastic zone
- E. Unconstrained segments are represented by the elastic zone

▸▸ Question 5

Mechanical back pain is characterized by the clinical triad of deep location, agonizing pain, and what additional finding(s)?

- A. Pain that radiates into the extremities
- B. Pain that is caused by trauma
- C. Pain that is worse with spinal loading and improved with unloading
- D. Pain associated with neurological deficit
- E. Pain that is dull/achy instead of lancinating/burning

▸▸ Question 6

Which intervention is able to shrink a pathologically widened neutral zone?

- A. Fusion
- B. First-generation TDA
- C. Second-generation TDA
- D. Dynamic stabilization device
- E. Interspinous spacer

▸▸ Question 7

Which of the following stress/strain curves (see ▶ Fig. 32.1, ▶ Fig. 32.2, ▶ Fig. 32.3, ▶ Fig. 32.4, ▶ Fig. 32.5) best represents that of a degenerated intervertebral disc (*orange line*) in comparison to a normal curve (*black line*)?

- A.
- B.
- C.
- D.
- E.

▸▸ Question 8

Regarding attributes of TDA devices, which of the following statements is correct?

- A. The “ball-in-socket” first-generation implants are similar in concept to the intervertebral disc, which is an amphiarthrodial joint
- B. None of the devices allow for adequate flexion/extension or lateral bending
- C. TDA devices adapt and change mechanically with time as the patient ages—an advantage over spinal fusion
- D. Despite limitations with flexion/extension and lateral bending, TDA devices have been able to closely replicate the IAR of the intervertebral motion segment
- E. Newer elastomeric devices provide for some axial load cushioning, whereas the first-generation metal-on-metal or metal-on-polymer implants do not cushion axial loads and are stiff under axial loads

▸▸ Question 9

Which of the following statements regarding TDA complications is true?

- A. TDA has been definitively shown to be associated with less adjacent segment degeneration—a major advantage over spinal fusion
- B. Soft bone, suboptimal geometry, and suboptimal footprint size/shape have been associated with implant subsidence
- C. Heterotopic ossification is not a concern with TDA as it is a nonfusion procedure, and the goal is to preserve motion by avoiding new bone formation
- D. If a TDA device fails, there are no revision options and patients should be counseled appropriately
- E. TDA has no effect on kyphosis or lordosis of the treated segment and thus there is no risk of deformity

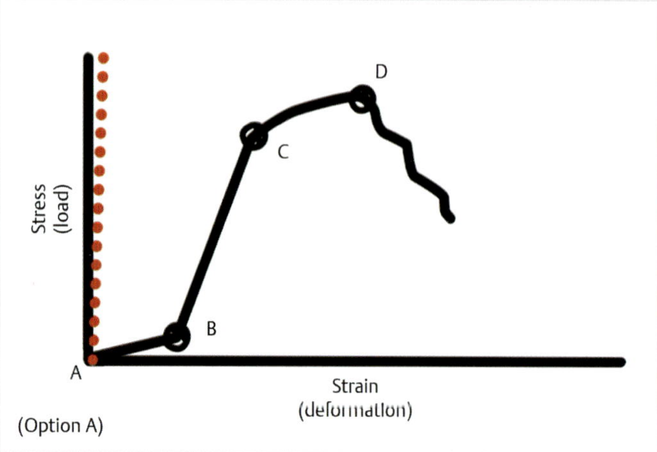

Fig. 32.1 A curve depicting nearly infinite stiffness (high stress/strain relationship) associated with fusion or solid instrumentation (*dotted line*). (Source: Biomechanics of Spine Stabilization: Third Edition, © 2015 Thieme Medical Publishers, Inc.)

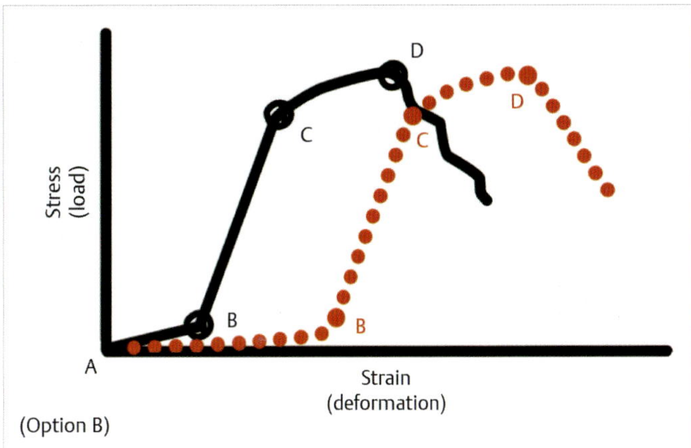

Fig. 32.2 Widening (a shift to the right) of the neutral zone, associated with instability of the motion segment (*dotted curve*). (Source: Biomechanics of Spine Stabilization: Third Edition, © 2015 Thieme Medical Publishers, Inc.)

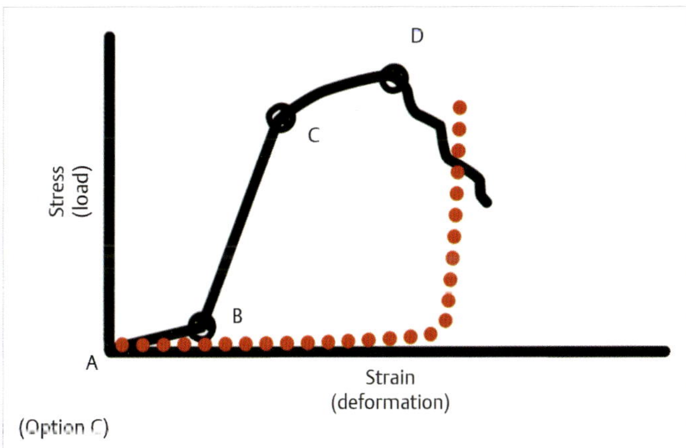

Fig. 32.3 The stress/strain curves of three widely disparate devices. A first-generation "ball-in-socket" device, in which no or little resistance is met until a "hard stop" is reached. (Source: Biomechanics of Spine Stabilization: Third Edition, © 2015 Thieme Medical Publishers, Inc.)

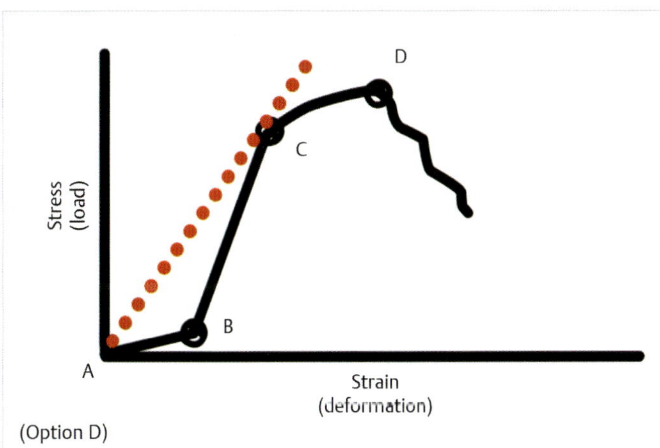

Fig. 32.4 The stress/strain curves of three widely disparate devices. An elastomeric total disc arthroplasty. Here, we see a "hybrid neutral zone and elastic zone" combination. In (A) and (B), the dotted lines and curves represent the stress/strain relationship of the device. (Source: Biomechanics of Spine Stabilization: Third Edition, © 2015 Thieme Medical Publishers, Inc.)

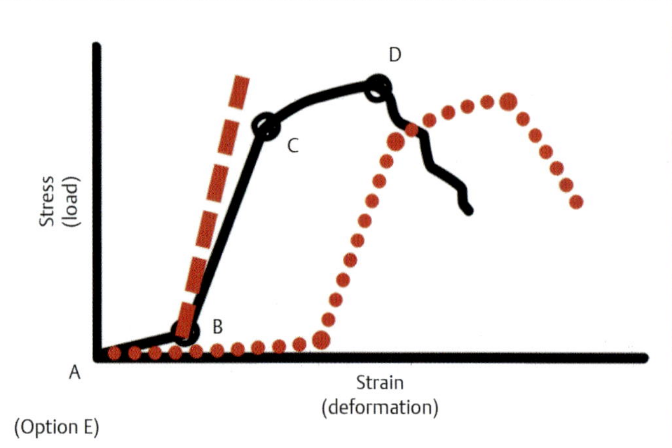

Fig. 32.11 The stress/strain curves of three widely disparate devices. A dynamic spine stabilization system should "stiffen" the spine from a mechanically unstable state (*dotted curve*) to a more normal situation (*dashed curve*). (Source: Biomechanics of Spine Stabilization: Third Edition, © 2015 Thieme Medical Publishers, Inc.)

Answers

▸▸ Answer 1

Correct answer is D

Surgical decompression always has a risk of destabilization and can thus result in an increase in motion. Spinal fusion serves to diminish or eliminate spinal motion. Either way, spinal mechanics are usually affected during surgery and can be detrimental. Avoiding surgery altogether avoids any iatrogenic changes to the spine and is thus the ultimate motion-preserving strategy. Interspinous spacers, dynamic stabilization, and nucleus replacement devices are not widely employed and are lacking evidence as far as clinical efficacy. Neural element decompression can indeed avoid any implants/devices but, as discussed earlier, there is always a risk of destabilization, however small. It is too early to tell how motion preservation will be utilized in the future. Similar to spinal fusion, motion preservation will likely become part of the surgeon's armamentarium and should be employed on a case-by-case basis.

▸▸ Answer 2

Correct answer is E

Stiffness is a function of both stress (applied load) and resultant strain (motion or deformation). Answer A is the equation for stress (θ), not stiffness. Stress is a function of bending moment (M) and section modulus (Z) or $\theta = M/Z$. Answers B, C, and D are incorrect equations using various incorrect physical parameters.

▸▸ Answer 3

Correct answer is E

In one report by Duggal et al, kyphosis was observed below the implant, while lordosis was observed at the index level.[1] Such differences in sagittal alignment can introduce the spine to nonnative distribution of stresses that could lead to adjacent segment degeneration and disease. Thus, adjacent segment degeneration and disease should be a concern for TDA, in addition to fusion procedures.

One drawback of TDAs, as they are currently constructed, is that they are not equipped to match the natural aging of intervertebral discs, characterized by progressive drops in internal pressures. This mismatch with adjacent levels can introduce altered intervertebral biomechanics and should be considered carefully. The subsequent clinical trials have not necessarily matched the early enthusiasm for TDAs. None of the currently available TDA implants replicate the normal or natural IAR motion characteristics.

Clinically, recent long-term studies have demonstrated that not only TDA may continue to function, but also the preservation of motion may reduce the rates of adjacent segment disc degeneration. A recent meta-analysis of 14 randomized controlled trials demonstrated that at up to 7 years out from surgery, TDA had significantly less adjacent segment disease compared with fusion patients. Additionally, long-term studies demonstrated the rates of reoperation were significantly reduced in TDA patients at 10 years out compared with fusion patients.[1,2,3]

▸▸ Answer 4

Correct answer is A

The slope of the elastic zone on a stress/strain curve represents functional stiffness. The preceding neutral zone represents unconstrained motion where it takes very little force to cause any motion or deformation. If there is additional load beyond the neutral zone and elastic zone, a plastic zone can be observed prior to failure. The progression of stress/strain curves involves the following: neutral zone → elastic zone → plastic zone → failure. Solid fusion is depicted by a straight vertical line (infinite stress with no motion) and not a horizontal line (low stress with a lot of motion).

▸▸ Answer 5

Correct answer is C

Mechanical back pain worsens with spinal loading and improves with unloading. Mechanical back pain does not need to be caused by trauma (it is often degenerative) and does not need to be associated with neurological deficit. Pain that radiates into the extremities is more consistent with radiculopathy. Patients can describe mechanical back pain using many descriptors, but lancinating/burning pain is usually associated with neuropathic pain.

▸▸ Answer 6

Correct answer is D

In theory, dynamic spine stabilization reduces spinal instability while maintaining some amount of motion, promoting more uniform load transfer compared with fusion and in turn reducing the risk of adjacent segment disease. The added stability of these devices helps shrink the neutral zone, while the preservation of some motion and load distribution prevents the infinite or nearly infinite stiffness seen following fusion procedures.

The Dynesys system, which is no longer in use, was shown to have comparable outcomes to traditional lumbar fusion surgery at both short-term and medium-term follow-up.[4,5,6] However, while comparative studies focusing on long-term outcomes are lacking, single-arm studies with long-term follow-up on the Dynesys system showed a high incidence of adjacent segment disease.[7,8,9] All in all, although an intriguing motion-sparing alternative to fusion, this dynamic spine stabilization system was eventually discontinued.

▸▸ Answer 7

Correct answer is B

The stress/strain curve shown in B where the neutral zone is widened and the elastic zone is shifted to the right best represents a segment with a degenerated disc. The widened neutral zone depicts increased laxity at that motion segment otherwise known as the "zone of disengagement." Answer A shows a nearly straight vertical line with little to no motion, which depicts a solid fusion or rigid instrumentation. Answer C is a typical stress/strain curve for first-generation TDA devices utilizing a "ball-in-socket" concept where there is little resistance until a "hard stop" is reached and then there is a sharp increase in stress once the device is engaged. Answer D best represents the stress/strain characteristics of newer elastomeric disc arthroplasties with a hybrid neutral–elastic zone. Answer E depicts the additional "stiffening" associated with dynamic stabilization devices—the stiffness achieved is less than achieved by a solid fusion, as depicted in answer A.

▸▸ Answer 8

Correct answer is E

TDA devices, even the first-generation ones, have always allowed for adequate flexion/extension as well as lateral bending[1] but have been very limited in regard to axial loading—thus answer B is incorrect. Answer E is correct in that newer generation elastomeric devices have better axial load properties than the first-generation devices. Answer A is incorrect as the first-generation "ball-in-socket" devices are more similar to a synovial joint, which is a diarthrodial joint. Regarding answer D, no device has yet been able to closely replicate the normal IAR of the intervertebral motion segment, although there is ongoing testing with both fixed and variable IAR devices. Lastly, answer C is incorrect as the *inability* of TDA devices to change/adapt with time is a notable limitation of these devices. The device does not change as adjacent segments and the spine around the device ages with the patient.

[1] It is of note that any motion has both quantitative and qualitative properties. TDA devices may have adequate *quantitative* flexion/extension as well as lateral bending but are unlikely to match the *qualitative* properties of the normal, physiologic, intervertebral motion segment.

▸▸ **Answer 9**

Correct answer is B

Although early studies touted a lower risk of adjacent segment degeneration with TDA, subsequent clinical data have not definitely shown this yet. Answer B lists the usual findings in patients that have failure of a TDA device and is correct. Heterotopic ossification is a known complication with TDA and has been associated with bone milling and/or other disc space preparation techniques. In cases of failure, there are methods to remove or replace the TDA device. Segments that underwent a TDA can also be salvaged by spinal fusion in many cases. Lastly, TDA can have a profound effect on kyphosis/lordosis and thus there is potential for changes in sagittal profile and a risk of spinal deformity.

▸▸ **Answer 10**

Correct answer is E

The normal physiologic aging of an intervertebral disc can be described as a progression from answer B → answer A → answer E. The intervertebral disc in youth has high intradiscal pressures that are relatively uniform across the span of the disc space. Over time, the central portion of the disc begins to degenerate with decreasing central pressures, although the pressure along the peripheral annulus remains relatively preserved (answer A). Vacuum disc phenomenon is not a sign of TDA failure. It is also not a contraindication to TDA—on the contrary, it could be an indication in favor of TDA as it can be a sign of degenerative disc disease.

▸▸ **Answer 11**

Correct answer is C

At this time (March 2024), there is still debate on which patients are good candidates for TDA. There are some guidelines on patient selection, but many patients would be poor candidates for TDA. So far, there are no clear data on the superiority of TDA over spinal fusion. Age over 45 years is not a contraindication for TDA. Bone quality is a significant factor to consider when selecting patients for TDA, as poor bone quality is a known risk factor for implant subsidence.

▸▸ **Answer 12**

Correct answer is E

Points A to B portray the neutral zone. Points B to C portray the elastic zone. Points C to D portray the plastic zone. Finally, the curve after point D represents failure where the motion segment has reached maximum loading capacity and has become incompetent.

▸▸ **Answer 13**

Correct answer is C

Interspinous spacers are one approach to decompression that are recognized for their ability to be placed with a minimally invasive technique. Interspinous spacers are inserted between the spinous processes and gently distracted to expand the lumbar neuroforamina. Its placement within the spine limits extension, but also invariably results in some degree of kyphosis due to its distraction. It is typically used for moderate lumbar stenosis. Devices that "stiffen" the spine and are used in practice to "enhance" fusion are referred to as dynamic spine stabilizers.

▸▸ **Answer 14**

Correct answer is B

Nuclear replacement devices can be used in the patient with discogenic pain and early nuclear degeneration with minimal to no signs of collapse, herniation, or instability. In theory, these devices replace only the nucleus pulposus, leaving the native annulus fibrosus intact to contain the prosthetic. However, rigorous evidence regarding the clinically utility of nuclear replacement devices is still lacking, and so currently this treatment is employed in a limited manner. TDA replaces both the annulus fibrosus and nucleus pulposus and represents the gold standard for motion preservation device technologies. Additionally, literature regarding the clinical benefit is mixed, with a significant discrepancy existing between enthusiastic early clinical and later clinical evaluations.

▸▸ **Answer 15**

Correct answer is A

Nearly all invasive surgical interventions affect motion to some degree in an adverse manner, either excessively destabilizing (decompression) or diminishing motion (fusion). Thus, if a patient's complaint can be adequately managed with conservative measures (i.e., gabapentin), in turn preserving native biomechanics, it should be chosen.

▸▸ Answer 16

Correct answer is A

Although TDAs represent the gold standard for motion preservation device technologies, significant gaps still exist from native biomechanics. TDAs only partially replicate flexion/extension, allowing for very similar quantitative range of motion, but lacking the fluidity and qualitative properties seen in a healthy spine. Additionally, the center of rotation for currently available TDAs has been seen to deviate from the norm. Further, first-generation TDAs do not allow for axial motion nor cushioning of the motion segment during axial loading. The nearly infinite stiffness observed in axial loading may theoretically cause these loads to be transferred to adjacent levels and to the facet joint complex at the index level, resulting in significant wear and tear over time. However, elastomeric and second-generation implants have been shown to better replicate normal intervertebral disc mechanics and provide more cushioning during axial loading.

▸▸ Answer 17

Correct answer is D

A "fully constrained" device implies no motion and infinite or nearly infinite stiffness, which would be characteristic of a fusion procedure. A "semicosntrained" device would be mechanically portrayed by the elastic zone of the stress/strain curve, while an "unconstrained" device would be mechanically portrayed by the neutral zone of the stress/strain curve. In general, unfortunately, there is a lack of consistency among authors and researchers with how these subtypes are defined and used. For example, a first-generation TDA might be considered a "semiconstrained" device by some and an "unconstrained" device by others. However, a fusion can reliably be understood as a "fully constrained" device.

▸▸ Answer 18

Correct answer is A

The zone of disengagement is the zone in which very little force (stress) is required to cause motion or displacement (strain) and thus refers to the neutral zone of a stress/strain curve. If a dysfunctional motion segment has an expansion of the zone of disengagement, the biomechanics of this area would be considered "sloppy."

▸▸ Answer 19

Correct answer is A

Especially for first-generation TDAs, implant loading mechanics vary widely depending on the plane of motion. In flexion/extension and lateral bending, they have a widened neutral zone until a hard stop is reached at the extreme of motion, which is represented by answer choice B. However, when axial loading, these implants are poor at effectively cushioning loads and result in an infinite or nearly infinite stiffness. Such mechanics are shared with a fusion procedure. It should be noted that later generations of TDAs, such as the elastomeric implants, respond better to axial loading and behave according to the stress/strain curve seen in answer choice D.

▸▸ Answer 20

Correct answer is B

Additional TDA-specific kyphosis has been observed in several studies[10,11,12] and has been thought to be secondary to surgical technique and/or device-specific issues. In the lumbar spine (most commonly L5–S1), Lee et al demonstrated that angular mismatch between the device and end plate reduced range of motion and affected outcomes.[10] Although the determination of candidacy for TDA is the subject of some debate, age has not been found to be an absolute contraindication for TDA. There are conflicting reports regarding the generation of wear debris following TDA, and so it cannot be ruled out as a potential adverse event. Available reports have found heterotopic ossification to be a particular problem with the Bryan cervical disc, not the lumbar SB Charité disc. Finally, less, not more, retraction of the esophagus is required to insert a cervical TDA compared with a fusion with plate.

▸▸ Answer 21

Correct answer is A

Although the success of cervical TDAs have been demonstrated in long-term studies compared with cervical fusions, there has been an increasing number of recent clinical reports on the failures of cervical TDAs. Most recently, a single-institution study evaluating 169 patients found clinical failure rate of 4.7% at 27.7 months from surgery. In that same study, a meta-analysis and review of prospective data in the literature was performed and the authors concluded six main types of failure mechanisms with associated subtypes (see ▶ Table 32.1).[13]

Table 32.1 Table Proposed classification system for mechanisms contributing to cervical TDA failure

Failure type	Description
Type I: stenosis	Central or foraminal stenosis
Type II: migration	
Gross extrusion	Migration with extrusion out of the disc space
End plate failure	Subsidence (> 3 mm) or acute end plate fracture
Type III: instability	
Mechanical loosening	Noninfectious loosening due to biomechanical stress or poor ingrowth
Septic loosening	Infectious end plate loosening
Device fracture	Device core or end plate fracture contributing to instability
Type IV: device motion loss	Loss of ROM (< 2 degrees) with the device "locked" in hyperlordosis or kyphosis
Type V: implantation error	
Malposition	Laterality, depth
Improper size	Too small or large
Type VI: wear	
Without osteolysis	Elevated ion levels, radiographic polyethylene wear
With osteolysis	Inducing osteolysis with/without pseudotumor formation

ROM, range of motion
(Biomechanics of Spine Stabilization: Third Edition),
© 2015 Thieme Medical Publishers, Inc.

Key Principles

- TDA represents the gold standard of motion preservation device technologies.
- The various motion preservation devices can be categorized and assessed by their stiffness characteristics: stiffness = stress/strain.
- Newer generation TDAs are able to replicate anatomy and quantitatively approach normal flexion/extension and lateral bending. However, center of rotation and qualitative motion may deviate from normal. First-generation TDAs do not allow for axial motion, but newer generation TDAs improve upon this cushioning effect.
- Reported complications following TDA have included facet joint pathology at the same level, degeneration of facet joints and discs at adjacent levels, subsidence, heterotopic ossification, vertebral body split fractures, and kyphotic deformation.

References

[1] Duggal N, Bertagnoli R, Rabin D, Wharton N, Kowalczyk I. ProDisc-C: an in vivo kinematic study. J Spinal Disord Tech 2011;24(5):334–339

[2] Findlay C, Ayis S, Demetriades, AK. Total disc replacement versus anterior cervical discectomy and fusion: a systematic review with meta-analysis of data from a total of 3160 patients across 14 randomized controlled trials with both short- and medium- to long-term outcomes. Bone Joint J 2018;100-B(8):991–1001

[3] Gornet MF, Burkus JK, Shaffrey ME, Schranck FW, Copay, AG. Cervical disc arthroplasty: 10-year outcomes of the Prestige LP cervical disc at a single level. J Neurosurg Spine 2019;31(3):317–325

[4] Zhang Y, Shan JL, Liu XM, Li F, Guan K, Sun TS. Comparison of the Dynesys dynamic stabilization system and posterior lumbar interbody fusion for lumbar degenerative disease. PLoS One 2016;11(1):e0148071

[5] Bredin S, Demay O, Mensa C, Madi K, Ohl X. Posterolateral fusion versus Dynesys dynamic stabilization: retrospective study at a minimum 5.5 years' follow-up. Orthop Traumatol Surg Res 2017;103(8):1241–1244

[6] Wu H, Pang Q, Jiang G. Medium-term effects of Dynesys dynamic stabilization versus posterior lumbar interbody fusion for treatment of multisegmental lumbar degenerative disease. J Int Med Res 2017;45(5):1562–1573

[7] Veresciagina K, Mehrkens A, Schären S, Jeanneret B. Minimum ten-year follow-up of spinal stenosis with degenerative spondylolisthesis treated with decompression and dynamic stabilization. J Spine Surg 2018;4(1):93–101

[8] Zhang Y, Zhang ZC, Li F, et al. Long-term outcome of Dynesys dynamic stabilization for lumbar spinal stenosis. Chin Med J (Engl) 2018;131(21):2537–2543

[9] Hoppe S, Schwarzenbach O, Aghayev E, Bonel H, Berlemann U. Long-term outcome after monosegmental L4/5 stabilization for degenerative spondylolisthesis with the Dynesys device. Clin Spine Surg 2016;29(2):72–77

[10] Lee CS, Chung SS, Oh SK, You JW. Significance of angular mismatch between vertebral endplate and prosthetic endplate in lumbar total disc replacement. J Spinal Disord Tech 2011;24(3):183–188

[11] Lazaro BCR, Yucesoy K, Yuksel KZ, et al. Effect of arthroplasty design on cervical spine kinematics: analysis of the Bryan Disc, ProDisc-C, and Synergy Disc. Neurosurg Focus 2010;28(6):E6

[12] Fong SY, DuPlessis SJ, Casha S, Hurlbert RJ. Design limitations of Bryan disc arthroplasty. Spine J 2006;6(3):233–241

[13] Zavras AG, Sullivan TB, Singh K, Phillips FM, Colman MW. Failure in cervical total disc arthroplasty: single institution experience, systematic review of the literature, and proposal of the RUSH TDA failure classification system. Spine J 2022;22(3):353–369

33 Minimally Invasive Spine Surgery

Jacob L. Goldberg, Joseph A. Carnevale, Ibrahim Hussain, Roger Härtl

Minimally invasive spine surgery refers to a rapidly growing set of techniques that aim to accomplish targeted surgical goals with less tissue invasion, supporting quicker recovery. Knowledge of the fundamentals of spine biomechanics is essential in the assessment of whether surgery can be accomplished via minimally invasive techniques without introducing iatrogenic instability.

Learning Objectives

- Understand the properties of intervertebral discs that lead to spinal degeneration.
- Understand the importance of preserving mechanically eloquent tissue.
- Understand the importance of avoiding overt disruption of spinal elements in preventing iatrogenic spinal destabilization.

Questions

▸▸ Question 1

The biomechanical and anatomic properties of intervertebral discs play significant roles in the degenerative pathology observed in the spine. Which of the following statements related to the biomechanical and anatomic properties of intervertebral discs is true?

- A. The biomechanical properties of intervertebral discs do not change from birth to end-stage senescence
- B. At birth, the intervertebral disc is best described as a desiccated nucleus fibrosis confined by a fibrocartilaginous annulus fibrosis
- C. The intervertebral disc is a diarthrodial joint
- D. The intervertebral disc is an amphiarthrodial joint
- E. The intervertebral disc is a ball-in-socket joint

▸▸ Question 2

Understanding the physiologic mechanics of intervertebral discs in the spinal column is essential in order to avoid iatrogenic destabilization of the spinal column. Which of the following statements about the stress/strain characteristics of amphiarthrodial joints is true?

- A. At a fixed stress, deformation increases with progressive degeneration
- B. Amphiarthrodial joints do not degenerate in response to repetitive loading
- C. A mechanically unstable motion segment is associated with a narrowing of the neutral zone
- D. A mechanically unstable motion segment results in a leftward shift of the stress/strain curve
- E. The intervertebral disc is a ball-in-socket joint

▸▸ Question 3

When surgically approaching a paracentral or foraminal disc, which condition can arise as a sequalae of disruption of facet joint integrity?

- A. Lumbar spinal stenosis
- B. Herniated disc
- C. Spondylolisthesis
- D. Spinal cord injury
- E. Central cord syndrome

▸▸ Question 4

Progressive slippage is noted in many patients with degenerative lumbar spondylolisthesis. Which of the following variables is associated with protection against slip progression in degenerative lumbar spondylolisthesis?

- A. Increased disc space height
- B. Bone spur/osteophyte formation
- C. Absence of vertebral body end plate sclerosis
- D. Absence of ligamentous ossification
- E. Trauma

▸▸ Question 5

The lumbar facet joints serve important roles in motion segment stabilization. Which of the following anatomic or biomechanical attributes of the lumbar facet joints is accurate?

- A. At all lumbar levels, the facet joints are oriented in the coronal plane

- B. At all lumbar levels, the facet joints are oriented in the sagittal plane
- C. The medial aspect of the lumbar facet joint presents a flat surface to the lateral aspect of the joint
- D. The three-dimensional orientation of the lumbar facet joints varies based on spinal level
- E. The lumbar facet joints are structurally analogous to the cervical facet joints

▸▸ Question 6

Avoidance of the introduction of iatrogenic spinal motion segment instability requires an understanding of the biomechanical and anatomic properties of the spine. Which of the following best describes the stabilizing function of the medial portion of the lumbar facet joint?

- A. Provide cushioning between vertebral bodies
- B. Provide the majority of spinal column support
- C. Prevent listhesis
- D. Prevent anterior and posterior flexion from occurring in the lumbar spine
- E. Prevent spinal cord injury

▸▸ Question 7

During the performance of minimally invasive laminectomy or discectomy, iatrogenic spinal segment instability can be introduced. Understanding the biomechanical and anatomic features of the spine is essential to avoid unnecessarily causing instability. In which spinal region are the facet joints relatively flat and shingled?

- A. Cervical
- B. Thoracic
- C. Lumbar
- D. Sacral
- E. Occipital

▸▸ Question 8

Tubular retractors are a muscle-sparing technique used in minimally invasive lumbar decompression. The orientation of the tubular retractor establishes the surgical trajectory. When performing a unilateral lateral recess decompression, the surgeon must decide the laterality to place the tubular retractor, which dictates the surgical trajectory. When performing a contralateral lateral recess decompression, what is the effect of a lower (less steep) trajectory angle to reach the lateral recess (rather than placing the retractor ipsilateral and taking a steeper angle)?

- A. Increased chance of medial facet joint integrity disruption
- B. Decreased chance of medial facet joint integrity disruption
- C. No effect on medial facet joint integrity
- D. Leads to spinal instability
- E. Leads to spondylolisthesis

▸▸ Question 9

Matsunaga et al observed progressive slippage in what percentage of patients with degenerative spondylolisthesis?

- A. 10%
- B. 24%
- C. 34%
- D. 48%
- E. 100%

▸▸ Question 10

Using a tubular retractor via minimally invasive means which trajectory for decompression of foraminal and lateral recess stenosis decreases the chance of medial facet joint integrity disruption?

- A. Right-sided L4–L5 retractor placement for decompression of right L4–L5 stenosis
- B. Left-sided L4–L5 retractor placement for decompression of left L4–L5 stenosis
- C. Midline L4–L5 retractor placement for decompression of right L4–L5 stenosis
- D. Right-sided L4–L5 retractor placement for decompression of left L4–L5 stenosis
- E. Cannot decrease the chance of medial facet joint disruption

▸▸ Question 11

The biomechanical and anatomic properties of intervertebral discs play significant roles in the degenerative pathology observed in the spine. Which of the following statements related to the

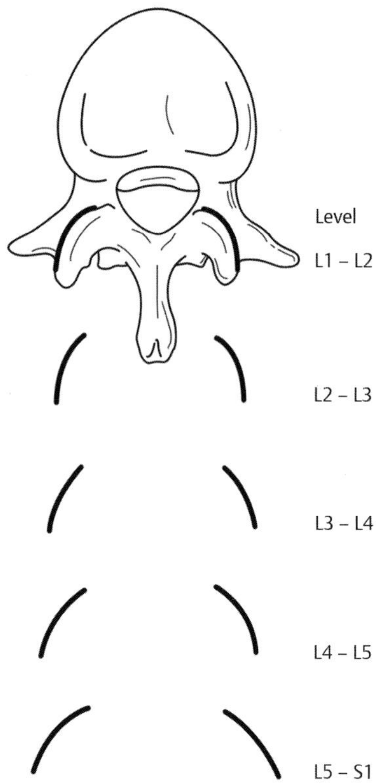

Fig. 33.2 The changes in lumbar facet joint morphology and orientation from level to level. (Data obtained from White and Panjabi.[1])

▸▸ **Answer 8**

Correct answer is B

A lower trajectory angle decreases the chance of medial facet joint integrity disruption, with preservation of the "mechanically eloquent" medial facet. See depiction of this concept in ▸ Fig. 33.3.

▸▸ **Answer 9**

Correct answer is C

Matsunaga et al observed progressive slippage in 34% of patients with degenerative spondylolisthesis. Preventing iatrogenic spondylolisthesis is important as it is a progressive process.[1]

▸▸ **Answer 10**

Correct answer is D

Placement of the tubular retractor contralateral to the foraminal or lateral recess stenosis allows for the surgeon to take a "less steep" trajectory and avoid medial facet joint disruption. Medial facet disruption is detrimental to spinal integrity in the lumbar spine as the medial portion of the lumbar facet joint functions as a "brake" preventing listhesis.

▸▸ **Answer 11**

Correct answer is D

An amphiarthrodial joint is not lined by synovium and does not contain synovial fluid. It is a stiff joint that degenerates in response to repetitive loading. It is not a "ball-in-socket" joint.

▸▸ **Answer 12**

Correct answer is B

Transfacet technique has theoretical biomechanical advantage over translaminar transfacet technique due to its ability to engage the pedicle with the screw, resulting in better purchase and potential restoration of lordosis. Answer choices C, D, and E do not describe transfacet screw techniques (see ▸ Fig. 33.4).

▸▸ **Answer 13**

Correct answer is E

The transsacral lumbar interbody screw fixation technique has fallen out of favor but is worth mentioning from a biomechanical perspective. The technique and device attributes listed are biomechanically unfavorable.

▸▸ **Answer 14**

Correct answer is E

Lumbar interspinous spacers are used as a minimally invasive strategy to address the symptoms of neurogenic claudication in patients with lumbar and lateral recess stenosis. The primary biomechanical effect of such technologies is the attainment of reduced extension. This reduces loading of the facet joints and decreases foraminal height loss with extension. Finally, the instantaneous axis of rotation is not substantially altered by this technique.

▸▸ **Answer 15**

Correct answer is A

LLIF cages are ideally placed ventrally within the disc space, providing a strong biomechanical

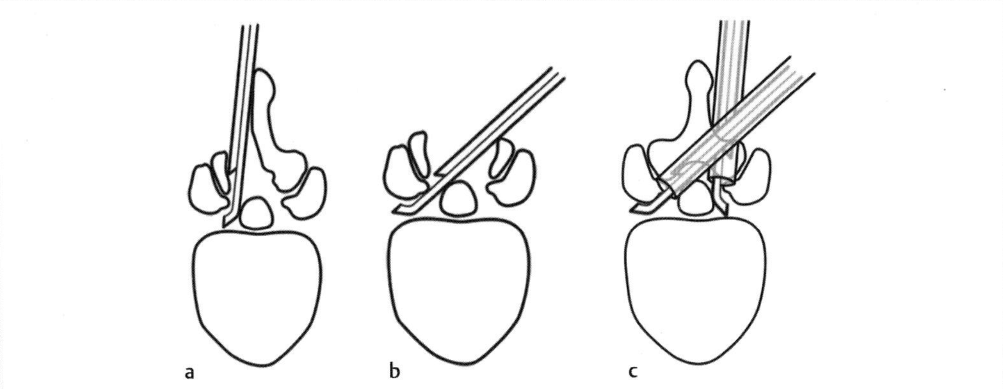

Fig. 33.3 The orientation of the surgical trajectory is critical to minimizing the resection of "mechanically eloquent" tissue. **(a)** A vertical trajectory, which may be used on the same side of a tubular minimally invasive spinal surgical procedure for lateral recess and foraminal decompression, can result in the excessive resection of such "mechanically eloquent" tissue and destabilize the spine. **(b)** A more horizontal trajectory provides access to the lateral recess and foramina without disrupting the "mechanically eloquent" medial facet joint. Even with the resection of midline structures (i.e., lamina, spinous process, ligamentum flavum, and interspinous ligaments), the preservation of facet joint integrity is associated with the preservation of adequate stability in most cases. **(c)** The tubular approach to both the same side and the opposite side is depicted. (Source: Data obtained from White AA, Panjabi MM. The basic kinematics of the human spine. A review of past and current knowledge. Spine 1978; 3: 12–20)

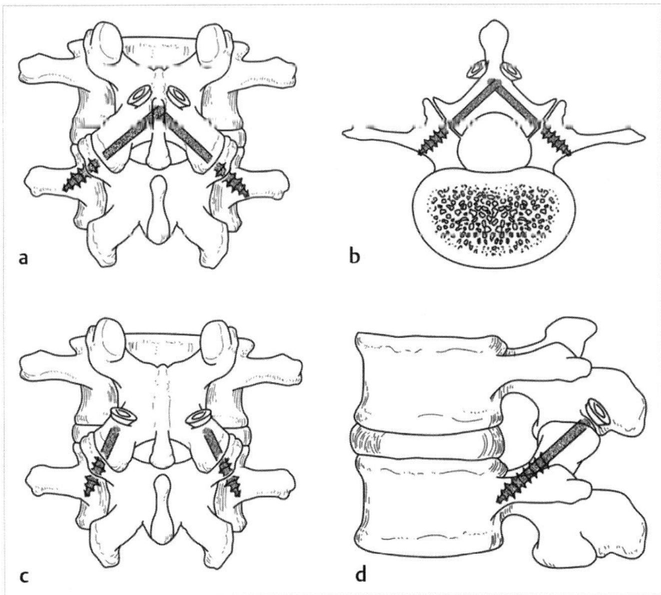

Fig. 33.4 Two techniques for lumbar facet screw fixation. **(a, b)** The Magerl translaminar transfacet fixation technique. **(c, d)** The Boucher transfacet technique. (Source: Biomechanics of Spine Stabilization: Third Edition, © 2015 Thieme Medical Publishers, Inc.)

foundation (apophyseal ring) and allowing for segmental lordosis. Less lordosis is achievable with a dorsally placed cage. LLIF cages have more contact with the vertebral body end plate than TLIF cages owing to their greater surface area. LLIF is a powerful technique for coronal deformity correction (both segmental and global).

Key Principles

- Intervertebral discs are stiff joints that degenerate over the lifespan with repetitive loading.
- Preservation of mechanically eloquent tissue is necessary to avoid spinal segment destabilization and iatrogenic instability.

References

[1] Matsunaga S, Ijiri K, Hayashi K. Nonsurgically managed patients with degenerative spondylolisthesis: a 10- to 18-year follow-up study. J Neurosurg 2000;93(2 Suppl):194–198

[2] White AA, Panjabi MM. The basic kinematics of the human spine. A review of past and current knowledge. Spine 1978; 3: 12–20

34 Construct Failure and Failure Prevention: The Decision-Making Process

David Freeman, Michael Wang

Preoperative, intraoperative, and postoperative decisions regarding spinal constructs heavily impact the success and/or failure of the construct. Understanding why constructs fail is essential to a successful spine surgery practice. This chapter examines specific examples of each type of failure and highlights key facets of the decision-making process that impact the success of the construct.

Learning Objectives

- Understand biomechanical and physical principles that can lead to construct failure.
- Understand how preoperative decision making can relate to construct failure.
- Understand how intraoperative decision making can relate to construct failure.
- Understand Wolff's law and subsidence-related construct failure.
- Understand implant–bone interface–related construct failure.
- Understand implant fracture–related construct failure.
- Understand postoperative decision making and how it can relate to construct failure.

Questions

▸▸ Question 1

What characteristics should be emphasized by a spine surgeon to help prevent construct failure?

- A. Foundation of knowledge
- B. Understanding of three-dimensional anatomy, biomechanics, and physical principles
- C. Utilization of a rigid postoperative orthosis
- D. Timely decision making
- E. Maintaining strict diagnostic criteria

▸▸ Question 2

What is the first and most critical factor that needs to be considered when deciding on a construct?

- A. Type of operation (approach)
- B. Technique employed
- C. Decision to operate
- D. Levels fused
- E. Back pain

▸▸ Question 3

Spine surgeons should be aware of other factors that may complicate the decision to operate. What are some of those factors?

- A. A lack of objective criteria to define good spine surgery candidates
- B. Surgeon-based decision making
- C. Suboptimal outcome instruments to assess postoperative success
- D. External influences such as hospital economics, relative value units (RVUs), and implant vendors
- E. Back pain

▸▸ Question 4

There are two types of intraoperative decision-making failures. What are they?

- A. Application of improper surgical principles; application of suboptimal surgical technique
- B. Application of improper biomechanical principles; application of suboptimal surgical technique
- C. Application of improper surgical principles; failure to follow Wolff's law
- D. Failure to follow Wolff's law; application of suboptimal surgical technique
- E. None of the above

▸▸ Question 5

The anterior cervical construct shown in ▸ Fig. 34.1 demonstrates an example of which type of construct failure?

- A. Improper surgical principles
- B. suboptimal surgical technique
- C. Failure to follow Wolff's law
- D. Error of assumption
- E. Materials failure

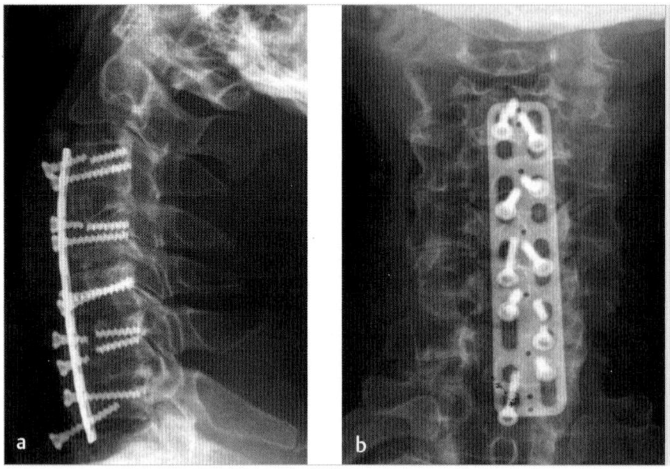

Fig. 34.1 A radiograph of a middle-generation Caspar plate, in which both slots and holes were provided for the nonfixed moment arm cantilever screws. **(a)** Lateral view. **(b)** Anteroposterior view. (Source: Biomechanics of Spine Stabilization: Third Edition, © 2015 Thieme Medical Publishers, Inc.)

▸▸ **Question 6**

Postoperative X-rays of a single-level minimally invasive transforaminal lumbar interbody fusion (MIS TLIF) demonstrate rods at strongly oblique angles to each other. What type of construct failure is this?

- A. Improper surgical principles
- B. Suboptimal surgical technique
- C. Failure to follow Wolff's law
- D. Error of assumption
- E. Material failure

▸▸ **Question 7**

A common manifestation of subsidence is _______.

- A. Error of suboptimal surgical technique
- B. Penetration of the vertebral body end plate
- C. Compression of abutting bone margins
- D. Loss of axial height and angular spine deformation
- E. Inevitable

▸▸ **Question 8**

A large multilevel anterior corpectomy cage is placed intraoperatively with violation of end plates. What long-term postoperative complication(s) should be expected?

- A. Suboptimal surgical principles
- B. Subsidence
- C. Implant failure
- D. Bone–bone interface failure
- E. Degenerated motion segment

▸▸ **Question 9**

What does Wolff's law explain?

- A. Mature bones remodel throughout life by employing interstitial growth
- B. Bone elongation is due to cartilaginous growth
- C. Bone thickness is a function of aging
- D. Explains the effect of mechanical stress on bone remodeling
- E. Hydroxyapatite is a critical part of bone matrix

▸▸ **Question 10**

Which of these pairings regarding implant–bone interface is correct?

- A. Hard implant + soft bone = failure
- B. Flexible implant + soft bone = failure
- C. Hard implant + hard bone = failure
- D. Flexible implant + hard bone = failure
- E. Bone implant interface is not important

▸▸ **Question 11**

What is the primary cause of the implant–bone interface–related failure depicted in ▸ Fig. 34.2?

- A. Subsidence
- B. Wolff's law
- C. Region of known low bone density
- D. Metastatic neoplasm
- E. Trauma

▸▸ Question 12

What are the factors underlying implant fracture?

- A. Fatigue fracture
- B. Low modulus of elasticity
- C. Osteoporosis
- D. Subsidence
- E. Wolff's law

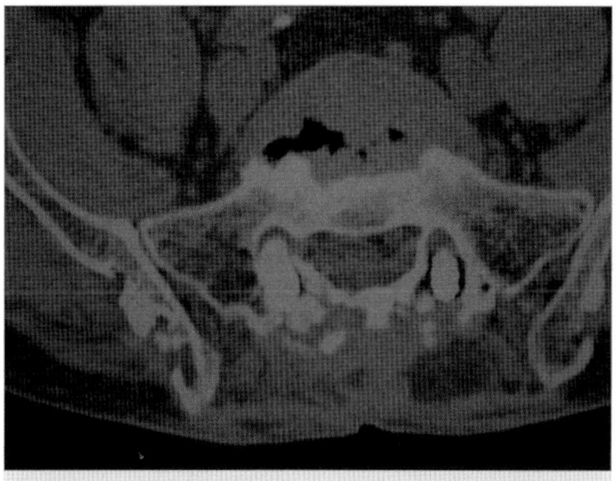

Fig. 34.2 Two examples of poor bone quality. Axial computed tomographic scan cut through the sacrum depicts cyclical loading–related degradation of the screw bone interface. Note the halos around the screws. (Source: Biomechanics of Spine Stabilization: Third Edition, © 2015 Thieme Medical Publishers, Inc.)

▸▸ Question 13

Where is the implant shown in ▸ Fig. 34.3 most likely to sustain a fracture?

- A. a
- B. b
- C. c
- D. a and c
- E. b and c

▸▸ Question 14

What is the mathematical definition of "stress" within the context of biomechanical principles?

- A. Section modulus/bending moment
- B. Bending moment/section modulus
- C. Arm length/force application
- D. Force application/arm length
- E. An integral part of Wolff's law

▸▸ Question 15

How should spine implants be selected?

- A. Identifying patient's unique risk factors for nonunion
- B. Recommendation of the sales representative
- C. Overall materials used in implant
- D. Strength of the implant at critical points
- E. Biomechanical principles

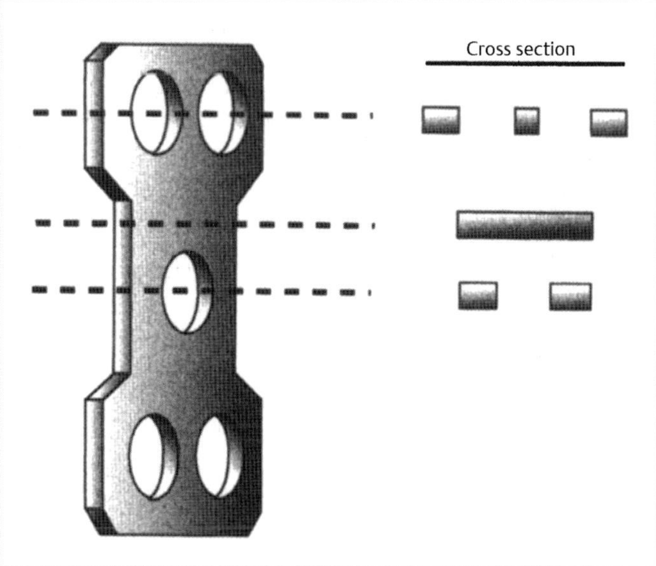

Fig. 34.3 The strength of a plate depends on its geometry, as well as its cross-sectional area. In regions of lesser cross-sectional area, the section modulus is less (in general) than it is in regions where the cross-sectional area is greater. Although a plate may appear to be very strong, it is no stronger than its weakest link. It is, indeed, most vulnerable at the site of greatest stress application. If it is weak (decreased strength or section modulus) at this point, failure by fracture may occur. (Source: Biomechanics of Spine Stabilization: Third Edition, © 2015 Thieme Medical Publishers, Inc.)

▸▸ Question 16

What is the *least* significant factor in construct failure?

- A. Preoperative management
- B. Postoperative management
- C. Intraoperative surgical technique
- D. Intraoperative strategy
- E. Wolff's law

▸▸ Question 17

How can two seemingly similar patients undergo the same operative procedure but have different clinical results?

- A. High bending moment/low section modulus
- B. Inappropriate early postoperative activity
- C. Unidentified adverse variables
- D. Strength of the implant at critical points
- E. Back pain is difficult to correctly diagnose

▸▸ Question 18

Why is a long bridging implant spanning a multilevel corpectomy likely to fail?

- A. Implant–bone interface failure
- B. Implant fracture failure
- C. Subsidence-related failure
- D. Preoperative decision making–related failure
- E. Postoperative decision making–related failure

▸▸ Question 19

Which of the following statements is true?

- A. Constructs do not fail. Surgeons fail
- B. Surgeons cannot fail. Constructs fail
- C. Wolff's law describes all constructs
- D. High bending moment/low section modulus = stress
- E. Force application/arm length = stress

▸▸ Question 20

Which factors of a screw are likely to precipitate failure?

- A. Thick and short screws
- B. Thin and long screws
- C. Tapered screws
- D. Thread pitch
- E. Material

Answers

▸▸ Answer 1

Correct answer is B

A mastery of surgical technique is a must for either orthopaedic or neurosurgeon who operates on the spine. This surgical mastery comes from understanding the three-dimensional anatomy, regional anatomy, and global alignment principles. Biomechanical principles and physical principles are also necessary to create successful constructs, which in turn lead to successful spine surgery.

▸▸ Answer 2

Correct answer is C

The decision to perform surgery in the first place is the most crucial decision made for both the surgeon and the patient. Responsibility lies with the surgeon to take into account the patient's symptoms, imaging findings, nonsurgical measures, and evaluating other causes of back pain that may not be surgically amenable. Operating on the wrong patient regardless of the stability or strength of construct will lead to unhappiness in both the patient and surgeon.

▸▸ Answer 3

Correct answer is A

There is a myriad of factors that must be weighed in order to make even the most basic but most important of decisions and that is whether or not to operate. Currently, there are no objective criteria to define who would be a good spine surgery candidate. This leaves much of the decision making to the surgeon, who must clearly evaluate all of the factors. In accord with the lack of objective criteria for candidacy, there are very few assessments capable of defining post–spine surgical success. We know what a successful patient looks like, but it has proven to be an objectively elusive set of criteria. Economic forces and human relationships can pervert the objectivity needed to make the correct decision.

▸▸ Answer 4

Correct answer is A

Surgical principle failure deals with the strategy used by the surgeon during the surgical case. This is the result of reading, planning, and preparing for the case. It requires knowledge of biomechanical principles. Surgical technique failure deals with the tactics implemented during the surgery. This is preventable and can be mitigated by reading and practicing complex and unfamiliar procedures, utilizing proven techniques, and working at becoming better. Knowledge of the implants and their characteristics is also critical.

▸▸ Answer 5

Correct answer is A

This is an intermediate-generation Caspar plate that utilizes both holes and slots in order to provide fixation. The screws placed in the holes failed due to fracture or back-out, and this was at least partially due to the curvature of the plate and the screw trajectories in this case. Multiple fixation points promote sharing of the overall load by a greater number of implant–bone interfaces. Symmetric and uniform loading of implant anchors and anchor implant interfaces decreases the possibility of biomechanical failure.

▸▸ Answer 6

Correct answer is B

This is a demonstration of an MIS TLIF in which the final tightening of the set screws was not performed in a sequential manner to minimize this oblique angle of both rods. Not only is this aesthetically displeasing, but also it places undue strain on the pedicle screws.

▸▸ Answer 7

Correct answer is D

While subsidence is inevitable due to the aging process and the compression of abutting bone margins and surgery often accelerates the process, it manifests as a loss of axial height. This can be accelerated or even caused by penetration of the vertebral body end plate. Subsidence must always be taken into account during preoperative planning.

▸▸ Answer 8

Correct answer is B

Subsidence of the vertebral bodies will lead to failure of the implant. Subsidence after corpectomy leads to the fracture of the plate screws.

▸▸ Answer 9

Correct answer is D

Julius Wolff, a German anatomist, created a theory in the 19th century that explains how bones respond to stress. This law is important in bony injury recovery and spinal fusion surgery and suggests that if bones are exposed to increasingly heavy loads, they with alter their composition to accommodate the increasing weight. This is an adaptive change and can be applied in both cases of increasing or decreasing weight.

▸▸ Answer 10

Correct answer is A

This question tests knowledge of Young's modulus of elasticity. It is the slope of the linear portion of the stress–strain curve for a material under tension. This correlates to the stiffness of the material. Placement of implants with a high modulus of elasticity in bone with a low modulus of elasticity often results in failure and degradation of the implant–bone interface.

▸▸ Answer 11

Correct answer is C

This is an example of poor bone quality, i.e., low bone density, leading to implant–bone interface–related failure. The sacrum is a region of known low bone density. Implant–bone interface failure is typically multifactorial. Other factors besides regions with low bend density are trauma, infection, tumor, and many other pathologies.

▸▸ Answer 12

Correct answer is A

Implant fractures predictably occur at the point of maximum stress application within the construct. This interplay between the implant and the surrounding bone helps to clarify the correlation to implant fractures. There are three components to this relationship:

1. Stress is the bending moment divided by the section modulus—providing proof of the importance of the material and design of the implant.
2. Implant vulnerabilities must be known as well: plates and screws areas exposed to shear stress are most likely to fail.

3. Failure of bony union results in continued stress being applied to the implant—further increasing the potential for failure/fracture within the construct.

▸▸ Answer 13

Correct answer is C

Implant fractures *are expected* to occur at the point of maximum stress application within the construct. These types of fractures occur as a result of repetitive loading and occur via a fatigue fracture (see ▶ Fig. 34.4).

▸▸ Answer 14

Correct answer is B

Stress is the bending moment divided by the section modulus (strength at the point of the applied bending moment). Implant fractures *always* occur at the point of maximum stress application.

▸▸ Answer 15

Correct answer is D

Implants should be selected on the basis of their strength at various points of vulnerability. This is detailed by the significant moment arm length and force application.

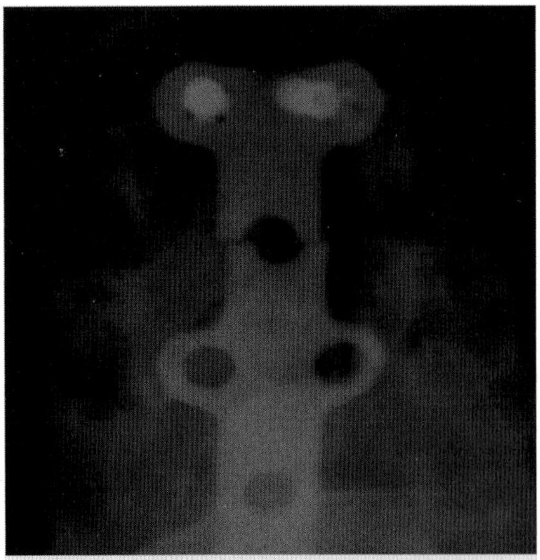

Fig. 34.4 A radiograph of a fractured plate. Implants always fracture at the point of maximum stress application. (Source: Biomechanics of Spine Stabilization: Third Edition, © 2015 Thieme Medical Publishers, Inc.)

▸▸ Answer 16

Correct answer is B

Postoperative care must be monitored and thoughtful, but it is the least significant factor in construct failure. Early postoperative activity, falls, poor nutrition, and immune compromise can all lead to insufficient autologous fusion. Despite ideal intraoperative surgical techniques and preoperative management, constructs can still fail due to a variety of factors—none of which are as important as the preceding decision making and actions.

▸▸ Answer 17

Correct answer is C

The difference in clinical results demonstrates a convergence of unidentified variables. The patients may have appeared similar, but they had significant underlying differences, and while operative procedures may be the same, the nuances of each operation are always varied.

▸▸ Answer 18

Correct answer is D

A long bridging implant after a multilevel anterior cervical corpectomy. Under loading conditions, the implant will move in desynchrony with the patient. Given this and the number of load cycles applied to the graft, the construct is most likely to fail at the implant–bone interface. However, this is really a failure of preoperative decision making. These stresses should have been taken into account and a three-point mode of fixation should have been attempted (i.e., more anchors in an intermediate fixation point in the native spine).

▸▸ Answer 19

Correct answer is A

Construct failure is a term that is very deeply embedded in spine surgeon's lexicon. However, a construct requires a surgeon to think about, operate, and implant the said construct. All spine surgeons need to recognize the limitations of the patient, the implants used, and the biomechanics.

▸▸ **Answer 20**

Correct answer is B

Screws with long and thin inner diameters that are exposed to shear stresses are most likely to fracture at the screw–implant or screw–plate interface. See Chapter 19 for further discussion.

Key Principles

- The decision to operate on a patient is the most important decision point.
- Stress = bending moment/section modulus.
- Biomechanical strength must be accounted for in each construct.
- Subsidence and Wolff's law must be taken into account for each patient.

Part VIII

Nonoperative Spine Stabilization

VIII

▸▸ Answer 4

Correct answer is C

Supine position results in pressure on the elbows, dorsal thoracic region, occiput, heels, scapulae, and sacral region.

▸▸ Answer 5

Correct answer is A

Lateral decubitus position results in pressure on the greater trochanter, ribs, shoulder, lateral knee, and the lateral malleolus of the ankle (see ▶ Fig. 35.2).

▸▸ Answer 6

Correct answer is C

The 45-degree sitting position is associated with greater integument interface pressures compared with other positions.

▸▸ Answer 7

Correct answer is A

Continuous-motion beds result in shearing pressures being exerted in the direction of gravitational forces.[6]

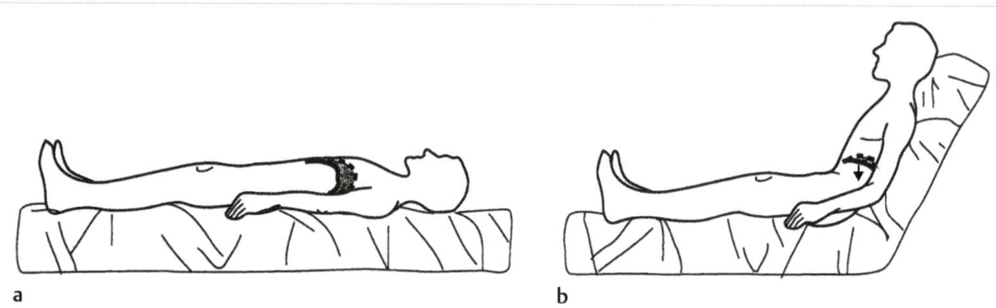

Fig. 35.1 The tidal volume of a quadriplegic patient is higher **(a)** in the supine position than **(b)** in the sitting position. This is related to gravitational effects on the abdominal cavity (*arrow*) and flailing of the chest wall, which results in paradoxical motion. (Source: Biomechanics of Spine Stabilization: Third Edition, © 2015 Thieme Medical Publishers, Inc.)

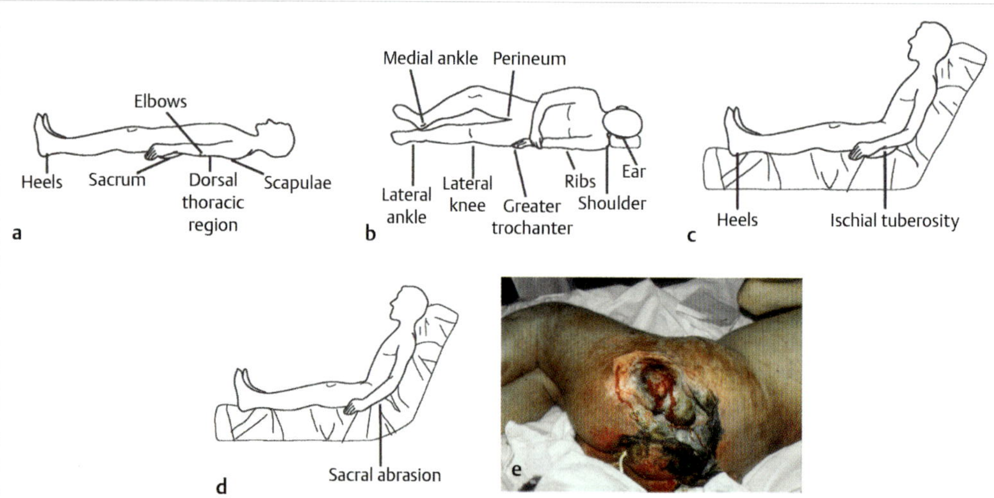

Fig. 35.2 Pressure points. **(a)** Supine position. **(b)** Lateral decubitus position. **(c)** Sitting position. **(d)** Traction related to a slumped sitting position. **(e)** The end result of relative or complete inattention to integument care in an insensate patient can be devastating. (Source: Biomechanics of Spine Stabilization: Third Edition, © 2015 Thieme Medical Publishers, Inc.)

▸▸ **Answer 8**

Correct answer is D

Uniform integument pressure beds (bead beds) use beads to equally distribute pressure and reduce the occurrence of pressure points.[7,8]

▸▸ **Answer 9**

Correct answer is E

Prone positioning if done incorrectly has resulted in worsening spinal deformity, spinal cord injury, respiratory arrest, and death. However, prone positioning results in increased distribution of pressure, leading to more possible pressure points.[9]

▸▸ **Answer 10**

Correct answer is C

Dependent leg extension in the lateral decubitus position decreases greater trochanter pressure. Nondependent leg should be flexed to help maintain lateral decubitus positioning (see ▸ Fig. 35.3).

▸▸ **Answer 11**

Correct answer is E

Almost all helmets have a coiled metal rim that requires bolt cutters to aid in the removal of the helmet.[10] While in the emergency department, radiographs can be obtained to determine the composition of individual helmets (▸ Fig. 35.4). On a positive note, these helmets can be utilized in cervical traction given their rigid nature.

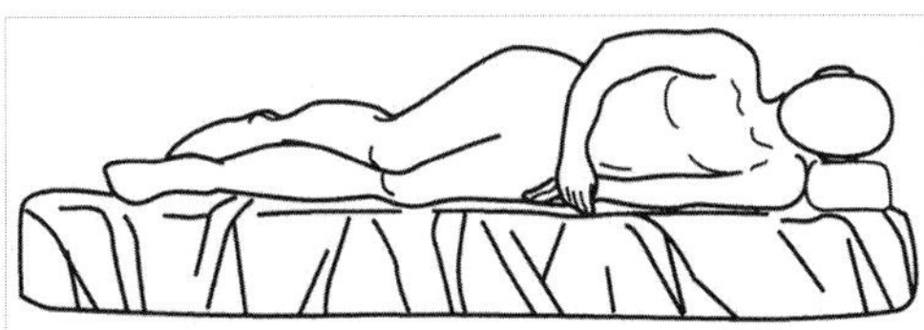

Fig. 35.3 Dependent leg extension in the lateral decubitus position decreases greater trochanter pressure. The nondependent leg is flexed to maintain the lateral decubitus position, as depicted. (Source: Biomechanics of Spine Stabilization: Third Edition, © 2015 Thieme Medical Publishers, Inc.)

▸▸ **Answer 12**

Correct answer is B

By placing the pins anterior to the cervical spine, a parallel backward force is applied and will result in extension. This can aid in patients with posteriorly translated fractures in the case of ankylosing spondylitis (▸ Fig. 35.5).[11]

▸▸ **Answer 13**

Correct answer is C

Ligamentous injury should be ruled out prior to the application of traction. If traction is applied in a patient with ligamentous disruptions, it can result in further injury through unexpected distraction with little weight.

▸▸ **Answer 14**

Correct answer is A

Friction of the patient's body against the bed absorbs most of the force of traction. Therefore, the effect of traction is not experienced by the vertebral bodies.

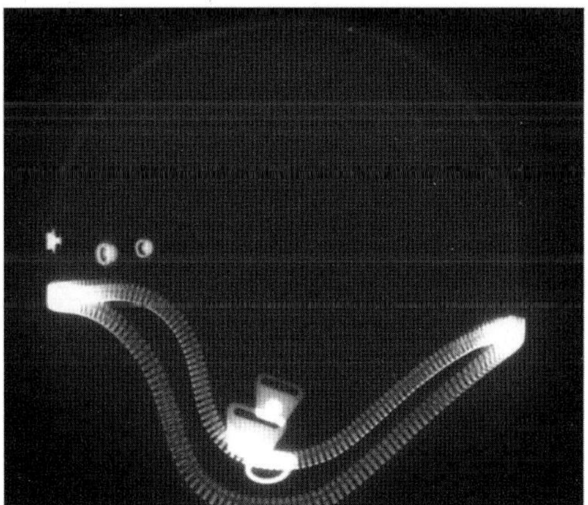

Fig. 35.4 Radiogragh of a helmet. Knowing that the helmet proper is made of composite that is amenable to cutting with a cast saw is relevant. Nearly all helmets have a coiled metal perimeter. A radiograph in the emergency room can be used to determine such helmet-related characteristics. This is relevant during cutting of the helmet proper. A wire cutter would therefore be necessary to complete helmet removal. (Source: Biomechanics of Spine Stabilization: Third Edition, © 2015 Thieme Medical Publishers, Inc.)

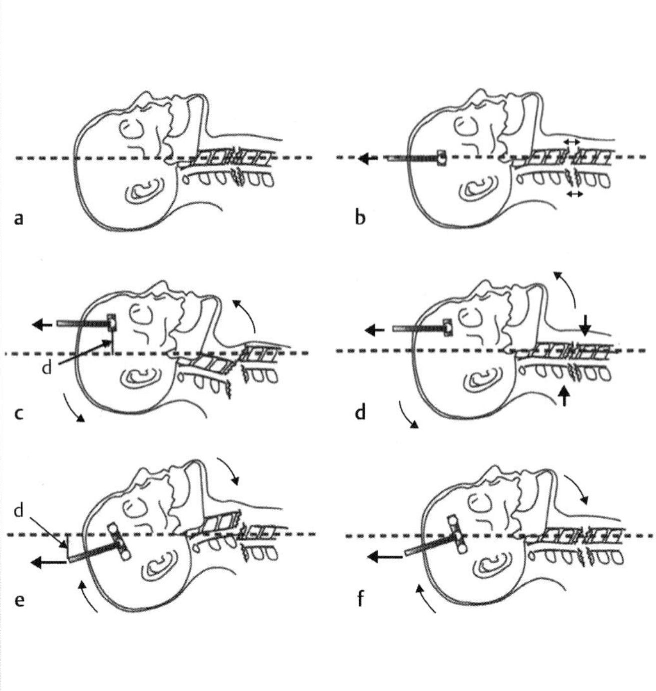

Fig. 35.5 Ankylosing spondylitis with a cervical spine fracture. **(a)** This is equivalent to a long-bone fracture (dotted lines). (Double-headed arrows, **b**) Traction applied "in line" with the spine (along its axis) results in spine distraction. Traction applied along an axis other than that of the spine causes a bending moment (curved arrows) to be applied. This can be used to reduce a deformity via the application of a force (load) to a moment arm, d. **(d)** Translational loads are then applied (straight arrows), thus reducing the deformity. The bending moment can be exaggerated by using three-point (or four-point) skull fixation to apply traction, thus eliminating loading of the tongs with respect to the skull. **(e, f)** This can be used to reduce a translational deformity. (Source: Bed Rest and Traction. In: Benzel E, ed. Biomechanics of Spine Stabilization. 3rd Edition. New York: Thieme; 2015. doi:10.1055/b-003-106374)

▸▸ Answer 15

Correct answer is B

Distractive forces can result in the retropulsion of disc fragments into the canal space. This may result in worsening spinal cord injury. Traction may also result in excessive traction.[12,13,14]

▸▸ Answer 16

Correct answer is E

Axillary rolls provide stress relief for the shoulder joint, helping to prevent patient discomfort and ligamentous stress that can predispose a patient to shoulder dislocation. The axillary roll also serves to relieve stress on the brachial plexus, reduce incidence of compartment syndrome, and increase circulatory return.[15] Risks of the roll include causing skin ulcers, bruising, and compromising circulation if malpositioned (▸ Fig. 35.6).[16]

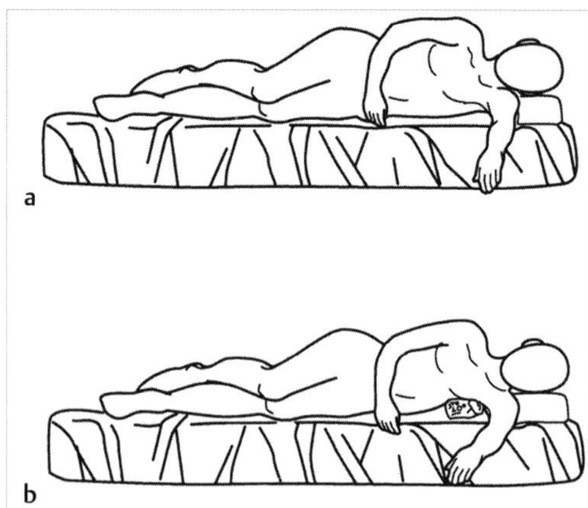

Fig. 35.6 Axillary rolls minimize shoulder dislocation and distortion. **(a)** Without axillary roll and **(b)** with axillary roll. (Source: Bed Rest and Traction. In: Benzel E, ed. Biomechanics of Spine Stabilization. 3rd Edition. New York: Thieme; 2015. doi:10.1055/b-003-106374)

▸▸ Answer 17

Correct answer is C

Fractures in the setting of ankylosing spondylitis are similar to long bone fractures, with a segment above and below the fracture site. Long bone fractures are highly unstable given the lack of ligamentous and adjacent bone support.[17] In these cases, traction can place significant forces on the proximal cervical spine depending on pin placement given it is a rigid construct. Therefore, low weight should be added slowly and via a vector that extends the neck.

▸▸ **Answer 18**

Correct answer is C

Turning a patient allows for the redistribution of pressure to various pressure points. Unfortunately, during turning, distraction, compression, torsion, shearing, and angular stresses can be applied to the spine. These forces represent a potential risk for exacerbating further neurologic injury.

▸▸ **Answer 19**

Correct answer is A

The sitting position results in decreased tidal volume due to the gravitational effects on the abdominal cavity. However, pneumonia, fluid retention, deep vein thrombophlebitis, and pressure sores all have clinical significance in a supine quadriplegic patient. Patients requiring supine bed rest should be carefully rotated to aid in the prevention of such clinical sequela.

▸▸ **Answer 20**

Correct answer is B

The forces applied by cervical tongs or halo screws degrade with time[18]. The force should be checked regularly to ensure adequate pressure is maintained. If this pressure is not maintained, then traction can fail. Ligamentous laxity and increased patient sedation may aid cervical traction. Muscle spasms may present a challenge to cervical traction but can be addressed with medications. Bone remodeling does not impact cervical traction in the traumatic setting.

Key Principles

- Bedrest and stabilization allows for spontaneous remodeling of bony injuries.
- Patient positioning can result in new injury. Care must be taken when positioning to avoid pressure ulcers and further injuries.
- Cervical traction allows for stabilization and reduction of fractures in the setting of traumatic injuries. Careful considerations must be taken with regards to pin placement, weight, and patient positioning.
- Varying placement of pins along the anterior skull allows the vector of traction to be adapted to aid in extension or flexion for reduction purposes.

References

[1] Cantor JB, Lebwohl NH, Garvey T, Eismont FJ. Nonoperative management of stable thoracolumbar burst fractures with early ambulation and bracing. Spine 1993;18:971–976
[2] Mumford J, Weinstein JN, Spratt KF, Goel VK. Thoracolumbar burst fractures. The clinical efficacy and outcome of nonoperative management. Spine 1993;18:955–970
[3] Chow GH, Nelson BJ, Gebhard JS, Brugman JL, Brown CW, Donaldson DH. Functional outcome of thoracolumbar burst fractures managed with hyperextension casting or bracing and early mobilization. Spine 1996;21:2170–2175
[4] Ball PA, Chicoine RE, Gettinger A. Anesthesia and critical care management of spinal cord injury. In: Benzel EC, Tator CH, eds. Contemporary Management of Spinal Cord Injury: From Impact to Rehabilitation. Park Ridge, IL: American Association of Neurological Surgeons; 2000:99–108
[5] Ball PA, Chicoine RE, Gettinger A. Anesthesia and critical care management of spinal cord injury. In: Benzel EC, Tator CH, eds. Contemporary Management of Spinal Cord Injury: From Impact to Rehabilitation. Park Ridge, IL: American Association of Neurological Surgeons; 2000:99–108
[6] Conrad BP, Horodyski M, Wright J, Ruetz P, Rechtine GR. Log-rolling technique producing unacceptable motion during body position changes in patients with traumatic spinal cord injury. J Neurosurg Spine 2007;6:540–543
[7] Conrad BP, Horodyski M, Wright J, Ruetz P, Rechtine GR. Log-rolling technique producing unacceptable motion during body position changes in patients with traumatic spinal cord injury. J Neurosurg Spine 2007;6:540–543
[8] Goetz LL, Brown GS, Priebe MM. Interface pressure characteristics of alternating air cell mattresses in persons with spinal cord injury. J Spinal Cord Med 2002;25:167–173
[9] Bearden BG, Conrad BP, Horodyski M, Rechtine GR. Motion in the unstable cervical spine: comparison of manual turning and use of the Jackson table in prone positioning. J Neurosurg Spine 2007;7:161–164
[10] Donaldson WF, Lauerman WC, Heil B, Blanc R, Swenson T. Helmet and shoulder pad removal from a player with suspected cervical spine injury. A cadaveric model. Spine 1998;23:1729–1732, discussion 1732–1733
[11] Alexander EJ, Davis CH, Forsyth HF. Reduction and fusion of fracture dislocation of the cervical spine. J Neurosurg 1967;27:588–591
[12] Benzel EC. Traumatic quadriplegia with dislocation and central disc herniation. J Spinal Disord 1991;4:497
[13] Berrington NR, van Staden JF, Willers JG, van der Westhuizen J. Cervical intervertebral disc prolapse associated with traumatic facet dislocations. Surg Neurol 1993;40:395–399
[14] Doran SE, Papadopoulos SM, Ducker TB, Lillehei KO. Magnetic resonance imaging documentation of coexistent traumatic locked facets of the cervical spine and disc herniation. J Neurosurg 1993;79:341–345

[15] Rozet I, Vavilala MS. Risks and benefits of patient positioning during neurosurgical care. Anesthesiol Clin 2007;25(3): 631–53, x
[16] Haldar R, Bhagat H, Toshniwal GR, Dash HH. Conventional axillary rolls in prolonged neurosurgical procedures: time for reconsideration. Asian J Neurosurg 2017;12(3):583–584
[17] Lazennec J-Y, d'Astorg H, Rousseau M-A. Cervical spine surgery in ankylosing spondylitis: review and current concept. Orthop Traumatol Surg Res 2015;101(4):507–513
[18] Lerman JA, Haynes RJ, Koeneman EJ, Koeneman JB, Wong WB. A biomechanical comparison of Gardner-Wells tongs and halo device used for cervical spine traction. Spine 1994;19: 2403–2406

36 Spine Bracing

Ian Connolly, Muhamed Hadzipasic, Theresa Williamson

Spinal bracing is an important component in the management of spinal instability. When applied properly, bracing serves predominantly as a supplemental treatment rather than a stand-alone solution due to its limited capacity in restricting spinal movements. The duration of spinal bracing, a key consideration, is tailored to individual patient needs and specific clinical contexts, balancing the benefits against potential complications. A snug chest fit is paramount in the efficacy of spinal bracing, especially in the thoracic region. This helps in maintaining the brace's biomechanical effectiveness, preventing deformations, and maintaining structural integrity. Understanding these dynamics is essential for optimizing spinal bracing strategies, making it a vital tool in the broader spectrum of spinal care management.

Learning Objectives

- Recognize the goals of spinal bracing.
- Identify the problems associated with spinal bracing.
- Understand the role of brace length and soft tissue thickness in the effectiveness of spinal bracing.
- Understand the materials used in spinal splints and their advantages.
- Understand the concept of the body shell in spinal bracing.
- Learn about the different types of spinal bracing, including cervical, thoracic, and lumbosacral spine bracing.
- Understand the complications associated with spinal bracing.

Questions

▸▸ Question 1

What is the relationship between the thickness of the soft tissue between the spine and the inner surface of the brace and the effectiveness of the brace?

- A. Direct relationship
- B. Inverse relationship
- C. No relationship
- D. Exponential relationship
- E. Logarithmic relationship

▸▸ Question 2

What is the usual effect of a longer brace?

- A. Less spinal stability
- B. More bracing-related respiratory complications
- C. Greater spine stability
- D. Less skin-related bracing complications
- E. No effect on spinal stability

▸▸ Question 3

What is a limitation of limited cervical bracing techniques?

- A. They provide improved outcomes due to decreased bracing stiffness
- B. Their length-to-width ratio is too high
- C. Their points of contact with the torso result in wound complications
- D. They do not provide sufficient cervical spine stabilization
- E. They restrict too much neck flexion–extension

▸▸ Question 4

What is the primary disadvantage of the Jewett brace?

- A. It promotes maintenance of the cylindrical body shell
- B. It provides a three-point bending biomechanical advantage
- C. It does not promote maintenance of the cylindrical body shell
- D. It does not provide a three-point bending biomechanical advantage
- E. It is too comfortable for the patient

▸▸ Question 5

What is a primary advantage of plastic polymer brace materials?

- A. Increased weight
- B. Difficulty in the doffing and donning of the brace
- C. Difficulty of fabrication

- D. Increased discomfort for the patient
- E. The use of ventilation holes to provide increased comfort

▸▸ **Question 6**

What is the primary disadvantage of cervical–shoulder bracing techniques?

- A. They provide more patient discomfort compared with limited cervical bracing techniques
- B. They minimally influence movement in the low cervical region
- C. They significantly influence movement in the low cervical region
- D. They do not limit low cervical and cervicothoracic motion
- E. They limit low cervical and cervicothoracic motion

▸▸ **Question 7**

What is the "snaking effect" in the context of spinal bracing?

- A. The serpentine movement of the spine in which a simple overall movement is accompanied by a combination of flexion and extension movements at each intervertebral level outside of the bracing region
- B. The effect of the brace's shape on its effectiveness
- C. The effect of the brace's material on its effectiveness
- D. The serpentine movement of the spine in which a simple overall movement is accompanied by a combination of flexion and extension movements at each intervertebral level within the bracing region
- E. The effect of the brace's size on its effectiveness

▸▸ **Question 8**

How is the "snaking" phenomenon calculated in the cervical spine?

- A. By measuring the overall movement from the head to C7
- B. By summing up all segmental movements between the head and C7
- C. By subtracting the overall movement from the head to the C7 from the sum of the absolute value of all segmental movements
- D. By adding the overall movement from the head to C7 to the sum of all segmental movements
- E. By dividing the overall movement from the head to C7 by the sum of all segmental movements

▸▸ **Question 9**

How can the "parallelogram effect" be corrected in a cervical brace?

- A. By adjusting the tension of the brace
- B. By adding a chest component to the brace
- C. By making the brace shorter
- D. By using a different material for the brace
- E. By making the brace lighter

▸▸ **Question 10**

What is a significant advantage of the Minerva jacket brace in spinal bracing?

- A. It is lighter than other braces
- B. It is more comfortable than other braces
- C. It is easier to put on and take off than other braces
- D. It provides significant reduction of segmental movement at all cervical spine levels
- E. It is less expensive than other braces

▸▸ **Question 11**

How does the Minerva jacket brace compare to the halo brace in terms of controlling segmental motion in the cervical spine?

- A. The Minerva jacket brace controls segmental motion better than the halo brace
- B. The halo brace controls segmental motion better than the Minerva jacket brace
- C. Both braces control segmental motion equally well
- D. Neither brace is effective at controlling segmental motion
- E. The Minerva jacket brace is only effective at controlling segmental motion in the upper cervical spine, while the halo brace is effective at all levels

▸▸ Question 12

Why is the lower lumbar region difficult to splint externally?

- A. It is due to the lack of flexibility in the lower lumbar region
- B. It is due to the limitations created by an inadequate caudal fixation point
- C. It is due to the high density of nerve endings in the lower lumbar region
- D. It is due to the high mobility of the lower lumbar region
- E. It is due to the lack of muscle mass in the lower lumbar region

▸▸ Question 13

Why is the thoracic region easier to splint compared with other regions of the spine?

- A. It has a larger surface area for the brace to attach
- B. It has less soft tissue separating the brace from the spine
- C. It has two axial mobile segments above and below for fixation
- D. It is less mobile than other regions of the spine
- E. It has more muscle mass for the brace to grip onto

▸▸ Question 14

What unique complications are associated with the use of a halo brace?

- A. Increased mobility and flexibility of the spine
- B. Decreased effectiveness in stabilizing the spine
- C. Increased comfort and ease of use
- D. Decreased need for adjustments and fittings
- E. Cosmetic problems, infection, osteomyelitis, and brain abscesses due to pin site complications

▸▸ Question 15

What is the Jewett brace?

- A. A brace that applies a dorsally directed force at the sternum and the pubic region and a ventrally directed force at the thoracolumbar junction
- B. A brace that applies a ventrally directed force at the sternum and the pubic region and a dorsally directed force at the thoracolumbar junction
- C. A brace that applies a dorsally directed force at the sternum and the thoracolumbar junction and a ventrally directed force at the pubic region
- D. A brace that applies a ventrally directed force at the sternum and the thoracolumbar junction and a dorsally directed force at the pubic region
- E. A brace that applies a dorsal force at the sternum and a ventral force at the pubic region

▸▸ Question 16

How do lumbar braces primarily function?

- A. They provide significant spinal stabilization
- B. They cause discomfort and serve as a reminder to restrict movement
- C. They increase the range of motion in the lumbar region
- D. They alleviate all load on the lumbosacral spine
- E. They provide substantial movement restriction of the upper lumbar and thoracolumbar spine

▸▸ Question 17

Which of the following statements best describes the difference in the mechanisms of the halo and Minerva braces?

- A. Both braces function primarily as a three-point bending fixator
- B. The halo brace functions primarily as a fixed moment arm cantilever beam fixator, while the Minerva brace functions primarily as a three-point bending fixator
- C. The Minerva brace functions primarily as a fixed moment arm cantilever beam fixator, while the halo brace functions primarily as a three-point bending fixator
- D. Both braces function primarily as a fixed moment arm cantilever beam fixator
- E. Neither brace functions as a three-point bending fixator or a fixed moment arm cantilever beam fixator

▸▸ **Question 18**

What are the goals of spinal bracing?

- A. Restriction of movement, achievement and maintenance of spinal realignment, and trunk support
- B. Increase of movement, achievement and maintenance of spinal realignment, and trunk support
- C. Restriction of movement, decrease of spinal realignment, and trunk support
- D. Restriction of movement, achievement and maintenance of spinal realignment, and trunk instability
- E. Increase of movement, decrease of spinal realignment, and trunk instability

▸▸ **Question 19**

What is one of the potential severe complications of body cast syndrome?

- A. It leads to an increase in the frequency of lumbar brace application
- B. Duodenal obstruction
- C. It causes the loosening of lumbar braces
- D. It promotes the frequent use of casts
- E. It is associated with the loose application of lumbar braces

▸▸ **Question 20**

According to the Lind group's study on the use of a halo vest for cervical spine stabilization, where is the motion greatest and how does it change as you move down the cervical spine?

- A. The motion is greatest in the lower part of the cervical spine and increases farther up
- B. The motion is greatest in the middle part of the cervical spine and remains constant throughout
- C. The motion is greatest in the upper part of the cervical spine and decreases farther down
- D. The motion is greatest in the upper part of the cervical spine and increases farther down
- E. The motion is uniform throughout the cervical spine

Answers

▸▸ **Answer 1**

Correct answer is B

The effectiveness of spinal bracing is inversely related to the thickness of the soft tissue between the spine and the inner surface of the brace. This means that the thicker the soft tissue, the less effective the brace is at stabilizing the spine.

▸▸ **Answer 2**

Correct answer is C

A longer brace usually provides more spinal stability than a shorter one. This is because a longer brace can cover more of the spine and provide better support and stability due to an increased length-to-width ratio (see ▸ Fig. 36.1).

▸▸ **Answer 3**

Correct answer is D

Limited cervical bracing techniques provide little cervical spine stabilization. Their length-to-width

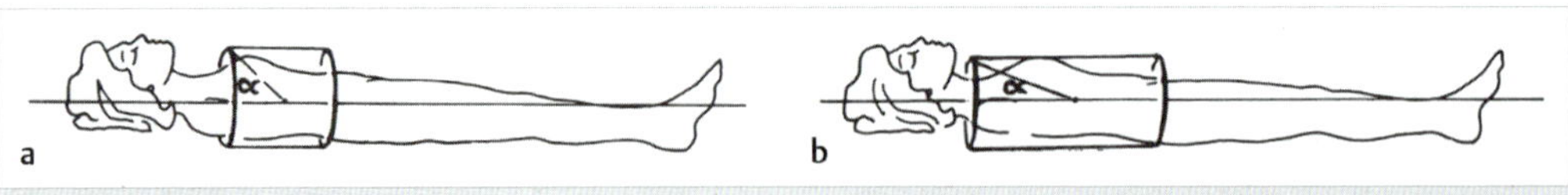

Fig. 36.1 The effectiveness of spinal bracing is inversely related to the axial distance between the spine and the inner surface of the brace. This is theoretically defined by the following relationship: efficacy of bracing is related to the cosine of α, in which α is the angle defined by the edge of the brace, the instantaneous axis of rotation at the unstable segment, and the long axis of the spine. This angle is determined by both the length of the brace and the thickness of tissue between the spine and the inner surface of the brace. **(a)** A short brace (α = 15 degrees; cosine α = 0.966). **(b)** A long brace (α = 45 degrees; cosine α = 0.707). Obviously, a significant reduction of efficacy comes with the use of a shorter, wider brace—that is, the length-to-width ratio of the brace is too small. (Source: Biomechanics of Spine Stabilization: Third Edition, © 2015 Thieme Medical Publishers, Inc.)

ratio is insufficient, and their points of contact with the torso are not solid. This means that they do not provide enough support or restriction to effectively stabilize the cervical spine.

▸▸ Answer 4

Correct answer is C

The Jewett brace does not promote maintenance of the cylindrical body shell. This is a disadvantage because maintaining the cylindrical body shell (as is done with the Minerva brace) can help to provide better support and stability to the spine.[1]

▸▸ Answer 5

Correct answer is E

Plastic polymer brace materials have several advantages, one of which is the use of ventilation holes to provide increased comfort. These holes allow for better airflow, which can help to keep the patient cool and comfortable while wearing the brace.

▸▸ Answer 6

Correct answer is B

Cervical–shoulder bracing techniques provide a slight advantage over limited cervical bracing techniques by extending the brace to include the neck base–shoulder region. However, this minimally influences movement in the low cervical region, which can have a significant impact on upper cervical segmental movement (see ▸ Fig. 36.2).[2]

▸▸ Answer 7

Correct answer is D

The "snaking effect" in spinal bracing refers to a serpentine movement of the spine in which a simple overall movement (e.g., flexion or extension) is accompanied by a combination of flexion and extension movements at each intervertebral level. Although overall movement from the head to the thorax may be minimal, the cumulative segmental movement between these points may be substantial. Therefore, snaking can be defined quantitatively

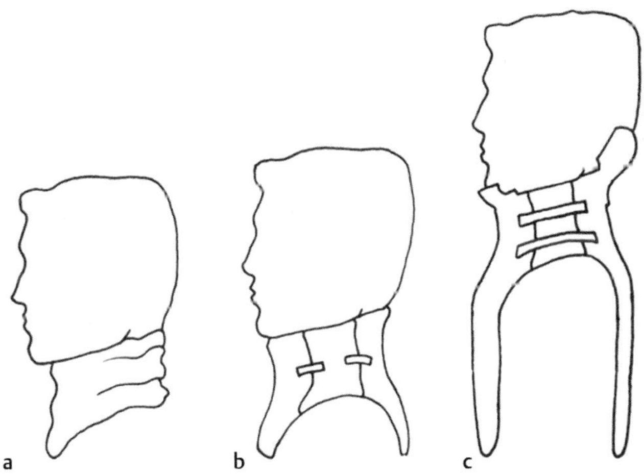

Fig. 36.2 **(a)** Limited cervical bracing techniques provide little cervical spine stabilization. Their length-to-width ratio is insufficient, and their points of contact with the torso are not solid. **(b)** Cervical–shoulder bracing techniques provide a slight advantage over limited cervical bracing techniques via extension of the brace to include the neck base–shoulder region. However, this minimally influences movement in the low cervical region, which in turn has a significant impact on upper cervical segmental movement (see Fig. 36.5 and Fig. 36.6). **(c)** Cervical–thoracic bracing techniques provide a biomechanical advantage by limiting low cervical and cervicothoracic motion and therefore compensatory higher cervical segmental movements. They are typified by the SOMI (sternal occipital mandibular immobilizer), four-poster, and cervicothoracic braces. (Source: Biomechanics of Spine Stabilization: Third Edition, © 2015 Thieme Medical Publishers, Inc.)

as the difference between the sum of all segmental movements (the sum of the absolute values of the segmental motions) between the head and the thorax and the overall movement between the head and the thorax.[3,4,5]

▸▸ Answer 8

Correct answer is C

The "snaking" phenomenon, a serpentine movement of the spine, is calculated as the difference between the sum of all segmental movements (the sum of the absolute values of the segmental motions) between the head and C7 and the overall movement between the head and C7. This calculation provides a quantitative definition of snaking. Although overall movement from the head to the thorax may be minimal, the cumulative segmental movement between these points may be substantial, leading to the snaking effect (see ▶ Fig. 36.3).

▸▸ Answer 9

Correct answer is B

The "parallelogram effect" in a cervical brace, which is a deformation of the brace itself due to a suboptimal fit between its halves, can be corrected by adding a chest component to the brace. This adjustment helps to prevent the parallelogram-like movements and enhances the brace's ability to stabilize the spine (see ▶ Fig. 36.4).[6]

▸▸ Answer 10

Correct answer is D

The Minerva jacket brace provides a significant reduction of segmental movement at all cervical spine levels. This is due to its design, which includes mandible, occipital, and chest points of attachment. These points of attachment help to minimize spinal snaking and provide an effective body shell. The Minerva jacket brace also provides greater segmental movement restriction compared with other braces, such as the halo brace.[7,8,9,10]

▸▸ Answer 11

Correct answer is A

The Minerva jacket brace controls subaxial sagittal plane segmental motion better than the halo brace. The Halo brace, however, is better at controlling capital flexion and extension. The Minerva jacket brace's advantage is due mainly to the extent of chest fixation, which provides a three-point bending biomechanical advantage. The major advantage of the Minerva jacket brace is its minimal amplification of snaking, a serpentine movement of the spine.

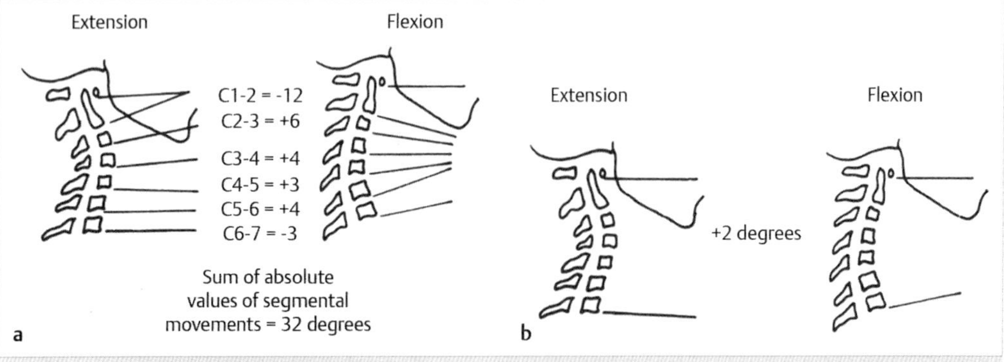

Fig. 36.3 Segmental movement at each individual level (in degrees) can be assessed, measured, and calculated from flexion and extension radiographs. The total movement is the sum of the angles. The overall movement between the cranium and the low cervical region (lowest segment assessed) is the measured movement. The difference is an objective assessment of snaking. **(a)** The differences at segmental levels are depicted in this hypothetical example. "Extension" identifies the extension intersegmental angles. "Flexion" identifies the flexion intersegmental angles. The sum of the angles is 32 degrees. **(b)** The overall movement between the cranium and the lowest segment assessed is 2 degrees. Therefore, in this case, the objective measure of snaking is 30 degrees. (Source: Biomechanics of Spine Stabilization: Third Edition, © 2015 Thieme Medical Publishers, Inc.)

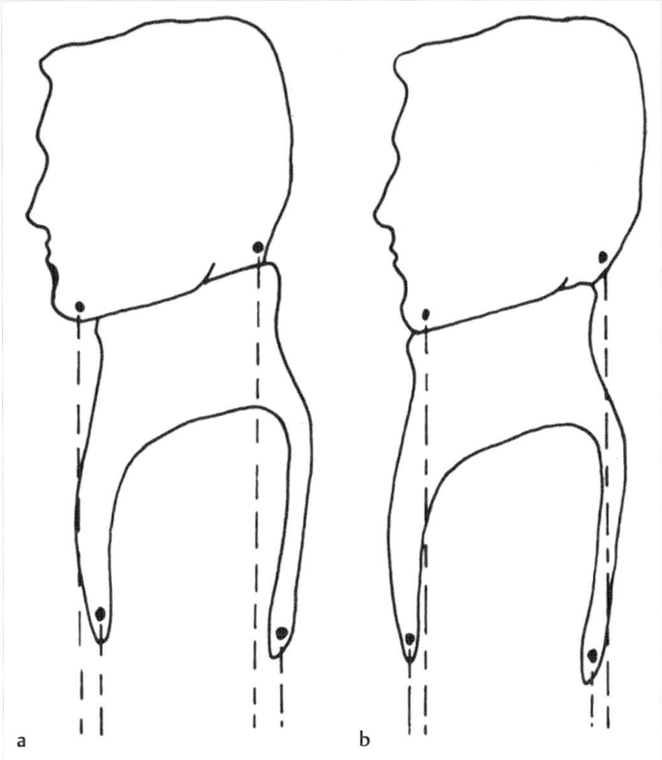

Fig. 36.4 (a, b) The parallelogram-like bracing effect can be significantly diminished by minimizing movement in the low cervical and cervicothoracic regions via a three-point bending mechanism. This significantly restricts true neck flexion–extension. (Source: Biomechanics of Spine Stabilization: Third Edition, © 2015 Thieme Medical Publishers, Inc.)

▸▸ Answer 12

Correct answer is B

The lower lumbar region is difficult to splint externally due to the limitations created by an inadequate caudal fixation point. For adequate fixation, two points that are at least four or five vertebral levels proximal and distal to the unstable segment, and that are amenable to immobilization by an external splint, are required. The pelvic region does not provide such an advantage; there is insufficient distance from the unstable segment to the pelvic points of fixation. In addition, hip flexion, even with hip spica application, allows unacceptable movement that may result in inadequate protection.

▸▸ Answer 13

Correct answer is C

The thoracic region is easier to splint compared with other regions of the spine due to the presence of two axial segments above and below for fixation. This allows for a more direct application of the brace's stabilizing force to the spine. Additionally, the smaller amount of soft tissue separating the brace from the spine itself and the substantial points of fixation available at the rostral and caudal termini of the cervical region, such as the cranium and the thoracic cage, aid in the effectiveness of the splint.

▸▸ Answer 14

Correct answer is E

The use of a halo brace is uniquely associated with pin site complications, which can lead to possible cosmetic problems, infection, osteomyelitis, and brain abscesses. These complications can occur despite appropriate torque and technique in affixing the device to the calvaria. Therefore, it is crucial to ensure the device is most effectively attached to the calvaria to minimize the risk of these complications.

▸▸ Question 13

What is one major disadvantage of spinal bracing?

- A. Bracing increases the strength of the supporting muscles of the spine
- B. Inadequate support for the spinal column
- C. Reduced spinal remodeling
- D. Atrophy of supporting spine muscles
- E. Increased pain of spinal origin

▸▸ Question 14

How does obesity adversely affect the biomechanics of the lumbar spine?

- A. Gained weight is predominantly dorsal to the C7 plumb line and increases axial loading
- B. Gained weight is predominantly ventral to the C7 plumb line and increases axial loading
- C. Obesity slows the degenerative process of discs
- D. Obesity creates a smaller movement arm on the lumbar spine
- E. Obesity improves distribution of axial loading

▸▸ Question 15

Injections into the region of spinal implants have been employed for what purpose?

- A. To treat pain of spinal origin
- B. To determine the potential efficacy of subsequent implant removal
- C. To manage radicular pain
- D. To treat osteoporotic vertebral collapse
- E. To strengthen spinous ligaments

▸▸ Question 16

Which of the following is true regarding patient education?

- A. Patient education prevents work-associated low back injuries
- B. Surgical outcomes are not impacted by the patient's participation in physical therapy for management of their pain
- C. A patient's self-assessment of his or her own health affects surgical outcomes
- D. Patient motivation does not affect back pain outcomes
- E. Surgeon involvement in patient education does not impact outcomes

▸▸ Question 17

Which of the following is true regarding general well-being augmentation?

- A. Smoking does not impact treatment outcomes for back pain
- B. Smoking decreases back pain
- C. Smoking decreases leg pain
- D. Cessation of smoking decreases back and leg pain
- E. Smoking is not a risk factor for back pain

▸▸ Question 18

Which of the following is true regarding aerobic exercises for treatment of low back pain?

- A. Decreases a patient's sense of accomplishment
- B. Decreases a patient's ability to increase activity without increasing pain
- C. Is not associated with an increased incidence of back pain
- D. Decreases endorphin release
- E. Results in mood dysregulation

▸▸ Question 19

Which of the following is true regarding stretching exercises and back pain?

- A. Stretching exercises can lyse adhesions
- B. Compared with toe-touching stretching, back extension is easier to monitor for progress
- C. Bouncing during toe-touching stretching is encouraged
- D. Aggressive stretching exercises are appropriate initially
- E. Lack of flexibility does not impact pain from mechanical instability

▸▸ Question 20

Why is muscle strength imbalance of the dorsal paraspinous muscles and abdominal muscles a concern in patients with spinal origin pain?

- A. It leads to an excessive ratio of load application to spine
- B. It results in weakened spinal ligaments
- C. It causes a reduction in spinal movement
- D. It increases joint flexibility
- E. The imbalance is not a concern

Answers

▸▸ Answer 1

Correct answer is D

Muscles, as well as associated fascial and tendinous attachments and ligaments, provide significant support for the spine. They create both a guy wire–like support system and a cantilever support system (see ▸ Fig. 37.1). (**a**) Increasing the tension of support muscles, tendons, and fascia increases axial loading of the discs and vertebral bodies. (**b**) This increases resistance to angular deformation (e.g., kyphosis or scoliosis). Strengthening either or both of these systems increases axial loading as well as angular deformity resistance. The associated multiplanar deformity resistance augments spinal stability.

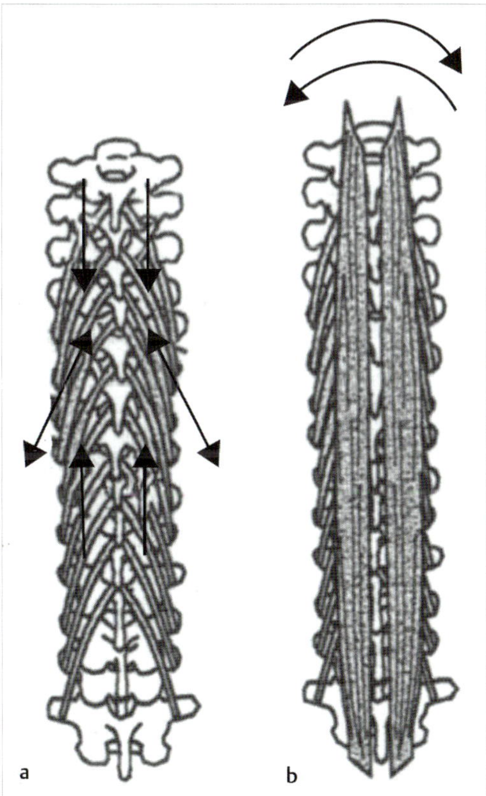

Fig. 37.1 (**a**) Increasing the tension of support muscles, tendons, and fascia increases axial loading of the discs and vertebral bodies. (**b**) This increases resistance to angular deformation (e.g., kyphosis or scoliosis). (Source: Biomechanics of Spine Stabilization: Third Edition, © 2015 Thieme Medical Publishers, Inc.)

▸▸ Answer 2

Correct answer is B

An exercise regimen is the predominant nonoperative strategy for the management of disorders of the spine. Immobility can cause motion segment stiffness by foreshortening ligaments and tendons and by causing fibrous adhesions. This can, in and of itself, be associated with pain. Increasing mobility by stretching may decrease pain. Stretching exercises can increase the range of motion and relax spasms; strengthening exercises can augment spinal stability. The other options may help with back pain but are not the best answer.

▸▸ Answer 3

Correct answer is D

Strengthening the paraspinal muscles occur via "guy wire" and cantilever mechanism. A guy wire is a tensioned cable designed to add stability to a freestanding structure (see ▸ Fig. 37.2). This consists of tightening the support system so that it may better resist applied loads and stresses. Strengthening paraspinal muscles and tendon support systems of the spine has been proven effective in back pain management. Adequate spinal mobility ensures proper distribution of forces across the spine, and a balanced approach to strengthening both spinal and abdominal muscles is key for maintaining spinal alignment and function. A is incorrect because immobility shortens ligaments and tendons. B is incorrect because strengthening abdominal core muscles will increase angular deformity resistance. C is incorrect because lower extremity laxity is associated with back pain. E is incorrect because strengthening the paraspinal muscles does increase angular resistance.

▸▸ Answer 4

Correct answer is C

If the patient cannot seek and find a position of relative comfort, the likelihood of achieving relief with stabilization surgery for mechanical back pain is significantly diminished. The triad of mechanical back pain includes (1) deep and agonizing pain (2) that is worsened with spine loading and (3) improves with spine unloading. Often, patients

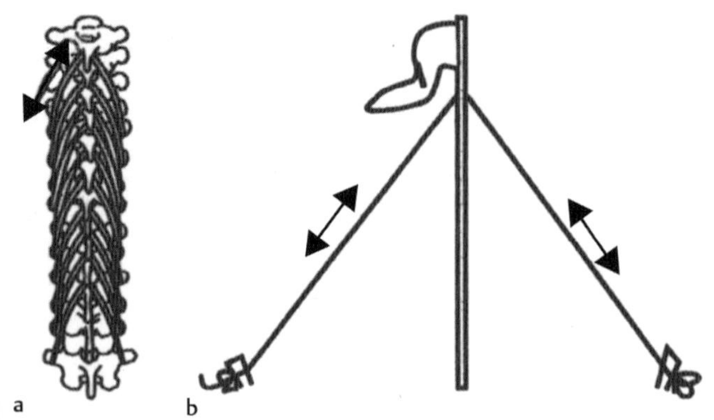

Fig. 37.2 (a, b) Muscles, fascia, and tendons may support the spine via a guy wire mechanism (e.g., erector spinae muscles). (Source: Biomechanics of Spine Stabilization: Third Edition, © 2015 Thieme Medical Publishers, Inc.)

are able to find comfort by lying down and thus unloading the spine. A is incorrect because it does not predict success from fusion surgery. B is incorrect because pain worsens with spinal loading. D is incorrect because it is not part of the triad of mechanical back pain. Answer E, radicular pain, is incorrect as it is not part of the triad of mechanical back pain.

▸▸ Answer 5

Correct answer is B

Lower extremity laxity, or overuse, is associated with back pain. This is thought to be due to the kinetic chain or link theory, in which abnormal forces that are applied caudally are transmitted rostrally. The other options are incorrect.[1]

▸▸ Answer 6

Correct answer is C

The patient is describing mechanical back pain. The triad of mechanical back pain includes (1) deep and agonizing pain that is (2) worsened with spine loading (activity) and (3) improved with spine unloading (inactivity or bed rest). Core-strengthening exercises may improve a patient's pain. Myofascial pain is akin to a "muscle pull." Neuropathic pain would be described as a shooting, stabbing, or burning sensation or as a sharp electric shock. Inflammatory pain is often worse in the morning and often improves after the patient arises and ambulates; it would not necessarily improve with rest.

▸▸ Answer 7

Correct answer is B

Greater trochanteric pain is a nonspinal masquerader of spinal pathology. Greater trochanteric pain can complicate both the diagnosis and treatment of leg pain in combination with back pain. It accounts for a substantial proportion of the patients referred to spine surgeons for evaluation of low back pain. The other answer choices can represent true spinal pathologies.

▸▸ Answer 8

Correct answer is C

Inflammatory back pain usually presents in younger patients and is worse in the morning. This is in stark contrast to mechanical back pain, which usually worsens throughout the day and is worsened with spinal loading. The differentiation between the two is critical. Unnecessary operations should be avoided, and early treatment of inflammatory back pain can retard the advancement of disease. The other answers are incorrect.

▸▸ Answer 9

Correct answer is A

Strengthening the pelvic floor and lower abdominal muscles is crucial in managing urinary continence, especially in patients with low back pain. These muscles provide direct support to the bladder and urethral structures. When strengthened, they improve the structural integrity and functioning of the pelvic region, which in turn enhances the control over urinary functions. This is particularly beneficial in patients with low back pain, where altered biomechanics may indirectly impact urinary continence.

▸▸ Answer 10

Correct answer is B

The decreased lumbar lordosis in flatback syndrome is often associated with the loss of thoracic kyphosis as a compensatory mechanism. Loss of lumbar lordosis may also cause excessive pelvic tilt, such that knee flexion and cervical extension are required to maintain forward vision. Pelvic incidence is a fixed spinopelvic parameter.

▸▸ Answer 11

Correct answer is A

The elevation of vertebral body height, reversal of kyphotic deformity, and elimination of vertebral body deformation restore structural support of the collapsed vertebral body and are the probable mechanisms of reported pain relief with vertebroplasty and kyphoplasty. The other answers are incorrect.

▸▸ Answer 12

Correct answer is D

Traction has been shown to lack efficacy for the management of back pain. The other modalities listed have been touted for the treatment for back pain, although high-level evidence may be lacking. Bracing has been shown to diminish pain of spinal origin (mechanical pain) by supporting the spinal column but may ultimately be deconditioning. Yoga has been associated with improvement of pain, but the cause-and-effect relationship for management of back pain is not clear. Acupuncture has been used for management of spinal disorders with mixed results. Muscle relaxants have been associated with diminution of spine pain symptoms.[2]

▸▸ Answer 13

Correct answer is D

A major disadvantage of bracing is the associated limitation of motion, as well as obligatory inactivity and subsequent atrophy of the supporting muscles of the spine. A is incorrect because supporting muscles of the spine are weakened during prolonged bracing. B is incorrect because the correct application of spinal bracing should adequately support the spinal column. C is incorrect because bracing increases spinal remodeling. E is incorrect because bracing can improve spinal pain of mechanical origin by supporting the spinal column.

▸▸ Answer 14

Correct answer is B

Obesity increases the axial loading of spine segments. The gained weight is centered ventral to the axis of the spine, thus creating a moment arm and a bending moment. Torso extension is necessary to maintain balance. This may cause disc bulging and exacerbate back pain.

▸▸ Answer 15

Correct answer is B

Injections into the region of spinal implants in patients with recurrent back pain after a failed degenerative lumbar spine operation have been employed to determine the potential efficacy of subsequent implant removal. The other answers are incorrect because this type of injection is diagnostic and does not have the therapeutic benefit described by answers A, C, D, or E.

▸▸ Answer 16

Correct answer is C

A patient's self-assessment of his or her own health and comorbidity has been shown to affect surgical outcomes. One study found that a patient's assessment of their own health and comorbidity is the most cogent outcome predictor of surgery for spinal stenosis. Patient education has been shown to lack efficacy in the prevention of work-associated low back injuries. A patient who refuses to participate in physical therapy or pain management is less likely to benefit from spinal surgery.[3]

▸▸ Answer 17

Correct answer is D

Smoking plays a major role in back pain, increases both back and leg pain, and is a risk factor for a negative outcome of treatment of back pain.[4]

▸▸ Answer 18

Correct answer is C

Aerobic exercise is not associated with an increased incidence of back pain, even in children or adolescents. Aerobic exercise enhances a patient's well-being and sense of accomplishment. It augments a patient's ability to further increase exercise without increasing pain. D and E are false because exercise does increase endorphins and there are mood-related benefits associated with physical activity.

▸▸ Answer 19

Correct answer is A

Stretching exercises can lyse adhesions and lengthen foreshortened ligaments and tendons. Toe-touching exercises are easily assessed and therefore easier to monitor for progress compared with back extension or other stretching exercises. Bouncing during toe-touching exercises is discouraged; instead, progress should be made slowly during the stretching exercise. Less aggressive exercises are more appropriate initially. Lack of flexibility is an integral part of pain associated with mechanical instability. The spine of a patient with mechanical instability should be thought of as akin to a joint frozen from long-term immobilization.

▸▸ Answer 20

Correct answer is A

It leads to an excessive ratio of load application to the spine. This increased ratio of load application to the spine results in an exaggeration of the dysfunctional nature of affected motion segments. This effect is exaggerated in aging patients because of the muscle laxity associated with diminished mechanical strength and integrity of the dorsal spinal ligaments.

Key Principles

- Pain of spinal origin is multifactorial, and exercises for spinal disorders are designed to diminish pain and increase stability.
- Strengthening the support systems of muscles—associated fascia, tendons, and ligaments—increases axial loading and angular deformity resistance, thus augmenting spinal stability.
- Traditional schemes for back pain management can be categorized into four groups: general well-being augmentation, aerobic exercises, stretching exercises, and strengthening exercises. A programmatic approach that incorporates the four above-mentioned essential components is effective for managing back pain.

References

[1] Nadler SF, Wu KD, Galski T, Feinberg JH. Low back pain in college athletes. A prospective study correlating lower extremity overuse or acquired ligamentous laxity with low back pain. Spine 1998;23:828–833

[2] Beurskens AJ, de Vet HC. Efficacy of traction for nonspecific low back pain. 12-week and 6-month results of a randomized clinical trial. Spine 1997;22:2756–2762

[3] Katz JN, Stucki G, Lipson SJ, Fossel AH, Grobler LJ, Weinstein JN. Predictors of surgical outcome in degenerative lumbar spinal stenosis. Spine 1999;24(21):2229–2233

[4] Leboeuf-Yde C. Smoking and low back pain. A systematic literature review of 41 journal articles reporting 47 epidemiologic studies. Spine 1999;24:1463–1470

Part IX

Synthesis: Putting it All Together

IX

38 Biomechanical Testing

John V. Wainwright, Guilherme Bastos Ferreira Porto, Kylee Shivok, James S. Harrop

Understanding the limitations and pitfalls of biomechanical testing is essential to interpreting and applying the results of biomechanics studies to the clinical practice of spine surgery.

Learning Objectives

- Understand the different testing methodologies employed in a biomechanical testing laboratory.
- Understand stress/strain curve responses relative to structures tested.
- Understand the limitations of biomechanical testing.
- Understand the sources of error in biomechanical testing.
- Select the appropriate biomechanical testing methodology for a given hypothesis.

Questions

▸▸ Question 1

Various methods for securing the specimen in the testing apparatus are available. What is a major pitfall during this process that can significantly impact the results of an experiment?

- A. The specimen must be centered in the pot
- B. Using a frozen specimen
- C. Not clearing nonstructural tissue
- D. Using a long specimen with multiple motion segments
- E. The use of a follower load

▸▸ Question 2

A PhD student would like to use animal specimens for the biomechanical study. What is/are the major benefit(s) to animal specimens over human cadaver specimens?

- A. Increased variability in bone quality and degenerative conditions
- B. Increase in uniformity in bone quality and ability to procure young specimens
- C. Increased anatomic variance
- D. Similar biomechanical properties to human spines
- E. Increased size of some nonprimate mammal spines compared with human specimens

▸▸ Question 3

A spinal motion segment is being deformed. A rapid loading rate, with several loading vectors, is being applied to the spine as part of a biomechanical study in degenerative spine cadaveric samples. Considering the above information, how would you classify the degree of stiffness at the end of the load, type of load being applied to the spine, and the effect on the validity of the study?

- A. Less stiffness, simple load, increased study validity
- B. Greater stiffness, simple load, decreased study validity
- C. Greater stiffness, complex load, decreased study validity
- D. Neutral stiffness, simple load, increased study validity
- E. Neutral stiffness, complex load, increased study validity

▸▸ Question 4

A PhD student is working on a project in a biomechanics lab. He is attempting to study the effect of pure axial loading on a cadaveric cervical spine specimen. He is concerned about the effect of "snaking" on the specimen during the application of axial loads. Which of the following models would minimize the effect of snaking?

- A. Long and kyphotic segment
- B. Long segment and lordotic segment
- C. Short segment, kyphotic segment
- D. Short and lordotic segment
- E. Short and neutral segment

▸▸ Question 5

A PhD student is attempting to create a fully accurate model for multiple segment axial load testing in the cervical spine. Which of the following variables is most important and needs to be

accounted for (which is present in vivo and difficult to replicate in vitro)?
- A. Amount of force applied
- B. Degree of degeneration of the segments in the specimen
- C. Snaking effect
- D. Intermediate muscle force application
- E. Bone quality

▸▸ Question 6

What are the four basic types of biomechanical testing procedures?
- A. Bone quality, physical, chemical, material
- B. Strength, fatigue, stability, mathematical
- C. Strength, fatigue, physical, chemical
- D. Bone quality, fatigue, mathematical, failure
- E. Fatigue, physical, mechanical, mathematical

▸▸ Question 7

A PhD student is performing strength testing on a new metal alloy rod for spine deformity correction. She plan on generating a load–deformation curve to better understand its biomechanical properties (see ▸ Fig. 38.1). What is the most appropriate way to calculate the stiffness of the new rod based on the data she collects?
- A. Measure the load applied in the elastic zone (B–C) minus the neutral zone (A–B)
- B. Measure the slope of the curve in the elastic zone (B–C)
- C. The load at the failure zone minus the plastic zone (C–D)
- D. Measure the slope of the curve in the plastic zone (C–D)
- E. Measure the maximal load at the time of failure zone (E)

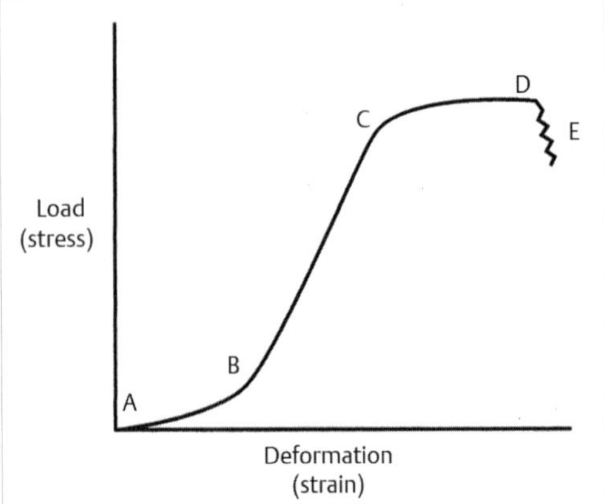

Fig. 38.1 A load–deformation curve. This test is used to measure the strength of an implant, which is determined by notation of the load applied at the time of failure. *A–B*, neutral zone; *B–C*, elastic zone; *C–D*, plastic zone; *E*, failure zone. (Source: Biomechanics of Spine Stabilization: Third Edition, © 2015 Thieme Medical Publishers, Inc.)

▸▸ Question 8

What is the primary principle in fatigue testing, which must be accounted for in the laboratory during biomechanical studies of instrumentation constructs?
- A. Maximal load should be applied to the construct
- B. An implant should be cycled at a minimum 10,000 to 30,000 times
- C. The load applied should be subclinical to that expected in vivo
- D. Bone quality must be assessed prior to any fatigue testing in vitro
- E. The cyclical nature of the submaximal loads should be applied until bony fusion is expected to occur

▸▸ Question 9

A PhD student would like to assess flexibility and stiffness of a construct. Which variables should she control for, respectively, to obtain this information?
- A. Submaximal load, failure load
- B. Load, displacement
- C. Displacement, failure load
- D. Loading rate, stability
- E. Motion, load

▸▸ Question 10

A PhD student would like to design a mathematical model to test a new construct's stiffness and flexibility. He searches the literature for relevant parameters and quickly realizes it is impossible to account for all parameters mathematically that are present in vivo, and therefore some would need to be calculated. What concept known to mathematical modeling does this represent?

- A. Input and output
- B. Boundaries and attributes
- C. Moment application
- D. Boundary conditions
- E. Assumption and error

▸▸ Question 11

A PhD student is trying to understand biomechanics of a spine construct. He would like to test the minimum amount of load required to result in construct failure. This can be accomplished by ________.

- A. Applying the load over a large surface area
- B. Applying the load rapidly, therefore increasing stiffness
- C. Applying the load slowly, therefore decreasing stiffness
- D. Applying the load over a small surface area, without affecting stiffness
- E. Applying the load with variable speed

▸▸ Question 12

What is the primary limitation of fatigue testing to evaluate the long-term integrity of the screw–bone interface in an implanted specimen?

- A. Assessment of the long-term fatigue life is precluded because the researcher cannot put the specimen through a meaningful number of cycles to provide clinically relevant information
- B. Assessment of the long-term fatigue life is precluded because the number of load cycles to apply cannot be determined
- C. The age and bone quality of human cadaveric specimens limit the applicability of the data to young patients
- D. The length of time the experiment will run will result in changes in the response to testing due to desiccation
- E. The number of cycles needed will lead to failure of the vertebra–pot junction

▸▸ Question 13

A PhD student wants to test a new disc replacement device by comparing stiffness with a human cadaveric motion segment. Which of the following is an approach to mitigate the effects of creep in the experimental model?

- A. Increase the load applied during testing to account for tissue deformation
- B. Apply a preloading step before testing to allow for viscoelastic deformation to occur prior to applying the experimental load
- C. Increase the loading rate to decrease the duration of the experiment to minimize the effects of creep
- D. Adjust the temperature of the testing environment to reduce the effects of tissue expansion on the results
- E. Use a time-dependent analysis technique to capture tissue deformation more accurately over time

▸▸ Question 14

An engineer would like to test the pullout strength of a new pedicle screw thread pattern for adolescent scoliosis correction. What is the major pitfall of using human cadaveric specimens for this experiment and how might this be mitigated?

- A. The ex vivo nature of the experimental model prevents the natural remodeling process of bone in response to an applied load from occurring, confounding the results. Using live animal models allow the remodeling process to occur and mitigate this
- B. Specimens are more frequently procured from elderly individuals. Degenerative changes in the discs and ligamentous structures and resultant changes in stiffness reduce the relevance of biomechanical testing to young patients. Using a young nonprimate mammal specimen would mitigate this
- C. Infectious disease transmission must be considered when cadaveric tissue is used and appropriate precautions should be taken including utilizing personal protective equipment
- D. Specimens are more frequently procured from elderly individuals and are often osteopenic or osteoporotic. Bone-density measurement (e.g., dual-energy X-ray absorptiometry [DEXA] scan) can be used to identify specimens with normal or near-normal bone density
- E. Standard uniaxial testing apparatus is not able to apply representative loads to the specimen. Robotic apparatus is able to apply multiplanar loads and better mimic physiologic conditions

▸▸ Question 15

An engineer wishes to study how a new material for spinal tethers for correcting adolescent scoliosis affects the flexibility of the implanted spine. What model/method would best accomplish this study?

- A. Use any available human cadaveric spine specimens
- B. Develop a mathematical model/perform a finite element analysis
- C. Implant the tethering system into a polyurethane block model
- D. Utilize only elderly human cadaveric spine specimens as they are more readily available
- E. Utilize nonprimate mammal spines (e.g., calf or sheep)

▸▸ Question 16

Which of the following is an appropriate method for testing the fatigue life of a new rod material?

- A. Apply a static load until failure occurs
- B. Measure the displacement of the implant under a static load
- C. Measure stiffness of the implant under a static load
- D. Apply a cyclic load to an implanted spine specimen and measure number of cycles until failure
- E. Apply a cyclic load to the implant and measure the number of cycles until failure

▸▸ Question 17

Which of the following is an appropriate method to determine the ability of an instrumentation construct to maintain a fracture in a fixed position under a physiologic load?

- A. Measure displacement while applying an increasing load until failure
- B. Measure displacement under a fixed load
- C. Create a mathematical model of the fracture and instrumentation construct
- D. Apply a repetitive loading and unloading cycle until failure
- E. Measure load necessary to reach a specified displacement

▸▸ Question 18

Specimen handling can affect the results of a biomechanical study. What is the major impact of temperature on a specimen's response to biomechanical testing?

- A. Freezing and thawing a specimen reduces the failure strength and total energy absorption of a specimen
- B. Freezing and thawing has no effect on the viscoelastic properties of a specimen
- C. The creep phenomenon has the most significant impact on results when testing at body temperatures
- D. Tissue permeability is unaffected by freezing and thawing a specimen
- E. The length of time a specimen spends at a certain temperature will change the results of testing

▸▸ Question 19

A researcher would like to study the properties of single spine motion segment, specifically the stiffness/flexibility of the intervertebral disc in a cadaveric model. Which of the following is a major factor that would impact the results?

- A. The environmental conditions of their testing setup
- B. Vertebral body bone quality of their specimen
- C. Intermediate muscle forces
- D. The total energy applied to the model
- E. The effect of snaking

▸▸ Question 20

An engineer would like to test a new device to prevent dynamic motion/worsening degree of slip of an isthmic spondylolisthesis under physiologic loads, in a single cadaveric motion segment compared with the native disc. What is the major limitation to this type of testing?

- A. The number of specimens harboring a spontaneous spondylolysis is limited and would preclude replication of the experiment
- B. Specimen bone quality and the bone–implant interface will not withstand repeated testing

- C. Replicating the forces on the spine and their complex interplay with currently available testing apparatus will be prohibitively difficult and limit the validity of the results
- D. It will not be possible to account for creep in the chronically loaded state
- E. The testing environment will have a significant impact on the results of the experiment

Answers

▸▸ Answer 1

Correct answer is A

Failure to center the specimen properly in the fixture (pot) can introduce unanticipated bending moments and load application with associated confounding of the results. Freezing a specimen prior to mounting can be beneficial as it can help prevent misalignment that can occur if mounting a thawed, flexible specimen. Nonstructural tissue should have no effect on the results of the experiment. A long specimen can increase the complexity of the data and analysis and reduce validity of the results but is not related to the mounting process. A follower load can be added to the experimental setup to simulate intermediate muscle forces but is not related to the mounting process.

▸▸ Answer 2

Correct answer is B

Although the data from human cadaveric specimens are the most direct way to assess human spine kinematics, animal specimens can be superior in that they can be more cost effective, have better and more homogenous bone quality that is similar to that of young adult humans, and can avoid the problems associated with degenerative disease and comorbidities in human specimens. This can allow an appropriately designed experiments to be replicated when assessing general biomechanical principles or implants. However, increased anatomic variance may confound experimental results, and specimens should be matched as closely as possible. Differences in biomechanical/kinematic properties relative to human spines reduce the relevance of the results. The increased size of some nonprimate spines is detrimental to experimental results, as the size of the vertebral body increases, its relative ability to resist load diminishes ("cube-square law").

▸▸ Answer 3

Correct answer is C

A spinal motion segment or vertebra becomes stiffer as it is progressively deformed. Rapid loading rates are associated with greater stiffness than slower loading rates. Multiple loading vectors may be applied to the spine during a biomechanical study. If more than one is used, loading is considered to be complex. An increase in complexity of spinal loading essentially decreases, in an exponential manner, the validity of the study.

▸▸ Answer 4

Correct answer is A

Pure axial loading is associated with unpredictable eccentric spinal element loading, particularly so if the normal spine posture is not used or multiple segments are studied. Snaking can occur during axial load applications. It can be focal and is minimized with normal cervical lordosis preservation and inclusion of short segments.[1]

▸▸ Answer 5

Correct answer is D

Intermediate muscle force application is of great biomechanical significance and is difficult to apply in vitro because unknown and oftentimes immeasurable variables are introduced. Furthermore, muscle forces apply diagonal and axial force vectors, which results in increased applied axial loading. Asymmetric diagonal load application can result in a rotational component. If the spine specimen is rigidly potted at each end, as it is usually the case, the rigid fixation at the termini of the specimen will resist the rotational component, therefore introducing significant error. Snaking effect is an effect present in in vitro biomechanical testing.

▸▸ Answer 6

Correct answer is B

There are four basic types of biomechanical testing procedures: strength, fatigue, stability, mathematical.

▸▸ **Answer 7**

Correct answer is B

Load failure testing generates a load–deformation curve, from which strength, stiffness, and failure can be documented. In a load–deformation curve, A–B is the neutral zone, B–C the elastic zone, C–D the plastic zone, and E the failure zone. Stiffness is measured as the slope of the tangent of the load–deformation curve, usually in the elastic zone (B–C), within which a nearly linear stress/strain relationship is usually present (see ▸ Fig. 38.2). Load–deformation data can be analyzed to obtain stiffness data (slope of the load–deformation curve, or load/deformation), as depicted. The slope is depicted by the *dashed line*. Stiffness data are derived from the load–deformation curve by calculating the slope of the curve in the elastic zone (between B and C; *dashed line*).

▸▸ **Answer 8**

Correct answer is E

With fatigue testing, the construct is usually cycled until it fails or until a clinically reasonable number of cycles have been applied. The number of cycles withstood defines the fatigue life for the load applied. The load should correspond relatively to the loads that the implant is exposed to clinically. Spine implants undergo approximately 3 million cycles per year; therefore, an implant should be expected to withstand 1 million to 3 million cycles before bony fusion occurs.

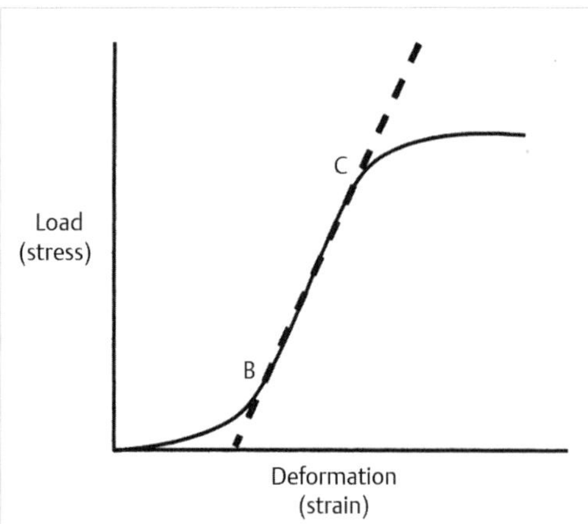

Fig. 38.2 Load–deformation data can be analyzed to obtain stiffness data (slope of the load–deformation curve, or load/deformation), as depicted. The slope is depicted by the dashed line. Stiffness data are derived from the load–deformation curve by calculating the slope of the curve in the elastic zone (between *B* and *C*; *dashed line*). (Source: Biomechanics of Spine Stabilization: Third Edition, © 2015 Thieme Medical Publishers, Inc.)

▸▸ **Answer 9**

Correct answer is B

Stability testing assesses stiffness and its converse, flexibility, in general, submaximal loads applied. If flexibility is to be tested, a load or moment is applied, and displacement is measured. If stiffness is to be tested, the construct is displaced and the load or moment measured. The loading rate can significantly affect the results of stability testing; hence, it should be carefully taken into consideration.

▸▸ **Answer 10**

Correct answer is E

Mathematical testing assesses a spinal construct or model via mathematical testing. In this technique, anatomical structure is geometrically divided into multiple elements, which are associated with boundaries and attributes. Loads (input) and resulting stresses (output) are calculated. Each element has well-defined borders and is associated with conditions for interactions with adjacent elements (boundary conditions). Mathematical models depend on boundary-derived assumptions, which come from cadaveric models, obligating some error. Simplifying assumptions are also made, leading to further error. The literature simply cannot provide all the biomechanically relevant parameters; therefore, each assumption compounds leading to the inaccuracy of the model and therefore error.

▸▸ **Answer 11**

Correct answer is B

Load application rate affects results. Rapid loading increases stiffness, predominantly because the creep phenomenon is not allowed to manifest (meaning the spine is not allowed to relax and creep) before ultimate failure. Therefore, a rapidly loaded spine fails earlier and with less load than a slowly loaded spine.

▸▸ Answer 12

Correct answer is A

Spine implants undergo approximately 3 million cycles per year. An implant should therefore be expected to withstand 1 million to 3 million cycles before fusion occurs. Age and bone quality do affect the applicability of data to young patients; however, the lack of the natural bone remodeling response to load in an ex vivo specimen severely limits the number of cycles the specimen can withstand (80,000–100,000 cycles) relative to the number of cycles a spine implant undergoes per year (3 million). Specimen hydration and desiccation can be mitigated with hydration schedules or barrier films and will not be as large a factor as the lack of remodeling. There are various methods of specimen mounting/potting and adjuncts that can increase stability and prevent failure of the vertebra–pot junction (e.g., screws and bolts into the end vertebra).

▸▸ Answer 13

Correct answer is B

Creep is a time-dependent viscoelastic deformation that can occur under a constant load in a cadaveric model. Preloading the specimen allows some of the creep to be dissipated before the experimental load is applied. During stiffness testing, the specimen is displaced and the required load is measured. Creep can impact the biomechanical properties of spinal tissues and confound the results by reducing the amount of load required over time as the tissues accommodate to the displaced position. Stiffness testing requires a fixed load, and increasing load would not allow for stiffness to be measured. Increasing the rate of displacement of the specimen would change the results by increasing the measured stiffness but does not mitigate the effect of creep and can result in earlier failure of the specimen with less load. If the testing environment temperature is controlled, the effect of tissue expansion should be similar between testing conditions. A time-dependent analysis technique may allow a measurement of the effect of creep but does not mitigate it.

▸▸ Answer 14

Correct answer is D

Human cadaveric specimens are procured from elderly individuals and are often osteopenic or osteoporotic. This reduced bone density reduces the strength of the screw–bone interface and would decrease the measured pullout strength in the biomechanical model. Bone density testing can mitigate this by controlling for bone quality. Infectious disease transmission is a concern but would not directly affect the results of the experiment. This experimental design is not testing cyclic loading; therefore, the in vivo remodeling process to repetitive load is not a consideration. Degenerative changes do affect the results of biomechanical testing, particularly stiffness/flexibility, and a nonprimate mammal specimen could mitigate this but is not relevant to this experimental design. However, nonprimate specimens are easier to control for bone quality and may ultimately be the most representative model for this experiment.

▸▸ Answer 15

Correct answer is E

While anatomically different than a human spine, nonprimate mammal (e.g., calf or sheep) spine specimens have more homogenous bone density and geometry, are more readily available, are significantly less expensive than nonhuman primate spines, and provide a structurally similar replication of the young adult human spine. Utilizing this approach, more repetitions of the experiment can be performed with more uniform results that are applicable to the nondegenerated young human spine. Human cadaveric specimens are not ideal as there is significant variability in the bone quality, amount of degenerative disease, and comorbidities that may affect flexibility (e.g., diabetes, smoking), making the data less relevant to the study question. There is also limited availability of young adult spine specimens that could generate more relevant data. Implanting the tethering system into a polyurethane block model would be a way to test the characteristics of the implant itself, not the effect the implant has on the flexibility of an implanted spine. The assumptions necessary to generate a mathematical model/perform a finite element analysis introduce significant error/inaccuracy into the model, making it difficult to generate clinically useful data.

▸▸ Answer 16

Correct answer is E

Fatigue testing involves subjecting a material to cyclic loading until failure occurs and is an appropriate method for testing the fatigue properties of an implant. Applying a cyclic load to an implanted spine specimen does not test the fatigue properties of the implant as the bone–implant interface will fail long before the fatigue life of the implant is reached. Applying a static load until failure would only assess the strength and stiffness of the implant to a single loading event. Measuring displacement under static load is a method to determine the flexibility of a material. The stiffness is measured by controlling the displacement of an implant and measuring the required load.

▸▸ Answer 17

Correct answer is B

Measuring displacement under a fixed load would measure the *flexibility* of the construct, e.g., its ability to stabilize a fracture and resist movement of the spine. Measuring displacement under increasing load to failure would generate a load–deformation curve, which can be used to determine the stiffness of the construct. Mathematical modeling of an implanted spine involves the modeling of a large number of boundary conditions, which results in a significant amount of error and inaccuracy in the model, limiting the clinical applicability of the results. Applying a cyclic load cycle tests the fatigue life of the construct–bone interface but not the ability of the construct to stabilize the spine. Measuring load to reach a specific displacement is a method to determine the *stiffness* of the construct, which does not evaluate the construct's ability to stabilize the spine at a specific load.

▸▸ Answer 18

Correct answer is C

Specimen temperature does not generally affect a specimen's response to testing with some exceptions. Ligaments expand at body temperature compared with room temperature. This results in changes to their viscoelastic properties, leading to the most significant effect form the creep phenomenon. The fatigue life of a specimen decreases at body temperature; however, the ultimate failure strength and the total energy absorption at failure are usually unaffected by temperature. Freezing and thawing changes the permeability of a specimen, which can alter its creep behavior (viscoelastic properties). The length of time a specimen spends at a given temperature does not affect the biomechanical characteristics, although the temperature at which testing is performed does.

▸▸ Answer 19

Correct answer is A

The temperature and humidity of a testing environment can significantly impact the results of testing, particularly flexibility testing. The effect of creep is most evident at body temperature. Additionally, intervertebral disc hydration significantly impacts the results as a hydrated disc is stiffer than a dehydrated disc. The hydrophilic nature of the disc leads to swelling and increased stiffness particularly in the unloaded, ex vivo state. While human cadaveric specimens often have poor bone quality, bone strength is not being tested. Conversely, the degenerative state of the specimen, comorbidity status of the specimen donor, and smoking status all would have a major impact on the results of the study. Total energy absorption of a biomechanical model pertains to strength testing, not flexibility testing as in this experiment. Snaking will not come into play as this experiment is specifically looking at a *single* motion segment. Snaking becomes a factor when multiple segments are included in a specimen. Similarly, the impact of intermediate muscle forces is more significant when multiple motion segments are included in the experiment.

▸▸ Answer 20

Correct answer is C

Isthmic spondylolisthesis is the result of a loss in the integrity of the spinal elements to withstand axial loading, translation, and flexion/extension moments. The complex nature of these forces cannot accurately be replicated with current testing apparatus, particularly the translational component. In order to increase the number of specimens available to study, a researcher-induced spondylolysis can be used to create the proper model motion segment. The aim of the experiment is not to determine the fixation strength/implant–bone interface of the device, and bone quality will not be a significant factor in the limited number of cycles typically used for stability testing. Creep can be accounted for by preloading specimens to dissipate some of the creep before the ultimate experiment. The environmental conditions of the test (e.g., temperature and humidity) do have an impact on the results of any biomechanical study; however, these effects can be mitigated by proper experimental design and control of the testing room.

Key Principles

- Specimen choice and size/length can have a significant impact on the results of a biomechanical study.
- Close attention to experimental design, down to such details as how the specimen is mounted, is critical to ensuring the validity of the results.
- A hypothesis to be tested (e.g., implant fatigue strength, implant pullout strength, flexibility of an injury model) must be formed prior to selecting a biomechanical model, and testing modes (strength, fatigue, stability) have different applications. Incorrect experimental design can invalidate the results of even a well-conducted study.
- Mathematical modeling/finite element analysis is fundamentally limited by the error inherent in the boundary property assumptions used to generate the model.

Reference

[1] Oktenoğlu T, Ozer AF, Ferrara LA, Andalkar N, Sarioğlu AC, Benzel EC. Effects of cervical spine posture on axial load bearing ability: a biomechanical study. J Neurosurg 2001;94(1 Suppl):108–114

39 The Decision-Making Process: A Reprise

Clayton L. Rosinski, Timothy C. Ryken

One of the most difficult parts of being a spine surgeon is not performing the actual operations, but determining which patient requires surgery and what the best operation for that patient will be. Through using a systematic approach, which is detailed in the chapter, a surgeon can consistently identify patients who will respond well to surgical intervention and routinely select surgeries that fully address a patient's needs while minimizing surgical risk.

Learning Objectives

- Describe the multiple causes of back pain and how they can be differentiated.
- Understand criteria that must be met prior to lumbar fusion.
- Define problem-based decision making. Describe how problem-based decision making can be employed clinically.
- Describe the selection of operative approaches.
- Understand how "practice hygiene" can be used to optimize quality of care.
- Determine the trajectory for decompression and how this consideration should affect the operative approach selection component of the decision-making process.
- Discuss how stereotactic radiosurgery (SRS) may alter surgical treatment paradigms for patients with spinal metastases.

Questions

▸▸ Question 1

A 34-year-old man presents with a 10-day history of low back pain. He notes that the pain is worse with bending and twisting motions. He is tender to palpation of his right paraspinal lumbar muscles. What is the most appropriate treatment paradigm?

- A. Core strengthening
- B. Epidural steroid injections
- C. Time, muscle relaxants, stretching
- D. Narcotics
- E. Two weeks of bedrest

▸▸ Question 2

Which of the following is a key distinguisher of chronic pain from other types of back pain?

- A. Dull, agonizing pain
- B. Chronic fatigue
- C. Significant impairment in quality of life
- D. Worsening with ambulation
- E. Unresponsive to analgesics

▸▸ Question 3

A 34-year-old man is evaluated in the clinic for low back pain, which is characterized as deep, dull, and agonizing, which is worse in the morning and gradually improves throughout the day. He notes that sometimes the pain is worse with movement but sometimes with rest. Which image should be obtained to evaluate for a pathology that will not respond to mechanical stabilization?

- A. Discography
- B. Flexion/extension films
- C. Computed tomography (CT) myelogram
- D. Lumbar magnetic resonance imaging (MRI)
- E. Plain X-rays (XR) of sacroiliac joint

▸▸ Question 4

A 67-year-old woman presents for a second opinion. She has been experiencing chronic low back pain for several years. She reports that the pain does not radiate in her back and has changed from a dull pain to now including burning pain. She notes that the pain is debilitating and has greatly impaired her sleep, resulting in a feeling of always being tired and low energy. She notes that the pain is no worse with movement than it is at rest. There is a grade 1 anterolisthesis at L4–L5 with diffuse, mild facet arthropathy throughout the lumbar spine. Her other surgeon recommended performing L4–L5 transforaminal lumbar interbody fusion. Why is this unlikely to provide symptomatic relief?

- A. Fusion construct will not address the remainder of lumbar degenerative disease

- B. The pain does not radiate down her legs
- C. Extensive nonoperative management has not been completed
- D. The patient is not motivated to recovery
- E. Lack of pain with motion

▸▸ Question 5

A 27-year-old man is brought to the emergency department following a car accident and noted to have some loss of sensation and strength in his legs. CT shows a T9 burst fracture with significant retropulsion and extensive comminution of the vertebral body but without obvious deformity. MRI shows severe thecal sac compression at T9. When deciding to perform surgery, what is the most important aspect of the patient's history and results to consider?

- A. Neurologic function
- B. Degree of destruction to the ventral column
- C. Degree of deformity
- D. Mechanism of injury
- E. Amount of fractured vertebral body retropulsion

▸▸ Question 6

A 27-year-old man is brought to the emergency department following a car accident and noted to have an incomplete spinal cord injury. CT shows an T9 burst fracture with significant retropulsion and extensive comminution of the vertebral body but without large kyphotic deformity. MRI shows severe thecal sac compression at T9 and disruption of the posterior ligamentous complex. What is the most appropriate treatment of the following options?

- A. Custom thoracolumbar sacral orthosis brace
- B. Laminectomy
- C. Decompression with ventral column reconstruction supplemented with short-segment posterior fusion
- D. Prolonged flat bedrest
- E. Ventral corpectomy alone

▸▸ Question 7

Which of the following activities is not part of good practice hygiene?

- A. Assessing reimbursement to ensure that the service provided was reimbursed
- B. Ensuring that you both code for and are billed for documented procedures
- C. Performing the best operative procedure
- D. Reviewing cases to determine ways to increase the number of cases performed
- E. Using a systemic approach to identify surgical candidates

▸▸ Question 8

A 63-year-old woman with a history of breast cancer presents with progressive low back pain and progressive instability and lower extremity weakness. She is found to have a metastatic lesion at T12 body resulting in significant stenosis. What, if found on evaluation, would necessitate supplementing a ventral reconstruction with a posterior long-segment fusion?

- A. Kyphotic deformity
- B. Increased pain with axial loading of the spine
- C. Evidence of additional, distant sites of spinal metastases
- D. Bladder dysfunction
- E. Clonus

▸▸ Question 9

A surgeon planned and performed a large, 360-degree procedure with the goal of a gross total resection of a radiosensitive metastasis in the lumbar spine, which resulted in both residual tumor, cerebrospinal fluid leak, and new foot drop. Which of Augustus White's maxims was broken in planning and performing this procedure?

- A. Carefully plan operations and frequently review anatomy
- B. Stick with preoperative plans and contingencies
- C. Beware of the tendency to choose an operation because it is difficult
- D. Greater force used during surgery increases the risk of a complication
- E. Continually rededicate to the practice of aseptic technique

▸▸ Question 10

Augustus White's maxim "do the least amount of surgery that will solve the problem" is important in surgical decision making for which reason?

- A. Maximize profit
- B. Limit risk of hardware failure
- C. Improve symptom relief

▸▸ Answer 4

Correct answer is E

Chronic pain can present similar to mechanical back pain and even have imaging findings of degenerative disease. However, if there is doubt that pain is related to motion, then immobilization of the joint through instrumentation is unlikely to improve pain, which is why chronic pain patients often do not respond to surgical intervention.

▸▸ Answer 5

Correct answer is A

The most important consideration for performing surgery is neurologic function. If there is neurologic function to be recovered, surgery should be performed as quickly as possible. In this case, with neurological injury, decompression is indicated, followed by stabilization.

▸▸ Answer 6

Correct answer is C

Given that the patient has neural compression from burst fracture, ventral decompression is indicated. Additionally, given the significant burst fracture with large spread of bone fragments, ventral body reconstruction is indicated as well to prevent future kyphotic deformity. An additional consideration, however, is that the posterior ligamentous complex is disrupted. Therefore, despite the need to perform anterior reconstruction, posterior supplementation is reasonable given concern for development of kyphosis with ambulation prior to formation of bony fusion. As there is no significant kyphotic deformity to reduce, a short-segment fusion will suffice.

▸▸ Answer 7

Correct answer is D

Good practice hygiene is not concerned with increasing the number of cases or revenues with performing surgery, but with just ensuring that services performed are appropriately documented and billed for.

▸▸ Answer 8

Correct answer is A

This patient's immediate concern is the neurologic compression anteriorly from the T12 mass lesion, which has resulted in a pathologic fracture. Therefore, surgery must involve anterior decompression and reconstruction to restore the anterior column integrity. Unfortunately, a significant kyphotic deformity has also developed, which is unlikely to be corrected with anterior reconstruction alone. This requires long-segment posterior fusion and fixation to reduce the deformity and prevent further progression and a minimum.

▸▸ Answer 9

Correct answer is C

There is a natural tendency to want to perform larger surgeries due to the challenge they propose. However, this may not be in a patient's best interest always, as in this case. Given that the mass is radiosensitive and not causing progressive deformity, a simpler separation surgery could have been offered and performed, which would have had much lower risk for surgical complications but likely similar oncologic outcome with the use of SRS.[2,3]

▸▸ Answer 10

Correct answer is D

Ultimately, the goal of surgery should be to provide the maximum benefit to a patient while minimizing surgical risk. By performing the least invasive surgery, which is clinically proven to solve the patient's problem, a good outcome can be achieved with minimal risk to the patient, where performing a more extensive surgery increases risk to the patient without proven proposed benefit. A patient can have similar symptomatic relief with a more extensive surgery if it includes what would be considered the "minimum" intervention.

▸▸ Answer 11

Correct answer is B

In this patient, adding ventral reconstruction will add significant length and complexity to the surgery, one in which the patient is already at high risk due to medical comorbidities. Therefore, it is important to determine if the patient truly needs ventral reconstruction. If there is evidence of progressive kyphosis as the spine is progressively loaded, the likelihood of successful posterior decompression and fusion alone is less likely, and anterior reconstruction may be indicated. In this instance, the progressive deformity on XR is evidence that the least amount of surgery to solve the patient's problem might involve anterior reconstruction.

▸▸ Answer 12

Correct answer is E

Regardless of the type of tumor, patient risk factors, or any other factors, posterior separation surgery cannot be performed if there is concern regarding the stability of the spine after separation surgery. Therefore, a surgeon must not have doubt regarding the stability of the anterior and middle columns of the spine before performing a posterior separation surgery; otherwise, the patient will develop progressive deformity and possibly neurological injury.

▸▸ Answer 13

Correct answer is A

As an approach becomes more lateral in the spine, it reduces the amount of thecal sac retraction required to reach the ventral pathology, but increasingly destabilizes the spine. It is likely with a lateral extracavitary approach where the rib head and facet are needed to be removed to destabilize the spine at that level, and serious consider ation should be taken to supplemental posterior instrumentation (see ▸ Fig. 39.1). (**a**) Laminotomy, (**b**) transpedicular, (**c**) ostotransversectomy, and (**d**) lateral extracavitary approach.

▸▸ Answer 14

Correct answer is A

It is critical to be assured that a patient is committed to the recovery process prior to performing surgery when the symptom is pain. Ultimately, if a patient is unwilling to change the factors in their life which have contributed to the development of spinal instability and degeneration, they are unlikely to have long lasting benefit from surgical intervention, which alters the proposed risk–benefit ratio.

▸▸ Answer 15

Correct answer is A

Commitment to recovery process is easily objectively measured. This can be demonstrated by a patient in several objective ways, such as smoking cessation, weight loss, exercise tolerance, physical condition, flexibility parameters, and many other methods. Spinal motion can be quantified by XR, but the degree of motion is not always correlative to a patient's symptoms. Additionally, there may be micromotion that is symptomatic but cannot be captured with dynamic XR. There are measurement tools for quality-of-life impairment from pain, but these are ultimately subjective and rely on patient's answering honestly. Relation of motion to pain is also relying on a patient's subjective experience.

▸▸ Answer 16

Correct answer is C

By starting with ventral discectomy, risk of further neurologic compression and injury when performing posterior decompression and fusion is minimized as there is no risk for injury from the ventral disc. Spinal stability is not influenced, as performing a 360-degree operation where posterior decompression and fusion is followed by anterior cervical discectomy (decompression) and fusion results in the same spinal construct

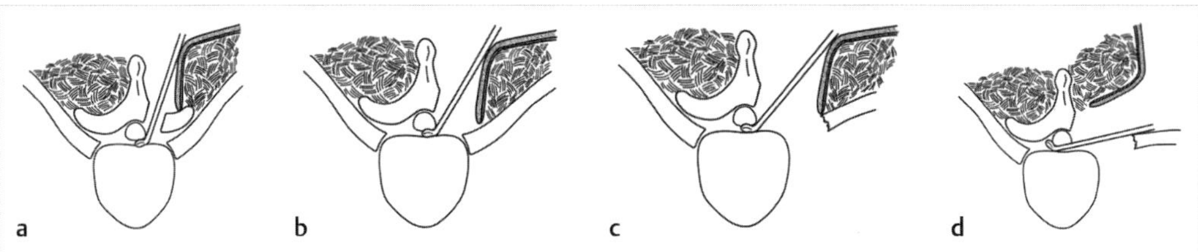

Fig. 39.1 The determination of the most appropriate trajectory for surgical intervention is a critical component of the decision-making process. The selection of a trajectory via which a pathology that is located ventral to the dural sac can be accessed is critical. **(a)** A laminotomy approach, **(b)** transpedicular approach, **(c)** costotransversectomy approach, or **(d)** lateral extracavitary approach can be used to address pathology that is positioned lateral or ventral to the dural sac. In descending order, each of these approaches may be effectively and safely employed for more ventrally positioned extradural pathologies. Note that the lateral extracavitary approach, by definition, approaches the spine from beneath the erector spinae muscle. (Source: Biomechanics of Spine Stabilization: Third Edition, © 2015 Thieme Medical Publishers, Inc.)

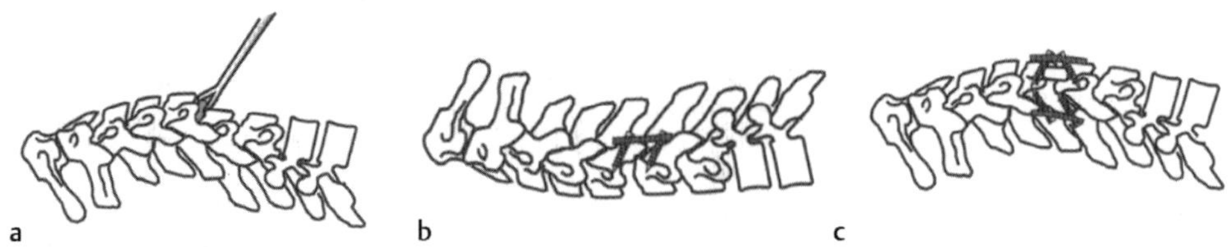

Fig. 39.2 A 540-degree operative strategy. **(a)** Bilateral locked facet joints may be surgically approached with a ventral discectomy and reduction. **(b)** If the ventral reduction cannot be achieved, a dorsal reduction, fusion, and instrumentation may be required. **(c)** A ventral interbody fusion with instrumentation may then be performed, if indicated. (Source: Biomechanics of Spine Stabilization: Third Edition, © 2015 Thieme Medical Publishers, Inc.)

and stability. Both cost and complications (other than risk of neural injury) are increased with a 540-degree procedure due to increased operative time. The degree of decompression is equivalent between both procedures. ▸ Fig. 39.2 shows 540-degree procedure to reduce fixed cervical subluxation first through (**a**) anterior discectomy, then (**b**) posterior reduction of locked facets and posterior instrumentation, then (**c**) anterior interbody placement and fixation.

▸▸ Answer 17

Correct answer is D

Regardless of the degree of neurologic compromise due to a fracture, if there are concerns regarding the patient's ability to tolerate a procedure, surgery cannot be performed in good conscious with too high of risk of surgical complications. This is often a serious consideration in polytrauma patients who may have considerable other injuries, which put the patient at too high of risk of life-threatening complication to undergo a spinal procedure. After a patient has been determined fit for a procedure, the most important aspect guiding surgical intervention and the mode of intervention is determining if there is neurologic compression and how it should be decompressed. Next, if the ventral column cannot support the spine under axial load, it must be restored immediately for the patient to be ambulated safely. Then, if there is concern for further deformity over time, consideration for a large segment dorsal instrumentation is necessary to prevent future deformity, which could require reoperation. Lastly, cost should be the last consideration after selecting the appropriate surgery by systemically evaluating each of the preceding factors.

▸▸ Answer 18

Correct answer is A

Neural compression is not an indication for performing a fusion, but rather a decompressive operation. Fusion should be performed when there is evidence of spinal segment motion that is causing quality of life–impairing pain in a patient who is motivated to recover.

▸▸ Answer 19

Correct answer is D

The pain due to mechanical instability stems from degeneration and irritation of the facet joints. Therefore, surgical removal of the joint from facetectomy should relieve pain. However, it is very infrequent where this can be done without compromising the stability of the spine, and thus instrumentation is often necessary.

▸▸ Answer 20

Correct answer is C

When evaluating a patient with a traumatic thoracolumbar injury, neurologic compression and function should be given the highest priority when deciding when and how to operate. Incomplete injury represents the most urgent neurologic injury to decompress as there is better recovery with earlier surgery, whereas complete injury is thought to represent permanent, irreversible injury.

Key Principles

- Differentiating the types of back pain is critical to a spine surgeon, and correlation of mechanical instability to a patient's symptoms must be done prior to fusion.
- Prior to lumbar fusion, there must be evidence that a patient has a spinal segment where motion exists, that the motion is related to the pain which significantly impairs their quality of life, and that the patient is dedicated to recovery.
- A surgeon should pursue the least amount of surgery that will address a patient's problem.
- When managing thoracolumbar trauma, neurologic function is the utmost important factor when evaluating the patient for surgery.
- The surgical approach and intervention should be at the site of pathology.
- When managing spinal metastases, the ability for a patient to receive SRS should be evaluated, and the patient should be considered for separation surgery if indicated.
- Maintaining good practice hygiene is important to deliver the best possible care.

References

[1] Raychaudhuri SP, Deodhar A. The classification and diagnostic criteria of ankylosing spondylitis. J Autoimmun 2014;48:128–133

[2] Conti A, Acker G, Kluge A, et al. Decision making in patients with metastatic spine. The role of minimally invasive treatment modalities. Front Oncol 2019;9:915

[3] Bate BG, Khan NR, Kimball BY, Gabrick K, Weaver J. Stereotactic radiosurgery for spinal metastases with or without separation surgery. J Neurosurg Spine 2015;22(4):409–415

Index

Note: Page numbers set **bold** or *italic* indicate headings or figures, respectively.

D

E

F

J

K

L

M

N

O

P

Q

R

S

T

U

V

W

Y

Z